Advances in Precision Medicine Oncology

Edited by Hilal Arnouk
and Bassam Abdul Rasool Hassan

Published in London, United Kingdom

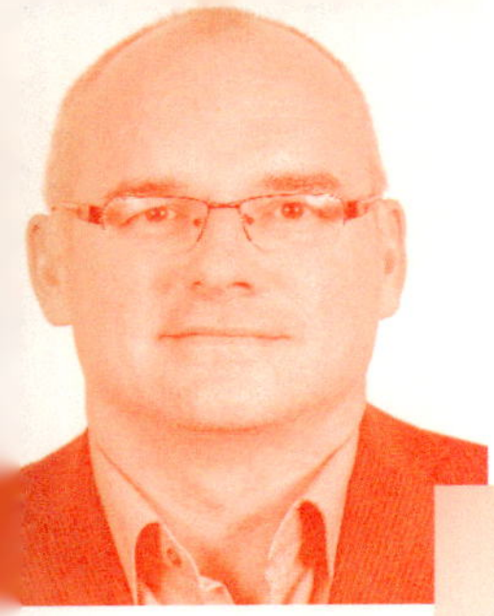
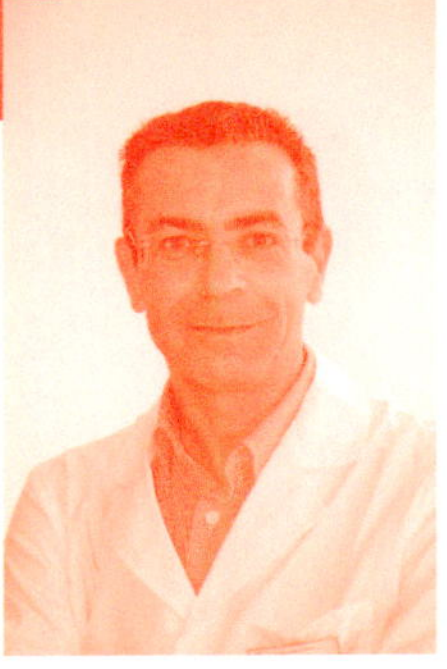
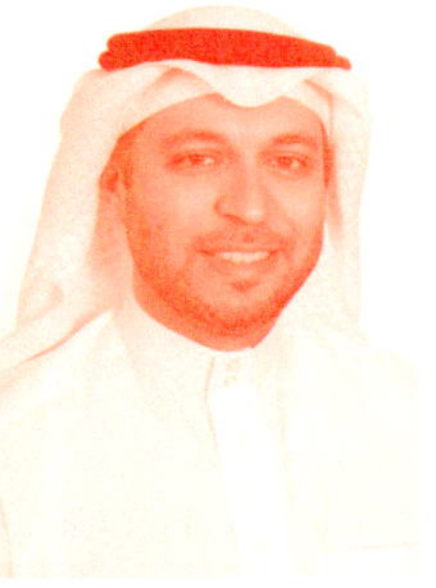
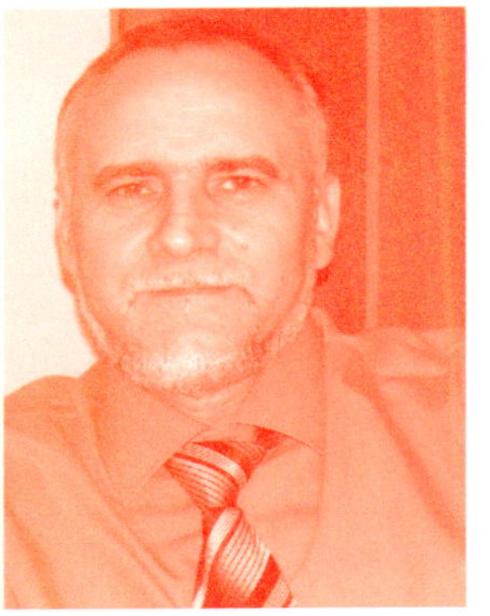
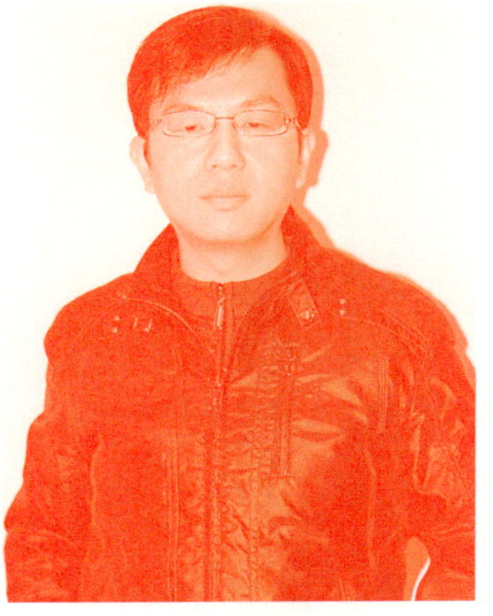
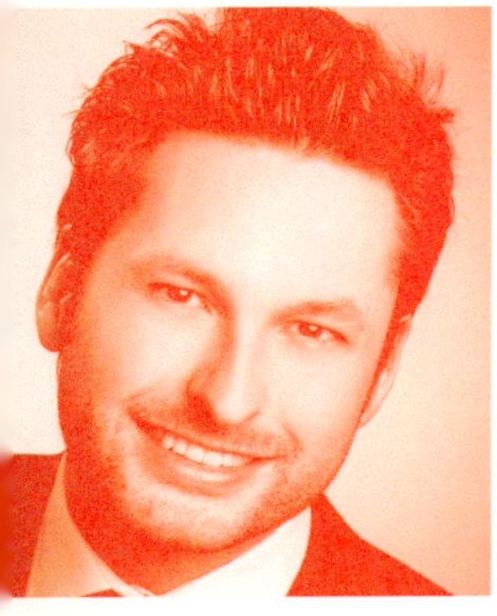
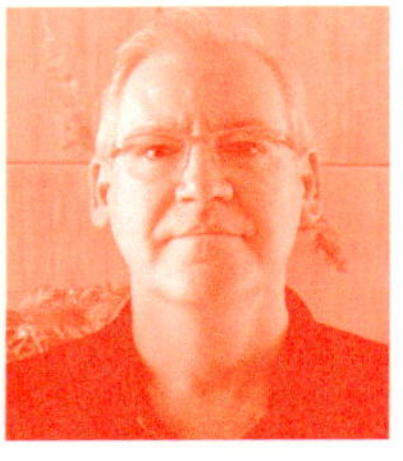

IntechOpen

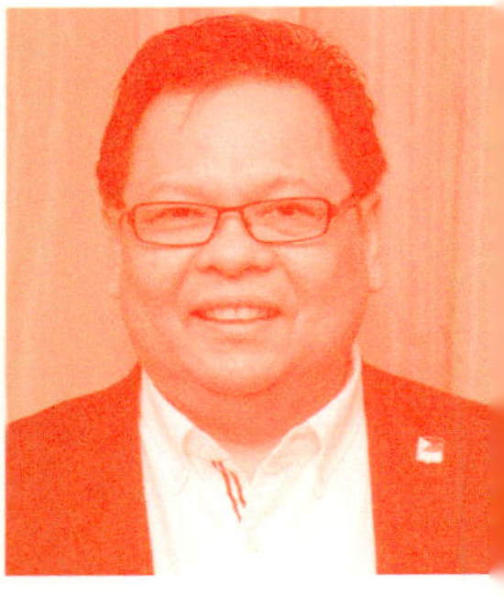
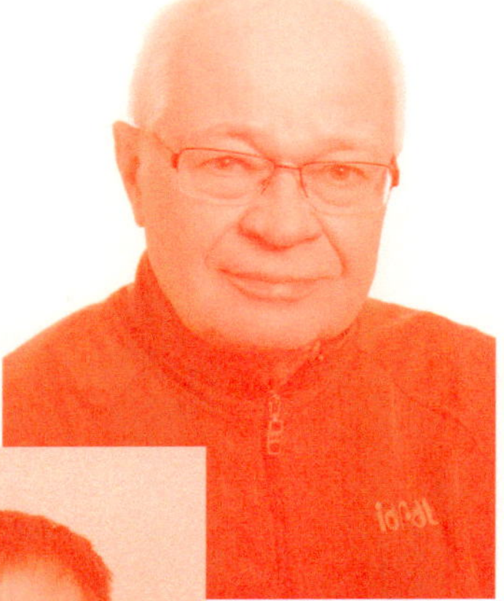
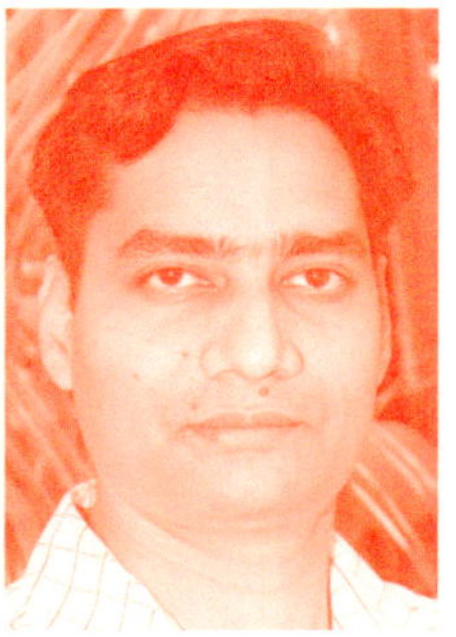
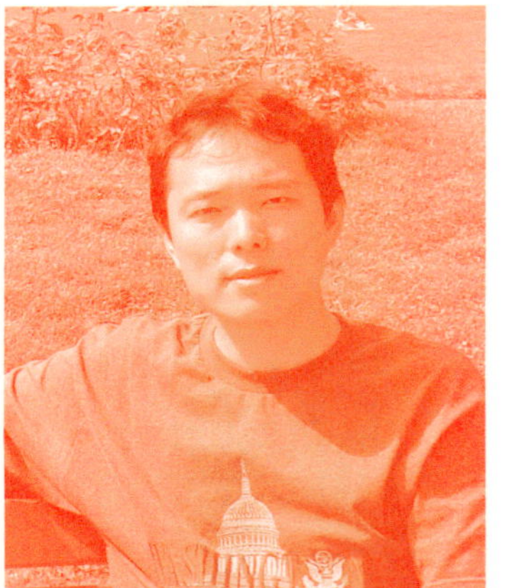
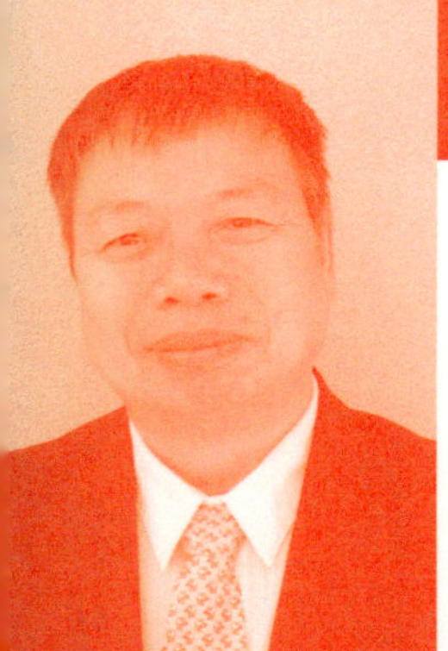
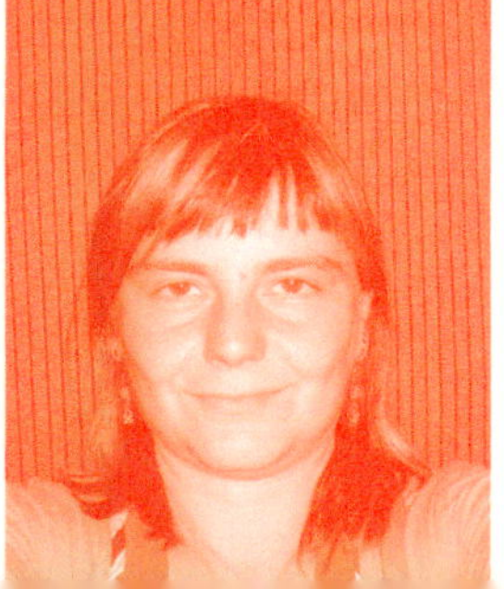

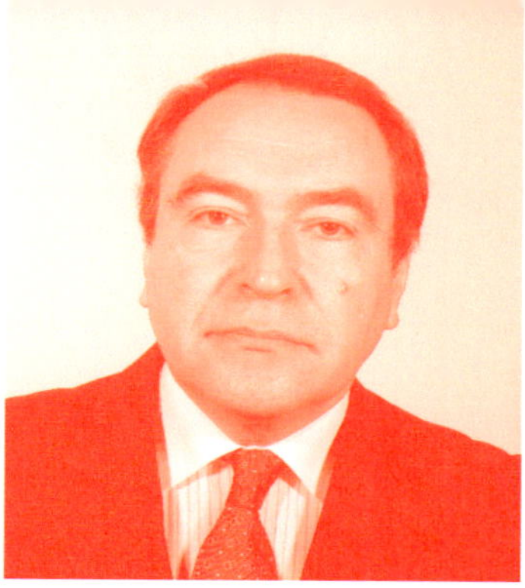
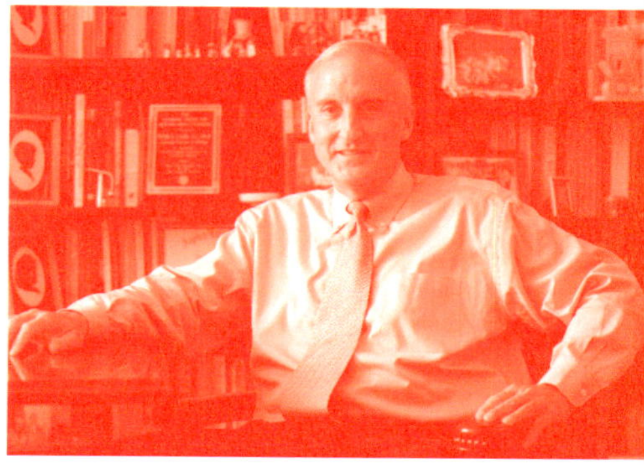
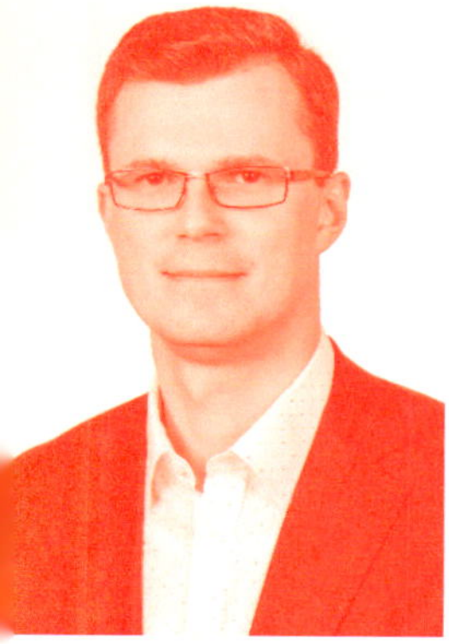
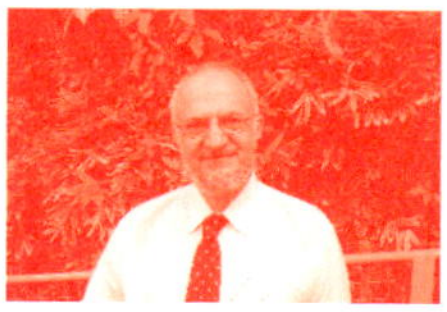
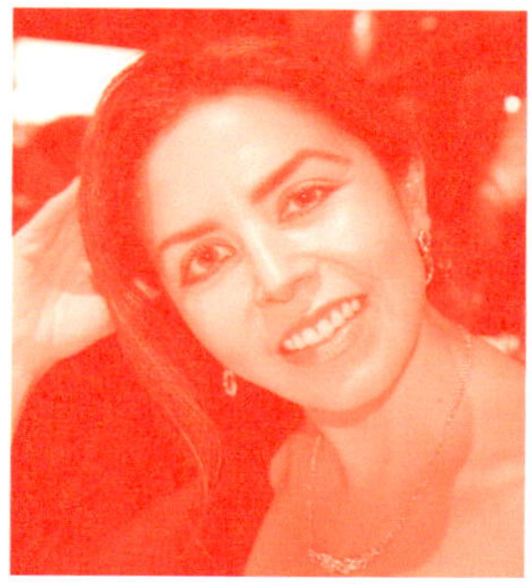

Supporting open minds since 2005

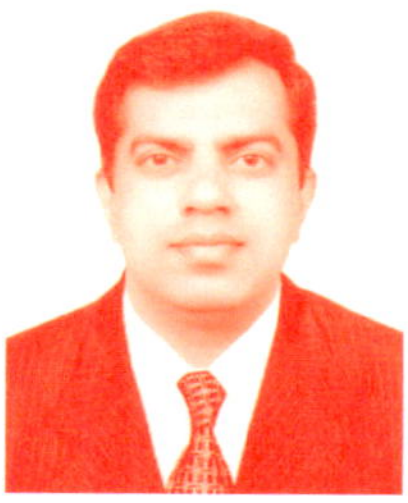
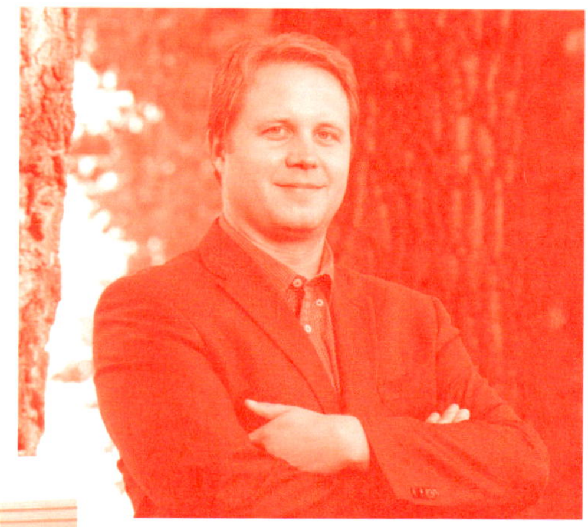
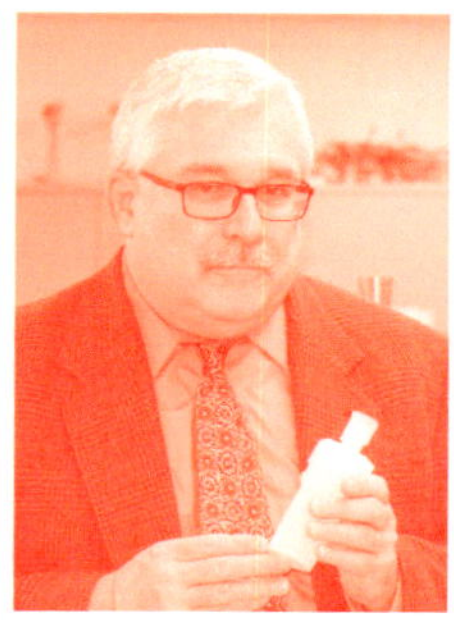
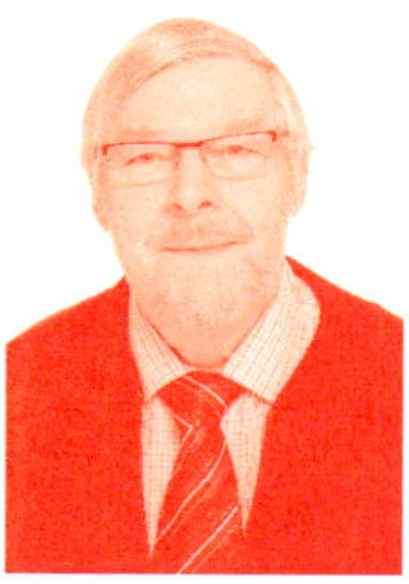
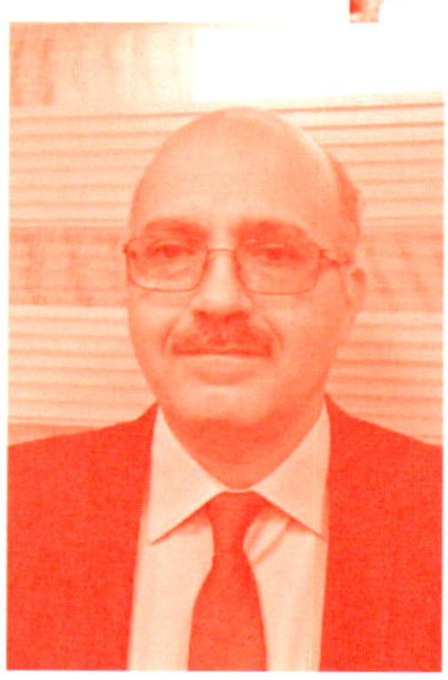
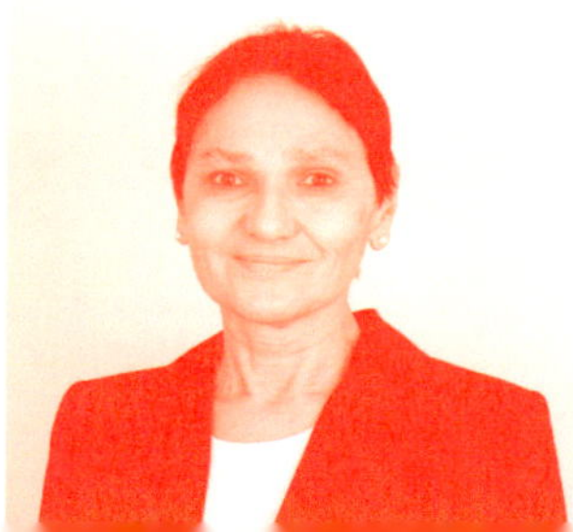
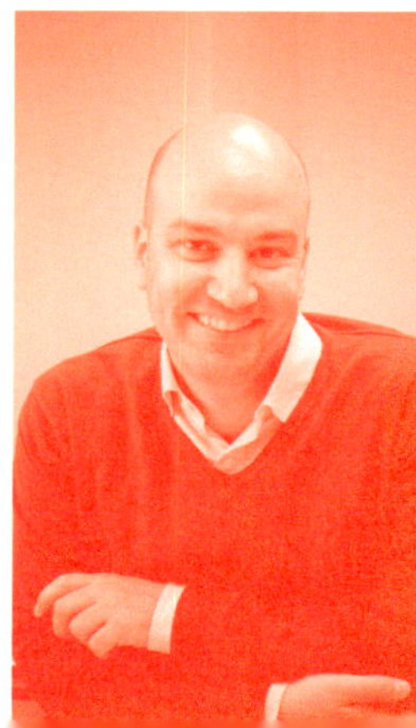

Advances in Precision Medicine Oncology
http://dx.doi.org/10.5772/intechopen.91507
Edited by Hilal Arnouk and Bassam Abdul Rasool Hassan

Contributors
Sonika Charak, Manish Shandilya, Shrutika Sharma, Prabhu Prasad Das, Anatoliy Parfentievich Maletskyy, Natalia Mikhailivna Bigun, Yuriy Markovich Samchenko, Suree Jianmongkol, Chittipolu Ajaykumar, Sadhana Sharma, Rajesh Kumar Yadav, Bandana Kumari, Asgar Ali, Pritanjali Singh, Krishnan Hajela, Anush Patel, Haisam Abid, Amrat Kumar, Said Dermime, Maysaloun Merhi, Queenie Fernandes, Afsheen Raza, Varghese Inchakalody, Shahab Uddin, Allan Relecom, Abdul Rahman Gul, Mohammed Al Homsi, Erlinda M. Gordon, Sant Chawla, Frederick Hall, Nicole Angel, Ted Kim, Don Brigham, Nobukazu Fujimoto, Asako Matsuda, Abdullah Abu-Rqayiq, Alvin Y. Liu, Tatjana Crnogorac-Jurcevic, James J. Lai, Hung-Ming Lam, Enrico Bracco, Giuseppe Saglio, Muhammad S. Ali, Stefano Magnati, Sankha Bhattacharya, Kapil Gore

First published in London, United Kingdom, 2021 by IntechOpen
IntechOpen is the global imprint of INTECHOPEN LIMITED, registered in England and Wales, registration number: 11086078, 5 Princes Gate Court, London, SW7 2QJ, United Kingdom
Printed in Croatia

British Library Cataloguing-in-Publication Data
A catalogue record for this book is available from the British Library

Additional hard and PDF copies can be obtained from orders@intechopen.com

Advances in Precision Medicine Oncology
Edited by Hilal Arnouk and Bassam Abdul Rasool Hassan
p. cm.
Print ISBN 978-1-83968-867-6
Online ISBN 978-1-83968-868-3
eBook (PDF) ISBN 978-1-83968-869-0

For EU product safety concerns:
IN TECH d.o.o., Prolaz Marije Krucifikse Kozulić 3, 51000 Rijeka, Croatia, info@intechopen.com or visit our website at intechopen.com.

Meet the editors

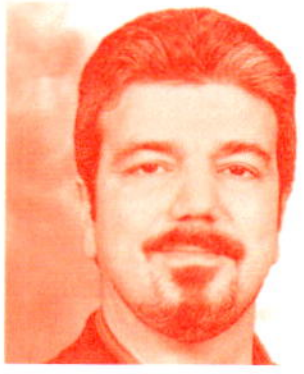

Hilal Arnouk, MD, Ph.D., is an associate professor at the Department of Pathology, Midwestern University, Glendale, Arizona. Dr. Arnouk received his education and post-doctorate training at Roswell Park Cancer Institute, the State University of New York at Buffalo, the Medical College of Georgia, and the University of Alabama at Birmingham. He has directed research studies in academia and biotech industry settings. His major areas of expertise include cancer immunotherapy, biomarker discovery, and precision medicine. Additionally, Dr. Arnouk tremendously enjoys being an educator and a mentor for professional students in the medical and biomedical sciences.

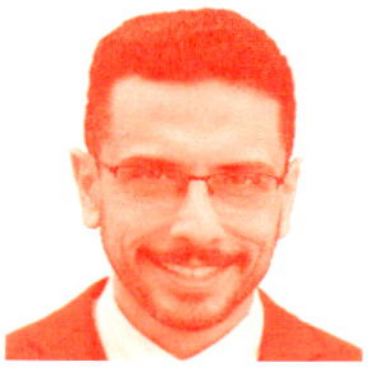

Bassam Abdul Rasool Hassan obtained a Ph.D. in Clinical Pharmacy from the School of Pharmacy, Universiti Sains Malaysia (USM). He worked as a senior lecturer at the Department of Pharmacy, Faculty of Medicine, Universiti Malaya (UM), in 2014–2017, and at the Department of Pharmacy Practice, Faculty of Pharmacy, Universiti Teknologi MARA (UiTM), Shah Alam, Malaysia, in 2017–2019. Dr. Hassan currently works as a senior lecturer at the Department of Pharmacy, Al-Rafidain University College, Baghdad, Iraq.

Contents

Preface

"In the depths of your hopes and desires lies your silent knowledge of the beyond; and like seeds dreaming beneath the snow your heart dreams of spring. Trust the dreams, for in them is hidden the gate to eternity."

– Kahlil Gibran-The Prophet

Recent advances in precision medicine and immuno-oncology have led to highly specific and efficacious cancer therapies. Most notably, immune checkpoint inhibitors (ICIs) are monoclonal antibodies engineered to release the brakes on the patient's own immune system so it can mount a robust immune response against cancer cells. ICIs have emerged as powerful treatments for patients with several types of solid tumors, such as melanoma, mesothelioma, lung, kidney, ovarian, and bladder cancers. Targets of ICIs include the programmed death-ligand 1 (PD-L1), the programmed cell death protein 1 (PD-1), and the cytotoxic T-lymphocyte-associated protein 4 (CLTA-4), which are major factors in tumor evasion of immune surveillance. It is crucially important to identify biomarkers to predict the response to ICIs as well as combination therapies with other targeted mechanisms such as targeted gene blockade and cell cycle checkpoint inhibitors. It is important to note, however, that the use of ICIs in cancer immunotherapy is frequently followed by inflammatory and autoimmune diseases, known as immune-related adverse events (irAEs), which include endocrine adverse effects. Other types of genetically engineered anti-cancer monoclonal antibodies work in a multitude of ways, including flagging cancer cells, blocking cell growth, directly attacking cancer cells, and bridging cancer and killer immune cells. Additionally, conjugated monoclonal antibodies exert their function by carrying a drug or radioactive substance that can destroy cancer cells.

In the field of chemotherapy, doxorubicin is considered one of the most powerful FDA-approved therapeutic agents. Doxorubicin is an anthracycline antibiotic extracted from the bacterium *Streptomyces peucetius*. It causes cancer cell death by intercalating with DNA leading to DNA breakage. It has been successfully used to treat patients with breast cancer, ovarian cancer, lung cancer, bladder cancer, sarcoma, and leukemia. However, the administration of doxorubicin is often limited because of its toxic side effects and drug resistance, which necessitate a clear understanding of the molecular mechanisms behind the emergence of doxorubicin's drug resistance and critical side effects.

It is an exciting time to be in the field of precision medicine and immuno-oncology, as the next generation of targeted therapies holds the promise of better survival rates for cancer patients.

I would like to thank everyone at IntechOpen publishing who helped with this publication. Finally, I dedicate this book to my family, my colleagues, my mentors, and students throughout my career.

Hilal Arnouk MD Ph.D.
Midwestern University (Department of Pathology),
Downers Grove, IL, United States

Bassam Abdul Rasool Hassan
Al-Rafidain University College,
Iraq

Section 1

Advances in Immuno-Oncology

Chapter 1

Immune and Cell Cycle Checkpoint Inhibitors for Cancer Immunotherapy

Erlinda M. Gordon, Nicole L. Angel, Ted T. Kim, Don A. Brigham, Sant P. Chawla and Frederick L. Hall

Abstract

The rational design of immunotherapeutic agents has advanced with a fundamental understanding that both innate and adaptive immunity play important roles in cancer surveillance and tumor destruction; given that oncogenesis occurs and cancer progresses through the growth of tumor cells with low immunogenicity in an increasingly immunosuppressive tumor microenvironment. Checkpoint inhibitors in the form of monoclonal antibodies that block cancer's ability to deactivate and evade the immune system have been widely indicated for a variety of tumor types. Through targeting the biological mechanisms and pathways that cancer cells use to interact with and suppress the immune system, immunotherapeutic agents have achieved success in inhibiting tumor growth while eliciting lesser toxicities, compared to treatments with standard chemotherapy. Development of "precise" bio-active tumor-targeted gene vectors, biotechnologies, and reagents has also advanced. This chapter presents ongoing clinical research involving immune checkpoint inhibitors, while addressing the clinical potential for tumor-targeted gene blockade in combination with tumor-targeted cytokine delivery, in patients with advanced metastatic disease, providing strategic clinical approaches to precision cancer immunotherapy.

Keywords: PD-1 inhibitor, CTLA4 inhibitor, DeltaRex-G, DeltaVax, NK cells, checkpoint inhibitors, cell cycle control, GMCSF

1. Introduction

The human immune system is an intricate network of cell types and signaling pathways that act in a concerted effort to ensure that when an immune response is elicited, it is directly proportional to the severity of the attack. Although this network exists to protect the body from foreign invasion, an overactive immune response can lead to immunopathogenesis and autoimmunity, thus it is crucial that there are mechanisms set in place to ensure this system remains tightly regulated [1]. The immune system achieves this strict regulation by engaging a complex system of checkpoint control pathways. These checkpoints act as metaphorical gateways that require a specific key, in the form of a protein or a small molecule, in order to initiate tightly regulated signaling pathways that prevent over-reactivity of an immune response through the binding of specific cell surface receptors. This process is known as peripheral tolerance [2]. Certain checkpoint pathways, including those involving transmembrane protein receptors cytotoxic t-lymphocyte antigen 4 (CTLA-4) and programmed death 1 (PD-1), play pivotal inhibitory roles in T-cell activation. Specifically, the CTLA-4 checkpoint is designed to inhibit T-cells from becoming autoreactive during the beginning stages of T-cell activation, while the PD-1 checkpoint is part of a family of costimulatory receptors that, when bound to its ligand, inhibits T-cell proliferation [2].

Tumor cells exploit the process of peripheral tolerance as a way to evade immunological surveillance by mimicking inhibitory receptors that are normally expressed on the surface of antigen presenting cells [3]. Expressing these inhibitory receptors allows cancer cells to effectively downregulate an immune response by deactivating the T-cells they come into contact with. The development of genetically engineered immune checkpoint inhibitors (ICIs) to treat malignancies therefore has the potential to revive pre-existing immune responses that would have otherwise been suppressed by the cancer [4]. Immunotherapies have been developed over the past decade using monoclonal antibodies as checkpoint inhibitors, binding the inhibitory receptor on T-cells and blocking tumor cells from binding to these sites.

The first immune checkpoint inhibition therapies to enter clinical trials for patients with advanced cancer were two fully human CTLA-4 blocking antibodies, ipilimumab and tremelimumab. Clinical activity of the CTLA-4 blockade was most significant in advanced melanoma patients, leading to a 15% response rate that, for some patients, persisted for over 10 years after discontinuing therapy [5]. In 2010, a large Phase III trial was published showing ipilimumab to have significantly improved overall survival rates in patients with metastatic melanoma, compared to treatment with standard gp100, a synthetic peptide cancer vaccine, alone [6]. Ipilimumab has since been FDA approved in combination for the treatment of advanced renal cell carcinoma, microsatellite instability high (MSI-H) or mismatch repair deficient (dMMR) metastatic colorectal cancer, hepatocellular carcinoma, non-small cell lung cancer (NSCLC), and malignant pleural mesothelioma.

The PD-1 checkpoint pathway was the next to be targeted with antibody therapy. Similar to ipilimumab, the first nivolumab trials were also shown to be most efficacious in melanoma patients, although it is now approved not only for the treatment of melanoma, but also of non-small cell lung cancer (NSCLC), small cell lung cancer, malignant pleural mesothelioma, renal cell carcinoma, Hodgkin lymphoma, squamous cell carcinoma of the head and neck, urothelial carcinoma, MSI-H or dMMR metastatic colorectal cancer, hepatocellular carcinoma, and esophageal squamous cell carcinoma. A study assessing the efficacy of anti-CTLA-4 and anti-PD-1 combined therapy in melanoma patients showed even more significant results, with 53% of patients achieving an objective response, and $\geq$ 80% tumor reduction was reported in all patients [7].

Thus far, the only two immune checkpoint inhibitors that have been successfully brought to market are those that involve the PD-1/PD-L1 checkpoint and CTLA-4 checkpoint. These targets are within the adaptive immune system, but scientists are looking at the potential anti-tumor effects of exploring checkpoint targets within the innate immune system. Another target currently being investigated involves immune checkpoint inhibition within natural killer (NK) cell-mediated immunity. Cancer cells frequently downregulate their MHC expression, rendering T-cell mediated immunotherapy insufficient for killing these tumor cells. NK cell-mediated treatment can, in theory, compensate for this. As a first line of defense within the immune surveillance system, NK cells are quicker to become activated and will indiscriminately induce apoptosis in any cell lacking MHC-receptors.

Similar to the immune system, a checkpoint control system is also used to control the distinct phases of the cell division cycle in order to regulate cellular proliferation. Unrestrained cell division is a fundamental characteristic of oncogenesis, therefore cell cycle checkpoint control is vital in preventing the development of cancer. The mechanism of action in this case of checkpoint control is site-specific protein phosphorylation executed largely by cyclin-dependent proline-directed protein kinases. For example, Cyclin D1 and CDK4/6 are downstream of growth-initiating signaling pathways which lead to cellular proliferation. Palbociclib, an inhibitor of cyclin-dependent kinases CDK4/CDK6 is approved for the treatment of HR-positive, HER2-negative advanced or metastatic breast cancer in combination with an aromatase inhibitor as initial endocrine based therapy in postmenopausal women or fulvestrant in women with disease progression following endocrine therapy [8].

Another example of an executive cell cycle regulatory protein is the cyclin G1 protein, product of the CCNG1 proto-oncogene: (i) identified as the prime molecular driver of "Cell Competence" (to proliferate), (ii) needed for quiescent cells to enter the G1 phase, subject to oncogene-addiction as a molecular survival factor [9]. Tumor-targeted gene therapy involving CCNG1 blockade was tested in a number of clinical trials over a decade ago, and has recently been revived for clinical use, upon analysis of long-term cancer-free survival data, as the first clinically validated tumor-targeted gene therapy vector of this kind. This genetic medicine, known as DeltaRex-G (Former names: Mx-dnG1, dnG1, Rexin-G), is a "retroviral expression vector displaying a cryptic/designer collagen-binding motif on its gp70 surface envelope, designed specifically for targeting abnormal (anaplastic) Signature (SIG) proteins in the tumor microenvironment and encoding a dominant-negative mutant construct (dnG1) of human CCNG1 (Cyclin G1)oncogene/survival factor [10]. Once administered intravenously, the DeltaRex-G nanoparticles (~100 nm) accumulate in cancerous lesions, where the transgene is expressed, using the tumor cell's replication machinery to translate a mutant, cytocidal protein that is specifically designed to block the Cyclin G1 pathways of cell competence and survival function, leading to active cancer cell death via apoptosis.

Herein, we discuss the current landscape of immune and cell cycle checkpoint inhibition by presenting a selected number of ongoing and past clinical research for advanced malignancies at the Cancer Center of Southern California (CCSC)/ Sarcoma Oncology Research Center (SORC) in Santa Monica, California, in context and collaboration.

2. Ongoing clinical research

Ongoing clinical research is either investigator-initiated or company sponsored. In the case of investigator-initiated research, CCSC/SORC serves as the sponsor, conceives and designs the clinical protocol, and manages the entire clinical trial with or without funding by a pharmaceutical company, the FDA or the NIH. Company-sponsored research is developed, monitored, and funded by a pharmaceutical company.

2.1 Investigator initiated research

2.1.1 SAINT: An Expanded Phase II Study Using Safe Amounts of Ipilimumab, Nivolumab, and Trabectedin as First-Line Treatment of Advanced Soft Tissue Sarcoma (NCT03138161). Erlinda M. Gordon, Principal Investigator

2.1.1.1 Background & rationale

Soft tissue sarcomas comprise a rare, heterogenous category of malignancies originating from connective tissue, blood vessels or lymphatic tissue [11].

This group accounts for only 1% of adult cancers in the United States, but it has a higher mortality rate than testicular cancer, thyroid cancer, and Hodgkin lymphoma combined [12]. The most commonly used modalities of treatment for sarcoma have been surgery, radiation and chemotherapy. Currently, chemotherapy treatment options have been shown to slow down disease progression but are ineffective in keeping most patients from eventually developing recurrent and metastatic disease [13]. Once unresectable or metastatic, the majority of soft tissue sarcomas remain incurable with chemotherapy. Immune checkpoint blockades do not act directly on the cancer cell, thus they can theoretically be applied to the treatment of any type of solid tumor, including the rarest and most aggressive malignancies. The precedent set by the approval of immune checkpoint inhibition for the treatment of numerous cancer types provides a strong rationale for studying their effects on soft tissue sarcoma. Studies with ipilimumab and nivolumab have since been done showing promising results when used in patients with advanced soft tissue sarcoma [14]. The third drug in this trial is a marine-derived alkaloid, trabectedin, an FDA approved chemotherapy treatment for leiomyosarcoma and liposarcoma [15]. A recently published retroactive analysis of 442 patients treated with trabectedin over a 10 year period confirms that trabectedin can prolong progression free survival (PFS) in patients with advanced sarcoma [16].

Gordon et al. designed the SAINT protocol based on the fact that sarcoma cells are most immunogenic early in the disease process [17] and prior to any other treatment, allowing immune checkpoint inhibitors to exploit this advantage and deploy the immune system to recognize and destroy them. This study was designed to evaluate the best objective response rates (BORR) assessed via CT scan or MRI and to assess the overall survival (OS) and progression-free survival (PFS) after 6 months of treatment.

2.1.1.2 Methods

Eligible patients for this Phase II clinical trial were treatment-naïve adult patients with advanced unresectable or metastatic soft tissue sarcoma. Trabectedin was administered to the study subjects at the maximum tolerated dose determined previously in the dose escalation phase of this trial. Ipilimumab and nivolumab were be administered at defined doses in order to assess the overall safety profile and potential efficacy of this treatment regimen. Patients continued on the treatment until they experienced significant disease progression or unmanageable toxicities. Best objective response was measured according to Response Evaluation Criteria in Solid Tumors (RECIST) v1.1 using CT scan or MRI. Median progression-free survival (PFS) and overall survival (OS) were also measured in months. Adverse events were assessed and categorized as related or unrelated to the treatment and listed by severity according to the Common Terminology Criteria for Adverse Events (CTCAE) version 5.0.

2.1.1.3 Preliminary results were presented at the Connective Tissue Oncology Society Meetings, November, 2020

Sixty subjects were evaluated using RECIST v1.1 for analysis of treatment efficacy. Twenty-five percent (25%) had either a complete response (11.7%) or a partial response (13.3%), and 37 patients (61.7%) had stable disease. Disease control rate was 86.6%. The median PFS was >6.7 months (6-month OS rate: 90%; 6-month PFS rate: 51%), while the median OS was >17.0 months.

Grade 3 TRAEs included fatigue (n = 6), adrenal insufficiency (n = 1), hyperglycemia (n = 1), dehydration (n = 1), hyponatremia (n = 2), bipedal edema (n = 2), increased AST (n = 6), increased ALT (n = 19), increased ALP (n = 1), port site infection (n = 2), psoriasis exacerbation (n = 1), anemia (n = 3), thrombocytopenia (n = 2), leukopenia (n = 1), and neutropenia (n = 3). Grade 4 TRAES include anemia (n = 1), neutropenia (n = 1), thrombocytopenia (n = 1), and increased CPK (n = 2). Grade 5 TRAES include rhabdomyolysis (n = 1). Therapy related AML occurred in one patient.

2.1.1.4 Conclusions/future directions

The positive results from this trial thus far strongly suggest that using combination therapy with ipilimumab, nivolumab, and trabectedin as first-line treatment in patients with advanced or metastatic sarcoma allows the treatments to engage synergistically without causing any additive toxicities. This combination may be superior to known therapies for STS. Overall, the adverse events experienced less severe than toxicities typically experienced with standard first line treatment (doxorubicin/ifosfamide) for metastatic soft tissue sarcoma. Future Phase 3 randomized studies are proposed to evaluate the safety and efficacy of first-line combinatorial therapy with ipilimumab, nivolumab and trabectedin in comparison to standard therapy for patients with advanced soft tissue sarcomas.

2.1.2 The TNT Protocol: A Phase II Study Using Talimogene Laherparepvec, Nivolumab, and Trabectedin as First, Second/Third Line Therapy for Advanced Sarcoma, including Desmoid Tumor and Chordoma (NCT03886311). Sant P. Chawla and Erlinda M. Gordon, co-Principal Investigators

2.1.2.1 Background & rationale

The significant immunotherapeutic potential of oncolytic virotherapy is due to its ability to induce a multifaceted anti-tumor response involving aspects of both the innate and adaptive immune systems [18]. A multitude of viral vectors have been explored for their potential oncolytic properties, particularly as a method of delivering targeted treatment to sites of malignant disease [19]. The ability to genetically modify these viruses to target and exploit essential oncogenic signaling pathways has kept them at the forefront of immuno-oncology research [20]. This particular vulnerability triggers selective replication of the viral genome and directly contributes to furthering the oncolytic process. Infected tumor cells secrete viral progeny composed in part by tumor-associated antigens and neoantigens in response to their infection, causing the innate immune system to activate an NK cell-mediated cytotoxic response. The tumor-associated antigens that are released into the tumor microenvironment are phagocytosed by antigen-presenting cells, thus initiating the process of T-cell-mediated adaptive anti-tumor immunity. In addition to the anti-tumor response, the presence of the oncolytic virus also triggers a concurrent anti-viral response, and regulatory mechanisms become crucial to ensuring a controlled immune response, including the upregulation of immune checkpoints [20].

Oncolytic viruses derived from Herpes simplex virus 1 (HSV-1) vectors are amongst the most frequently investigated in pre-clinical trials and have been shown to encompass the combined ability to induce oncolysis and anti-tumor immune responses simultaneously [21]. Talimogene Laherparepvec (T-VEC) is an injectable live, attenuated, oncolytic HSV-1 virus that has been genetically engineered to express human granulocyte-macrophage colony-stimulating factor (huGM-CSF), a known immune modulator and hematopoietic growth factor that stimulates the differentiation of multipotent progenitor cells and plays a key role in the functional abilities of many different circulating lymphocytes, including T-cells [22].

The objective of this ongoing study is to evaluate the potentially synergistic effects T-VEC may evoke when used in combination with anti-PD-L1 monoclonal antibody, nivolumab and marine derived alkaloid, trabectedin. The study is ongoing.

2.1.2.2 Methods

This open-label Phase II study is designed to assess the safety and efficacy of this combination treatment. This will be accomplished by determining the median month of progression-free survival, median duration of response, and best overall response rates based on each patients' percent of change in their tumor sizes. This study plans to enroll 40 participants with advanced disease who have at least one tumor that is easily accessible for intratumoral injection with T-VEC. Regarding the statistical analysis, continuous variables will be summarized by the sample size (n) and measures of central tendency and variation will be calculated including mean, standard deviation, first and third quartiles, maximum and minimum. Categorical variables will be summarized by the sample and by the percent in each category. "Point estimates for efficacy endpoint incidences will be accompanied by a 2-sided 95% exact binomial CI. Time to event endpoints will be summarized descriptively using the KM method. Safety (incidence and severity of adverse events and significant laboratory abnormalities) will be performed on all patients (ITT population). Patient incidence of all treatment emergent AEs will be tabulated by system organ class and preferred term" [23].

2.1.2.3 Preliminary results presented at the Connective Tissue Oncology Society meetings, November, 2020

Efficacy analysis (n = 31): There were 6.5% partial responses, 80.6% disease control rate, with 74.1% PFS rate and 92.6% OS rate at 4 months.

Safety Analysis (n = 41): Grade 3 TRAEs include fatigue (n = 2), decreased ejection fraction (n = 1), anasarca (n = 1), dehydration (n = 1), decreased cortisol (n = 1), anemia (n = 9), thrombocytopenia (n = 4), neutropenia (n = 4), gastroenteritis (n = 1), increased ALT (n = 8), increased AST (n = 1), and increased GGT (n = 1). Grade 4 TRAEs observed were thrombocytopenia (n = 2). There was no conversion from unresectable to resectable tumor. There were thirty-one evaluable subjects for efficacy analysis.

2.1.2.4 Conclusions/future directions

Second- or third- line combinatorial therapy with talimogene laherparepvec, nivolumab, and trabectedin.

1. may be equal or better than standard second/third line therapy in achieving disease control.

2. may be safer than standard therapy for patients with advanced soft tissue sarcoma with no unexpected toxicities.

2.1.2.4.1 Future directions for research

Studies are proposed to evaluate the efficacy and safety of first, second/third line combinatorial therapy with talimogene laherparepvec, nivolumab and trabectedin vs. standard therapy (doxorubicin/ifosfamide) in randomized studies for advanced soft tissue sarcomas.

2.1.3 A Phase Ib investigation of safety/efficacy of nivolumab and ABI-009 (nab-rapamycin) in advanced undifferentiated pleomorphic sarcoma (UPS), liposarcoma (LPS), chondrosarcoma (CS), osteosarcoma (OS) and Ewing sarcoma (NCT03190174). Erlinda M. Gordon, Principal Investigator

2.1.3.1 Background & rationale

Aberrant mTOR signaling, typically due to either an activating mutation in oncogenes related to the mTOR pathway or a loss of function mutation in an upstream tumor suppressor gene, has been found to play a significant, multifaceted role in oncogenesis [24, 25]. Originally discovered while investigating the targets of the drug rapamycin, a potent immunosuppressive agent, in the early 1990's, the protein kinase, mammalian target of rapamycin (mTOR), is a major signaling hub for directing cellular growth, metabolism, and proliferation [26]. While studying the mechanism of action behind rapamycin's inhibitory effects on mTOR signaling, the drug was also found to be involved in the inhibition of T-cell proliferation, specifically between the G_1 and S phases of the cell cycle. This finding launched a multitude of studies to better understand the role of mTOR signaling in T-cell activation and proliferation [27], culminating in the discovery that T-cells are also highly dependent on mTOR signaling to maintain normal T-cell activation and proliferation [28]. When t-cells receive immune stimuli, they then rely on signals from mTOR to promote t-helper cell differentiation while simultaneously inhibiting the induction of regulatory T-cells. Thus, mTOR exerts control over essential regulatory signals in both adaptive and innate immunity.

Initial clinical studies investigating the anti-cancer effects of single agent mTOR inhibitor, were disappointing, reporting its limited effects, thus leading to the investigation of rapamycin in combination with various chemotherapy agents where it was successful in inhibiting cancer growth in prostate cancer patients [29]. However, the experimental drug, ABI-009 or nab-sirolimus, a novel albumin-bound mTOR inhibitor, has been shown to be effective and safe for the treatment of malignant perivascular epithelioid cell tumors (PEComa) [30]. A phase 1/2 trial is currently ongoing to investigate the potential synergistic activity of nab-sirolimus when administered with an immune checkpoint inhibitor, nivolumab, in improving clinical outcomes for patients with advanced sarcoma.

2.1.3.2 Methods

The original objectives of the study are: (1) To investigate the maximum tolerated dose (MTD) of ABI-009 when given with nivolumab, a PD-1 inhibitor, in previously treated advanced undifferentiated pleomorphic sarcoma, liposarcoma, chondrosarcoma, osteosarcoma and Ewing sarcoma; (2) To investigate the disease control rate (DCR), progression-free survival (PFS), and overall survival (OS) of this combination therapy in the aforementioned patient group, and (3) To correlate PFS with PD-L1 and other biomarker expression in patients' tumors.

This is an IRB approved protocol with 2 parts. The phase 1 part is a dose-finding study using the "cohort of three design", wherein a standard dose of nivolumab 240 mg is given IV every 3 weeks (day 1 of every 21-day cycle). Escalating doses of ABI-009 are given IV on days 8 and 15 of each cycle starting in Cycle 2 following the 2nd nivolumab dose. The starting dose of ABI-009 is 56 mg/m^2, and sequentially escalating doses are 75, and 100 mg/m^2. Phase 2 of the study will enroll 31 additional patients to further assess efficacy and safety at the MTD.

2.1.3.3 Preliminary results presented at the ASCO annual meeting in June, 2019

The Phase I part of study included 9 patients who were treated successfully at 3 dose levels. No dose-limiting toxicities (DLTs) were observed, the MTD was not reached, and 100 mg/m^2 ABI-009 was designated as the recommended Phase II dose. Safety analysis: At Dose 1 (n = 3): Grade 3 treatment-related adverse events (TRAEs) included dyslipidemia (n = 1) and hyperglycemia (n = 1). At Dose 2 (n = 3): Grade 3 TRAEs included increased ALT (n = 1). At Dose 3 (n = 3): Grade 3 TRAEs included hypophosphatemia (n = 1).

2.1.3.4 Conclusions/future directions

The primary endpoint has been met with no DLTs, the MTD was not reached and Dose 3 (100 mg/m2) of ABI-009 has been designated as the phase 2 dose which is on-going.

2.2 Company sponsored clinical research

2.2.1 Phase I Study of INBRX-109 in Subjects With Locally Advanced or Metastatic Solid Tumors Including Sarcomas (NCT03715933) Sant P. Chawla, Principal Investigator

2.2.1.1 Background & rationale

The initiation of the extrinsic apoptosis pathway is mediated by several death domain receptors including death receptor 5 (DR5), a transmembrane protein receptor activated by the tumor necrosis factor-related apoptosis-inducing ligand (TRAIL) [31]. The DR5 apoptosis pathway naturally occurs to rid the body of neoplastic cells and is known to be crucial in immune system surveillance against cancer growth and metastasis. Normally, when an anchorage-dependent cell becomes detached, the cell will undergo a process of detachment-induced apoptosis called anoikis, initiated by a death receptor-mediated apoptotic pathway. A reduction in DR5 expression was found in melanoma tumor samples, strongly implying the TRAIL/DR5 pathway is associated with the prevention of tumor metastasis [32]. In 1999, Walczak et al. observed tumor cells to have a significantly higher sensitivity to TRAIL than normal cells, emphasizing its potential as a therapeutic cancer agent [33]. The subsequent development of agonistic antibodies against DR5 (i.e. recombinant human TRAIL proteins) was shown to be successful in stimulating apoptosis when tested in various tumor cell lines, and was later also shown to enhance the efficacy of chemotherapy and radiotherapy [34].

INBRX-109 is a tetravalent DR5 agonist antibody designed to initiate the DR5 apoptosis pathway and precisely engineered to avoid unnecessary crosslinking to lower the risk of hepatotoxicity.

2.2.1.2 Methods

This is the first in-human, open-label, non-randomized Phase I clinical trial for INBRX-109. Eligible patients had metastatic or unresectable solid tumors refractory to standard treatment or for which there is no FDA approved standard treatment. Phase I consists of two parts, part 1 being a 3 + 3 dose escalation cohort and part 2 being a dose expansion cohort. Safety, tolerability and dose-limiting toxicity were measured and analyzed using the National Cancer Institute's Common Terminology

Criteria for Adverse Events (CTCAE) criteria to assess the severity of adverse events experienced. This study's exploratory objective is an assessment of anti-tumor activity and was reported according to RECIST v1.1 standard.

2.2.1.3 Preliminary results presented at the CTOS meeting, November, 2020

Overall, INBRX-109 was well tolerated and approximately 90% of patients showed no signs of hepatotoxicity. The pharmacokinetics of INBRX-109 were approximately dose proportional across all doses tested and thus support dosing every 3 weeks without administration of any premedications. All patients have thus far tested negative for anti-drug antibodies. Maximum tolerated dose was not reached in the dose escalation cohort and only one dose-limiting toxicity was experienced. Very few serious adverse events that occurred were attributable to the drug being studied. One patient with mesothelioma has been reported to have experienced acute hepatic failure leading to death that could possibly be related to the study drug. Evidence of anti-cancer effects were observed in patients with chondrosarcoma, resulting in durable partial responses and stable disease.

2.2.1.4 Conclusions/future directions

NBRX-109, a precisely engineered tetravalent DR5 agonist antibody, showed promising results that warrant further exploration. The pharmacokinetics of INBRX-109 were essentially dose-proportional across all three dose levels, supporting dosing every three weeks with no premedications necessary. Specifically, the chondrosarcoma cohort of this Phase I study has been expanded to include twenty patients and is currently ongoing.

2.2.2 An Open-labeled, Phase I Study to Evaluate the Safety and Tolerability of Apatinib with Nivolumab in Patients with Unresectable or Metastatic Cancer (NCT03396211) Sant P. Chawla, Principal Investigator

2.2.2.1 Background & rationale

Unregulated angiogenesis is one of the key characteristics of malignant tumors [35]. In addition to creating neovasculature, tumor angiogenesis plays a key role in creating an immunosuppressive tumor microenvironment by causing an accumulation of pro-tumor immune cells and a decrease in the abundance and function of anti-tumor immune cells. Anti-angiogenic cancer treatments have been shown to reverse this process, essentially 'reprogramming' the tumor microenvironment by converting it from an immunosuppressive to an immunogenic one. This has been accomplished by targeting and inhibiting vascular endothelial growth factor (VEGF), a well-known cell surface-signaling proangiogenic protein that becomes stimulated when bound to tyrosine kinase receptors. With the use of antiangiogenic small molecule tyrosine kinase inhibitors (TKIs), VEGF can be blocked from binding its receptor, stopping the tumor from being able to continue to create neovasculature [36]. However, cancer has been able to circumvent this blockade using multiple other pathways, suggesting the use of antiangiogenic therapies that inhibit more than one signaling pathway simultaneously.

The experimental drug, apatinib, is a highly selective VEGFR-2 TKI, administered orally, that has already been approved in China for ≥3rd-line treatment for advanced gastric cancer. The potential benefit of combining TKI and PD-1 therapies has been demonstrated in preclinical murine models, suggesting that combining ICIs with antiangiogenesis therapy could have the synergistic antitumor effects needed to enhance the efficacy of the individual therapies [37]. This phase 1 single-center clinical trial beginning in 2018 evaluated the safety and tolerability of TKI, apatinib, and PD-1 inhibitor, nivolumab, in patients with unresectable or metastatic cancer.

2.2.2.2 Methods

All subjects enrolled had cancer that was refractory to prior lines of treatment. Specifically, patients were required to already be at least three cycles into nivolumab treatment and must be planning to continue this treatment throughout the trial period. Thirty patients in total were enrolled, ten of which were in part 1 of this study, where they were treated with apatinib using a classic 3 + 3 dose escalation method in order to determine the maximum tolerated dose. Part 2 of this study included twenty subjects and was an expansion phase using the MTD. The percent of change in tumor responses and amount of time until progression were measured and analyzed using RECIST v1.1 and iRECIST criteria.

2.2.2.3 Preliminary results presented at the Connective Tissue Oncology Society meetings, November, 2020

The overall response rate reported was 13.3% (95% CI: 3.8% to 30.7%) and the median PFS was 7.2 months (95% CI: 5.3 to 9.0 months). No complete responses occurred although four patients achieved a partial response and the majority of patients achieved stable disease. Seven patients from part 1 and six patients from part 2 experienced ≥ grade 3 treatment emergent adverse events including fatigue (10.0%), hypertension (10.0%), nausea (10.0%), anemia (16.7%) and asthenia (10.0%). Two patients experienced fatal adverse events, although there were no noted treatment related deaths. Nine patients eventually discontinued the study due to toxicity, and nine patients also received a dose reduction. No unexpected side effects were noted as a result of the combined treatment.

2.2.2.4 Conclusions/future directions

The results of this study demonstrate an acceptable safety profile and clinical benefit of combination treatment with nivolumab and apatinib that is worth exploring further in additional clinical studies.

2.2.3 Phase 1, Open-Label, Safety Study of Escalating Doses of Ex Vivo Expanded, Autologous Natural Killer Cells in Patients With Pathologically Confirmed Cancer Refractory to Conventional Therapy (NCT03941262). Sant P. Chawla, Principal Investigator

2.2.3.1 Background & rationale

Natural killer (NK) cells are the cytotoxic lymphocytes of the innate immune system [38]. As a rapid, first line of defense, NK cells are able to lyse tumor cells independent of the expression of tumor-associated antigens and/or the presence of major histocompatibility complex class I (MHC-I) molecules. This ability is crucial as cancer cells have been shown to downregulate the expression of MHC-I on their cell surface as a way to evade detection by immunosurveillance mechanisms [39].

Since the expression of MHC-I on cancer cells is needed for their detection and destruction by T-cells, evolving a loss of MHC-I expression has been a way for tumor cells to remain undetectable and this loss has therefore been reported "as a mechanism of resistance to anti–PD-1 therapy" [40]. In order to avoid the development of resistance to PD-1 checkpoint inhibition therapy, exploration of NK cell therapy is warranted, especially because of the NK cell's specific role in the recognition and destruction of cancer cells that display a loss of MHC-I. Additionally, the broad ability of NK cells to destroy tumor cells irrespective of prior sensitization or immunization therapy make them ideal candidates for engineered cell therapies.

Discoveries regarding the NK cell's role in anti-tumor immunity coupled with advancements in the field of hematopoietic stem cell transplantation have brought to light the potential in using NK cell-mediated immunotherapeutic strategies to fight cancer [41]. Adoptive immunotherapy using donor-derived autologous NK cell products can be engineered by using monoclonal antibodies alone, or in combination with in vivo and ex vivo NK cell activation techniques [42]. This is done by obtaining a patient's NK cells and incubating them as highly active NK cells, giving them the ability to mass produce NK cells which are then infused back into the patient. This study explores the safety and tolerability of treating cancer with SNK01 (autologous natural killer cells).

2.2.3.2 Methods

This study is a nonrandomized, multicenter safety study of adoptively infused, ex vivo expanded autologous NK cells to treat male and female adult patients with advanced or metastatic, intractable cancer. Study subjects were placed in one of three cohorts and received SNK01 in an open-label fashion according to a 3 + 3 Phase 1 dose-escalation method. Patients received 5 weekly infusions for a period of 5 weeks, and restaging imaging was performed on week 6. The primary objective of this study was a safety assessment based on the incidence and severity of dose-limiting toxicities and other adverse events observed by evaluating vital signs, clinical laboratory findings and physical examination abnormalities. The adverse events were graded according to the CTCAE v5.0 criteria. Subjects' performance status was assessed and recorded using ECOG criteria. The secondary objective is to evaluate the efficacy of the treatment by measuring the objective response rate of target lesions observed via CT scan using iRECIST criteria.

2.2.3.3 Preliminary results

Not yet available.

2.2.3.4 Conclusions/future directions

In order to effectively achieve immune surveillance, immunosuppressive signals within the tumor microenvironment must be interrupted. The PD-1/PD-L1 signaling blockade was developed in accordance with this principle. Tumors have been shown to secrete cytokines associated with suppression of T-cells and NK cells, and past murine studies have shown circulating IL-18 in low levels originating from tumor cells can suppress NK anti-tumor activity [41]. The principles of checkpoint blockade can be applied here with the development of a neutralizing antibody to IL-18, suggesting the potential of checkpoint inhibition to improve in vivo NK cell activity.

3. Past clinical research

3.1 Immune Design: A Randomized, Open-Label, Phase II Trial of CMB305 (Sequentially Administered LV305 [lentiviral vector expressing NYESO-1 gene] and G305[NY-ESO-1 recombinant protein plus GLA-SE]) and Atezolizumab in Patients with Locally Advanced, Relapsed, or Metastatic Sarcoma Expressing NY-ESO-1 (NCT02609984) Sant P. Chawla, Principal Investigator

3.1.1 Background & rationale

NY-ESO-1 is a protein that is normally expressed in fetal and testicular tissues, although some solid malignancies have been known to express an abnormal NY-ESO-1 protein that has become a target for emerging antigen-directed cancer therapies [43, 44]. Previous studies looking at NY-ESO-1 expression in cancer cells have reported its presence in the majority of synovial sarcomas tested, as well as sporadic expression in a number of other sarcoma subsets [45]. The immunogenicity of NY-ESO-1 has been demonstrated by the discovery of receptors against NY-ESO-1 on $CD8^+$ T-cells. A 2011 clinical trial conducted by the National Cancer Institute was the first to report promising anticancer effects of NY-ESO-1-targeted immunotherapy in patients with metastatic synovial sarcoma using adoptively transferred autologous T-cells containing a T-cell receptor against NY-ESO-1 [46], suggesting its potential to be effective in other sarcomas as well. Since then, numerous trials targeting NY-ESO-1 in various cancer types using both adoptive T-cell therapy and vaccination approaches have concluded that there is a clear clinical benefit in pursuing NY-ESO-1 as an immunotherapeutic target [47].

The drug being studied is CMB305, a prime-boost immunotherapeutic vaccine regimen developed to prime the immune system and enhance its subsequent response to immunotherapeutic agents. The priming component of CMB305 is an integration-deficient, replication-incompetent lentiviral vector containing RNA coding for NY-ESO-1. The boost component contains a recombinant E. coli-produced NY-ESO-1 protein that, as a single agent, can initiate anti-NY-ESO-1-specific $CD4^+$ T-cell and antibody responses. The combination of the primer and the booster was designed with the intention of eliciting an enhanced T-cell response.

The goal of this study was to investigate the ability of a prime-boost immunotherapy regimen that is able to elicit NY-ESO-1-specific $CD8^+$ T-cells to synergistically enhance the efficacy of PD-L1 checkpoint inhibition therapy in advanced or metastatic sarcoma patients whose tumors are positive for NY-ESO-1 expression.

3.1.2 Methods

The primary objective of this study was to compare the progression-free survival in locally advanced or metastatic sarcoma patients whose tumors expressed NY-ESO-1 when treated with CMB305 in combination with atezolizumab versus patients treated with atezolizumab alone. The secondary objectives of this study were to evaluate the safety of this combination treatment, as well as to evaluate the best overall response rate using RECIST v1.1 modified to use immune-related response criteria. The overall survival of the two groups will be evaluated.

Twelve patients were randomized 1:1 in a safety run-in evaluation. Next, 80 patients were randomized and stratified by disease. Tumor samples from all patients were tested for levels of PD-L1 and NY-ESO-1 expression prior to treatment, and again on Day 42 in order to assess the extent of successful immune cell invasion in the tumor. Re-staging imaging studies were performed every six weeks for the first twelve months, followed by staging every twelve weeks until the patient displayed symptomatic progression. CMB305 treatment was administered in seven doses over a three-month period, while atezolizumab was administered intravenously every three weeks, and was continued up to two years or until toxicities began to develop. An additional booster dose was also given every six weeks for the first year or until the patient displayed disease progression. Blood samples were collected to test for lentivirus vector persistence at baseline, six, twelve and twenty-four months following the initial treatment. Adverse events were recorded as related or unrelated to the study drug and graded based on CTCAE c4.03 criteria.

3.1.3 Published results

Not Available.

3.1.4 Conclusions/future directions

Phase I of this trial was the first of its kind to test a prime-boost vaccination regimen to treat patients with advanced cancer. In 2018, Immune Design released information stating that an early analysis of the Phase II clinical trial results showed the combination treatment of atezolizumab with CMB305 suggested that it is unlikely this regimen will show enhanced survival time of patients with recurrent synovial sarcoma [48]. A Phase III trial has not yet been pursued.

3.2 A Phase I-II Study Using DeltaRex-G (Former name:Rexin-G)Tumor-Targeted Retrovector Encoding a Dominant-Negative Cyclin G1 Inhibitor for Advanced Pancreatic Cancer (NCT00504998) Sant P. Chawla, Michael Morse, Howard Bruckner, Principal Investigators

3.2.1 Background & rationale

Advanced pancreatic adenocarcinoma is the third most common cancer type in the Unites States, although diagnostic tests are non-specific which leads to early-stage disease frequently going undetected [49, 50]. Once pancreatic adenocarcinoma reaches an advanced stage, it has likely become intractable and there is no cure. Previous targeted therapies revolved around the epidermal growth factor receptor (EGFR) signaling pathway, one of the most significant factors regulating cell growth, survival, differentiation and proliferation, making it a promising target for precision medicine [51]. EGFR signaling has been identified as an oncogenic driver in multiple cancer types, and EGFR inhibitors have been used as targeted therapy for pancreatic cancer [52].

DeltaRex-G is the first injectable tumor-targeted gene delivery system to be developed for cancer that blocks the G1 checkpoint of the cell division cycle of cancer cells by inhibiting the CCNG1 gene. DeltaRex-G includes a mutant construct of the CCNG1 gene that inhibits human cyclin G1, a proto-oncogene that promotes cell competence, cell survival, and stem cell proliferation. When administered systemically, DeltaRex-G seeks out and accumulates in tumor tissues by binding abnormal collagenous signature (SIG) proteins that are characteristically exposed as anaplasia during tumor invasion. Once the DeltaRex-G retrovector is incorporated in rapidly dividing cells, a cytocidal CCNG1 inhibitor protein is expressed that effectively blocks the cell division cycle, resulting in apoptosis and subsequent eradication of cancer cells, proliferative vasculature, and stroma.

Clinical data from DeltaRex-G trials conducted initially in the Philippines showed promising results for patients with advanced pancreatic adenocarcinoma.

This prompted USFDA Orphan Drug status, leading to progressive clinical trials in the United States, using DeltaRex-G to treat chemotherapy-resistant advanced pancreatic adenocarcinoma, soft tissue sarcoma, osteosarcoma, and breast cancers. This study reports the results compiled from a Phase I-II clinical trial using intravenous infusions of DeltaRex-G as treatment for advanced pancreatic cancer.

3.2.2 Methods

Twenty patients with chemotherapy-resistant metastatic pancreatic cancer were enrolled in the trial. Target lesions were identified in each patient and changes in tumor size were measured using RECIST v1.0 criteria. Patients were grouped and treated at 3 escalating doses of DeltaRex-G, with six patients at Dose 0-I, seven patients at dose level II, and seven patients at dose level III. Fifteen patients completed at least one full 4-week treatment cycle and had a follow-up PET-CT scan. These fifteen subjects comprised the modified intent-to-treat (mITT) population and were evaluated in terms of their response to the treatment, months of progression-free survival and months of overall survival.

3.2.3 Published results

The safety analysis revealed no clinically significant dose-limiting toxicities at any of the 3 dose levels, with no serious adverse events related to the study drug. None of the patients tested positive for vector neutralizing antibodies, replication-competent retrovirus in peripheral blood lymphocytes, antibodies to gp70, or vector integration into the genomic DNA of peripheral blood lymphocytes. According to the RECIST v1.0 evaluations of tumor responses, one patient achieved a complete response, two patients, partial response, and 12 patients, stable disease with 100% disease control rate. The median progression free survival by RECIST v1.0 was 2.7 months, 4.0 months, and 5.6 months at Dose levels I, II, and III, respectively. Median overall survival was 4.3 months, 9.2 months, and 9.2 months at Dose levels I, II, and III, respectively. A dose response relationship was shown between duration of survival and DeltaRex-G dosage ($p = 0.03$). Consequently, fast track designation was given by the USFDA for a planned Phase 2/3 study using DeltaRex-G as second line therapy for advanced pancreatic adenocarcinoma.

3.2.4 Conclusions/future directions

DeltaRex-G is a potent cytotoxic cell cycle checkpoint inhibitor. Complete and partial responses were observed at dose levels II and III, suggesting a significant dose–response relationship between the dose of DeltaRex-G given and the level of response seen in the tumors. This relationship is further implied by the increase in months of progression free survival as the dosages were increased. Additionally, CCNG1 is expressed in over 50% of various different malignancies other than pancreatic cancer, suggesting DeltaRex-G's potential efficacy in other cancer types [10].

3.3 Immune cell trafficking in the tumor microenvironment of human cyclin G1 (CCNG1) inhibitor-treated tumors

3.3.1 Background & rationale

Cell cycle checkpoint pathways that govern uninhibited cell proliferation can be rendered ineffective by a variety of cancer-induced immunosuppressive mechanisms [53]. The experimental cancer gene therapy, DeltaRex-G, is a pathotropic (disease-seeking) retrovector designed to disrupt the cell cycle machinery of proliferative tumor cells, forcing them to undergo apoptosis. This is accomplished through "precise" tumor-targeted gene delivery to block the Cyclin G1/Cdk/cMyc/Mdm2/p53 Axis, effectively arresting the dividing tumor cell in G1 phase of the cell cycle undermining CCNG1 oncogene addiction. Clinical trials using DeltaRex-G to treat cancers that are unresponsive to traditional therapy have shown remarkable efficacy in evoking long term cancer-free survival with monotherapy (>10 years) in a number of patients with pancreatic cancer, osteosarcoma, soft tissue sarcomas, breast cancer, and B-cell lymphoma [54]. Although DeltaRex-G is involved in cell cycle checkpoint inhibition, it has also been shown to reduce extracellular matrix production by tumor cells and increase immune cell entry into the tumor microenvironment, which raises the clinical potential for DeltaRex-G to work synergistically with specific immune checkpoint inhibitors.

One persistent thought is that blanket recruitment of immune cells to the tumor microenvironment may not always be advantageous in creating an effective anti-tumor response. Certain tumor-infiltrating immune cells of myeloid origin have been shown to aid in tumor metastasis [55]. Cancers often progress and metastasize using immunosuppressive mechanisms that includes production and secretion of molecules that recruit cells involved in immune responses to the tumor microenvironment, and by exploiting checkpoint altering pathways [56]. Alternatively, and plausibly, this is how the innate immune system works in a healthy individual, with its molecular start and stop switches to prevent exaggerated immune responses and autoimmune disease. This study reviews published literature on the specific tumor-infiltrating immune cells seen in tumors of patients treated with DeltaRex-G.

3.3.2 Methods

A review of published literature was conducted on articles pertaining to the efficacy of DeltaRex-G in influencing the tumor microenvironment. The tumor types identified throughout the literature review included pancreatic adenocarcinoma metastatic to the liver, melanoma metastatic to the inguinal lymph node, colorectal cancer metastatic to the lungs, pancreatic B-cell lymphoma metastatic to the liver and cervical lymph nodes, recurrent breast ductal adenocarcinoma, and non-small cell lung carcinoma metastatic to the adrenal gland. The presence of tumor-infiltrating lymphocytes in excised tumors of patients treated with DeltaRex-G was assessed using immunohistochemical staining, and anti-tumor immune cells were differentiated from pro-tumor immune cells by their cytological characteristics. Agents included in the category of anti-tumor immune cells included dendritic cells, helper T-cells, natural killer cells, and killer T-cells. Regulatory T-cells and B-cells have the ability to encourage tumor growth by preventing antigen presentation and killer T-cell activation, thus were categorized as possibly pro-tumor immune cells. M1 macrophages were categorized as anti-tumor, although M2-type tumor-associated macrophages can promote tumor pathogenicity by overpowering M1-type tumor-infiltrating macrophages that elicit anti-tumor inflammation and were therefore categorized as pro-tumor. Results were reported based on cancer type.

3.3.3 Published results

Killer T-cells were identified in the tumor microenvironment of all cancers analyzed and helper T-cells were identified in all tumor types except for pancreatic B-cell lymphoma metastatic to the liver and cervical lymph nodes. Dendritic cells were found in metastatic pancreatic adenocarcinoma, metastatic melanoma, breast ductal adenocarcinoma and metastatic non-small cell lung cancer. Natural killer cells were seen in metastatic pancreatic adenocarcinoma and metastatic non-small cell lung cancer. M1 macrophages were seen in breast ductal adenocarcinoma.

B-cells, possible pro-tumor cells, were seen in metastatic pancreatic adenocarcinoma, metastatic colorectal cancer, breast ductal adenocarcinoma and metastatic non-small cell lung cancer. Leukocyte common antigen was seen in metastatic pancreatic adenocarcinoma, metastatic melanoma, and non-small cell lung cancer. Pro-tumor macrophages were seen in breast ductal carcinoma.

3.3.4 Conclusions/future directions

Activating and optimizing the body's own immune system is at the core of precision medicine. Pathologic review showed evidence of **enhanced immune cell trafficking in the tumor microenvironment of patients treated with DeltaRex-G, suggesting that this treatment activates the innate immune response**. This implies that DeltaRex-G may enhance the performance of an immunotherapy agent when used simultaneously. Three patients identified in the literature with metastatic pancreatic cancer, B-cell lymphoma and metastatic osteosarcoma, respectively, have survived over 10 years following treatment with DeltaRex-G, no cancers have recurred, and no additional treatments have been needed. This clinical evidence strongly suggests that **DeltaRex-G has the ability to promote cancer immunization in situ through CCNG1 inhibition without causing deleterious immune suppression** [9]. Therefore, further evaluation of the role of DeltaRex-G in enhancing immune cell trafficking in the tumor microenvironment is warranted.

3.4 The Genevieve Protocol: Phase I/II Evaluation of a Dual Targeted Approach to Cancer Gene Therapy/Immunotherapy. Jorge G. Ignacio, Principal Investigator

3.4.1 Background & rationale

Patients whose cancer has recurred or progressed after therapy have likely exhausted their treatment options [57]. This is where the need for research towards the development of personalized targeted treatments becomes both vital and urgent. The GeneVieve (Genes for Life) Protocol was a dose-seeking study for chemoresistant solid malignancies and B-cell lymphoma, that evaluated the efficacy and safety profile of a dual targeted gene therapy regimen using DeltaRex-G and DeltaVax (Former name: Reximmune-C), two personalized vaccination strategies aimed to augment immune cell trafficking within the tumor microenvironment for in situ autoimmunization. DeltaRex-G is a retrovector encoding a cytocidal "dominant-negative" mutant construct of the human CCNG1 (Cyclin G1) oncogene. This retrovector is designed to destroy cancer cells, its tumor vasculature and tumor associated fibroblasts, expose neoantigens created by the tumor debris, inhibit the production of the extracellular matrix and enable immune cells to safely enter the tumor microenvironment. DeltaVax is a retrovector encoding the human GM-CSF gene, used for evoking T-cell proliferation, dendritic cell maturation and polarization of M1 macrophages. United States- and Philippine-based Phase I/II studies using DeltaRex-G for sarcoma, pancreatic cancer, and breast cancer led to its accelerated approval in the Philippines for all chemoresistant solid malignancies and subsequent USFDA approved Orphan Drug status for pancreatic cancer, soft tissue sarcoma and osteosarcoma. In 2009, DeltaRex-G received Fast Track designation for a pivotal Phase II/III trial for pancreatic cancer in the United States. The GeneVieve protocol added a second retrovector strategically to the DeltaRex-G treatment that encoded a GM-CSF gene to examine the role localized GMCSF might play in further improving treatment outcomes and inducing long lasting anti-tumor immunity.

3.4.2 Methods

The patient population consisted of 16 adults with unresectable advanced or metastatic disease. All subjects had an ECOG score between 0 and 1, adequate hematological, kidney and hepatic function, and an estimated survival of 3 months or more. A chemistry panel and complete blood count were assessed weekly during treatment. DeltaRex-G was administered with escalating doses of DeltaVax, five patients at Dose Level I, four patients at Dose Level II, and seven patients at Dose Level III. All patients received a minimum of two cycles of treatment over an 8-week period. Toxicity was assessed prior to each infusion and subsequent treatment cycles using NCI CT-CAE version 3.0 criteria. A staging assessment was performed every 4 weeks with an FDG PET-CT scan. All images were performed and reviewed independently by the radiologists and RECIST v1.0 and International PET criteria were used to assess overall tumor response and progression-free survival.

3.4.3 Published results

No dose-limiting toxicities were observed at any of the three Dose Levels of DeltaVax, and no deaths that occurred were considered to be related to the treatment. None of the patients tested positive for vector neutralizing antibodies, replication-competent retrovirus in peripheral blood lymphocytes, antibodies to gp70 or vector integration into genomic DNA of peripheral blood lymphocytes. Using RECIST v1.0 criteria, three patients achieved a partial response, nine patients achieved stable disease, and two patients had progressive disease. The median progression free survival was 4.5, 9.0, and 13.0 months for Dose Levels I, II, and III respectively, and the median overall survival was 17, 13 and > 21 months for Dose Levels I, II, III respectively.

Histopathologic examination of patients' residual tumor tissues showed vector localization as well as GM-CSF transgene expression in necrotic tissue, displaying the accuracy in delivery of both treatments. Safety and tolerability are displayed by the lack of adverse reactions associated with the study drugs. The one-year survival rate of 86% in patients who received higher doses of DeltaVax suggests that the combination regimen of DeltaRex-G and Deltavax has significant anti-tumor activity in patients with chemoresistant solid malignancies and B-cell lymphoma. In addition, the substantial increase in progression free survival with each increased dosage of DeltaVax suggests a trend towards a positive dose–response relationship between the two treatments.

3.4.4 Conclusions/future directions

DeltaRex-G has displayed through numerous clinical trials its cytocidal effect on cancer cells. This effect introduces neoantigens from the tumor into the tumor microenvironment to be recognized by the immune system and targeted for destruction through T-cell mediation. Nevertheless, these cytotoxic immune responses may not be significant enough to overcome the suppressive signals from surrounding regulatory T-cells that may also be recruited to the tumor microenvironment. The addition of DeltaVax is hypothesized to heighten the development of dendritic cells and increase proliferation and activation of T-cells, thereby improving the potency of tumor-targeted DeltaRex-G. These activated T-cells can then go on to recognize and destroy the newly introduced tumor neoantigens. This has the potential to further tumor regression and evoke long-lasting antitumor immunity.

This data therefore strongly suggests that the advancement of personalized cancer vaccination treatment has the potential to gain control of tumor growth and increase overall survival time in patients with advanced or malignant chemoresistant solid malignancies, as well as B-cell lymphomas.

4. Discussion/conclusion/summary

Targeted Immunotherapy has revolutionized the way scientists and physicians conceptualize their approaches to cancer treatment and cancer checkpoint controls. Mechanistic understanding of innate and adaptive mechanisms of immunity are considered important aspects of both physiological cancer surveillance and tumor eradication, as seen in immune checkpoint control and in precision blockade of cell cycle control elements. The low immunogenicity of cancer cells, as well as the tendency of advanced cancers to create an immunosuppressive tumor microenvironment presents a technical problem of precision tumor-targeted drug delivery for both immune checkpoint antibodies and cell cycle control elements, which form a rational basis for emerging treatments. The precision of monoclonal antibodies as checkpoint inhibitors targeting cancer cells has allowed research to advance in a direction that moves away from the untoward toxicities associated with chemotherapy towards treatments that enhance the naturally powerful cytotoxic responses of the immune system. The use of checkpoint inhibitors as cancer immunotherapy has been validated in 16 indications; however, immune checkpoint inhibition is still only considered appropriate for a specific subset of patients [58], and is often confounded by serious immune-related Adverse Events (imAEs). The significance and durability of response to treatment with checkpoint inhibitor therapy is generally dependent on tumor cells having a high mutational burden or microsatellite instability that creates an increased amount of neoantigens to be recognized and eliminated by the adaptive immune system [59]. Based on the documented physiological tumor-seeking behavior and demonstrated survival value of the tumor-targeted gene therapy vectors, DeltaRex-G and DeltaVax, in treating advanced metastatic cancers, the successful adaptation of bioactive gene-targeting biotechnologies to (i) target FDA-approved off-the shelf checkpoint monoclonal antibodies to tumors, and/or (ii) recombinant "tumor-targeted" adaptor proteins have been developed, in anticipation of precisely targeting immune checkpoint inhibitors and immunostimulatory cytokines against tumors to improve clinical outcomes.

Another strategic approach is enhancing the anti-tumor properties of innate immunity. The innate immune system is also regulated by its own activating and inhibitory pathways that can be investigated as future targets for NK cell-based immunotherapy. One important characteristic to consider when making the case for focusing on boosting innate immunity is the fact that innate immune cells play a major role in immunosurveillance, acting as the first line of defense. Engaging the innate immune system is a necessary prerequisite for antigen-specific T-cells to respond, although innate immune cells such as NK cells do not require activation of T-cells to kill tumor cells [58]. NK cell activation occurs through their direct interaction with target cells, bypassing the need for antigen presentation and processing. Innate immunity is always activated prior to adaptive immunity, however, once activated, adaptive immunity has the advantage of higher specificity and lower probability of self-harm.

In recent years, the human Cyclin G1 (*CCNG1*) gene was established as a central executive element of a Commanding Cyclin G1/Cdk/Mdm2/p53 Axis: representing a strategic locus for restoring cell cycle checkpoint control through precision gene transfer. With the development of the first tumor-targeted cancer gene therapy, DeltaRex-G [60], it became possible for patients to (i) benefit clinically, (ii) enjoy good quality of life and (iii) survive appreciably longer without experiencing the debilitating toxicities of chemotherapy. The tumor-targeted DeltaRex-G vector consists of bioactive nanoparticles displaying a high-affinity targeting motif on its surface for "pathotropic" (lesion-seeking) targeting by binding to abnormal signature (SIG) proteins found abundantly in invading tumors, and then delivering a cytocidal genetic payload, a CCNG1 cell cycle checkpoint inhibitor gene, into rapidly dividing cancer cells, tumor associated microvasculature and tumor-associated fibroblasts, without collateral damage to normal cells and non-target organs. The observed reduction in tumor matrix production and tumor destruction paved the way for enhanced innate immune cell entry into the tumor microenvironment. The enhanced immune cells consist of cytotoxic T cells, NK cells, and dendritic cells for cell recognition, destruction and autoimmunization, as well as regulatory immune cells to prevent exaggerated immune responses that cause cytokine release syndrome or cytokine storm.

Hence, DeltaRex-G eradicates cancer cells without causing immune-mediated adverse events, an unwanted complication of immune checkpoint inhibitors such as ipilimumab, nivolumab, pembrolizumab, atezolizumab, etc. Conceivably, DeltaRex-G could also be used in combination with reduced doses of immune checkpoint inhibitors to minimize off-target toxicity (imAEs) and maximize anticancer efficacy.

A second tumor-targeted retrovector, DeltaVax, displaying the same high-affinity tumor-targeting motif as DeltaRex-G, but this immuno-vector—encoding both the GM-CSF gene and the pro-drug regulated HSV-tk gene, and allowing for personalized "pulsed" *in situ* vaccinations—demonstrated promising results in a small Phase I/II study conducted in Manila, Philippines with considerable clinical benefit: good quality of life and an 86% one year survival rate in patients with advanced chemotherapy-resistant Stage 4 malignancies and a uniformly poor prognosis.

In the era of precision medicine, with tumor-targeted cancer gene therapy and immunotherapy coming of age, these recent advances bring great optimism to the medical and scientific communities around the world and the patients that they serve.

Acknowledgements

The authors are grateful to J Isaacs Charitable Trust (UK), Thomas Makin Family, James B. Finn Memorial, ArtistsforAveni, Capital Group, Trader Joes, Holmes Family Trust, Ronald and Linda Chelsky, Ritchie and Keri Tuazon, Lance S. Ostendorf, Norma Yaeger, Lawrence Yaeger Memorial, Martin Berwitt, Adolf Weinberger Foundation, Jun and Alice de Guzman, Dr. and Mrs. Antonio Ong for their generous donations.

Conflict of interest

Drs. Gordon and Hall are co-inventors of the targeted gene delivery system represented by DeltaRex-G and DeltaVax which was originally developed at the University of Southern California Keck School of Medicine, and are co-founders of Delta Next-Gene, LLC. Dr. Gordon is founder and president of the Aveni Foundation, a 501c3 public charity. NLA, TTK, DAB and SPC have no competing interest.

Ethics approval and consent to participate

The clinical protocol was approved by the USFDA, the Western IRB, and the Institutional Biosafety Committee. A written informed consent was obtained from each patient prior to treatment with an investigational agent.

Author details

Erlinda M. Gordon[1,2,3]*, Nicole L. Angel[1], Ted T. Kim[1], Don A. Brigham[2], Sant P. Chawla[1] and Frederick L. Hall[3]

1 Cancer Center of Southern California/Sarcoma Oncology Center, Santa Monica, CA, USA

2 Aveni Foundation, Santa Monica, CA, USA

3 Delta Next-Gene, LLC, Santa Monica, CA, USA

*Address all correspondence to: erlinda.gordon@gmail.com

References

[1] Dyck L, Mills KHG. Immune checkpoints and their inhibition in cancer and infectious diseases. European Journal of Immunology. 2017;47:765-779. DOI: 10.1002/eji.201646875

[2] Buchbinder EI, Desai A. CTLA-4 and PD-1 pathways. American Journal of Clinical Oncology. 2016;39:98-106. DOI: 10.1097/COC.0000000000000239

[3] Gonzalez H, Hagerling C, Werb Z. Roles of the immune system in cancer: from tumor initiation to metastatic progression. Genes & Development. 2018;32:1267-1284. DOI: 10.1101/gad.314617.118

[4] Chawla SP, Sankhala KK, Ravicz J, et al. Clinical experience with combination chemo-/immunotherapy using trabectedin and nivolumab for advanced soft tissue sarcoma. Journal of Clinical Oncology. 2018;36:e23568-e23568. DOI: 10.1200/JCO.2018.36.15_suppl.e23568

[5] Ribas A, Wolchok JD. Cancer immunotherapy using checkpoint blockade. Science. 2018;359:1350-1355. DOI: 10.1126/science.aar4060

[6] Hodi FS, O'Day SJ, McDermott DF, et al. Improved survival with ipilimumab in patients with metastatic melanoma. The New England Journal of Medicine. 2010;363:711-723. DOI: 10.1056/NEJMoa1003466

[7] Wolchok JD, Kluger H, Callahan MK, et al. Safety and clinical activity of combined PD-1 (nivolumab) and CTLA-4 (ipilimumab) blockade in advanced melanoma patients. The New England Journal of Medicine. 2013;369:122-133. DOI: 10.1056/NEJMoa1302369

[8] www.accessdata.fda.gov/drugsatfda_docs

[9] Al-Shihabi A, Chawla SP, Hall FL, et al. Exploiting oncogenic drivers along the CCNG1 pathway for cancer therapy and gene therapy. Molecular Therapy - Oncolytics. 2018;11:122-126. DOI: 10.1016/j.omto.2018.11.002

[10] Chawla SP, Bruckner H, Morse MA, et al. A phase I-II study using Rexin-G tumor-targeted retrovector encoding a dominant-negative cyclin G1 inhibitor for advanced pancreatic cancer. Molecular Therapy - Oncolytics. 2019;12:56-67. DOI: 10.1016/j.omto.2018.12.005

[11] Sarcoma Oncology Research Center, LLC. SAINT: A Phase 1/2 Study of Safe Amounts of IPLIMUMAB, NIVOLUMAB and TRABECTEDIN as First Line Treatment of Advanced Soft Tissue Sarcoma (STS). Clinical Trial Registration NCT03138161, clinicaltrials.gov, https://clinicaltrials.gov/ct2/show/NCT03138161 (31 August 2020, accessed 11 January 2021)

[12] Morrison BA. Soft tissue sarcomas of the extremities. Proceedings (Baylor University Medical Center). 2003;16:285-290. DOI: 10.1080/08998280.2003.11927915

[13] Tseng WW, Somaiah N, Engleman EG. Potential for immunotherapy in soft tissue sarcoma. Human Vaccines & Immunotherapeutics. 2015;10:3117-3124. DOI: 10.4161/21645515.2014.983003

[14] Zhou M, Bui N, Bolleddu S, et al. Nivolumab plus ipilimumab for soft tissue sarcoma: a single institution retrospective review. Immunotherapy. 2020;12:1303-1312. DOI: 10.2217/imt-2020-0155

[15] Demetri GD, von Mehren M, Jones RL, et al. Efficacy and Safety of Trabectedin or Dacarbazine for Metastatic Liposarcoma or

Leiomyosarcoma After Failure of Conventional Chemotherapy: Results of a Phase III Randomized Multicenter Clinical Trial. Journal of Clinical Oncology. 2015;34:786-793. DOI: 10.1200/JCO.2015.62.4734

[16] Syed I, Sudan M, Tseng W, et al. Trabectedin for advanced soft-tissue sarcoma: A single-center experience of over 10 years. Journal of Clinical Oncology. 2016;34:11052-11052

[17] Schreiber RD, Old LJ, Smyth MJ. Cancer immunoediting: Integrating immunity's roles in cancer suppression and promotion. Science. 2011;331:1565-1570. DOI: 10.1126/science.1203486

[18] Sarcoma Oncology Research Center, LLC. The TNT Protocol: A Phase 2 Study Using Talimogene Laherparepvec, Nivolumab and Trabectedin as First, Second/Third Line Therapy for Advanced Sarcoma, Including Desmoid Tumor and Chordoma. Clinical Trial Registration NCT03886311, clinicaltrials.gov, https://clinicaltrials.gov/ct2/show/NCT03886311 (7 July 2020, accessed 11 January 2021)

[19] Filin IY, Solovyeva VV, Kitaeva KV, et al. Current trends in cancer immunotherapy. Biomedicines. 2020;8:621. DOI: 10.3390/biomedicines8120621

[20] Müller L, Berkeley R, Barr T, et al. Past, present and future of oncolytic reovirus. Cancers (Basel). 2020;12:3219. DOI: 10.3390/cancers12113219

[21] Koch MS, Lawler SE, Chiocca EA. HSV-1 oncolytic viruses from bench to bedside: An overview of current clinical trials. Cancers (Basel). 2020;12:3514. DOI: 10.3390/cancers12123514

[22] Shi Y, Liu CH, Roberts AI, et al. Granulocyte-macrophage colony-stimulating factor (GM-CSF) and T-cell responses: what we do and don't know. Cell Research. 2006;16:126-133. DOI: 10.1038/sj.cr.7310017

[23] Chawla SP, Chua VS, Kim K, et al. The TNT protocol: A phase II study using talimogene laherparepvec (TVEC), nivolumab (N) and trabectedin (T) as first, second/third line therapy for advanced sarcoma, including desmoid tumor and chordoma. Journal of Clinical Oncology. 2020;38:TPS11572-TPS11572. DOI: 10.1200/JCO.2020.38.15_suppl.TPS11572

[24] Sarcoma Oncology Research Center, LLC. A Phase 1/2 Study Using Nivolumab and ABI-009 for Advanced Sarcoma, Advanced Carcinoma Treated With PD1 Inhibitors, and Tumors With Genetic Mutations Sensitive to mTOR Inhibitors. Clinical Trial Registration NCT03190174, clinicaltrials.gov, https://clinicaltrials.gov/ct2/show/NCT03190174 (27 August 2020, accessed 11 January 2021)

[25] Rad E, Murray JT, Tee AR. Oncogenic signaling through mechanistic target of rapamycin (mTOR): A driver of metabolic transformation and cancer progression. Cancers (Basel). 2018;10:5. DOI: 10.3390/cancers10010005

[26] Li J, Kim SG, Blenis J. Rapamycin: one drug, many effects. Cell metabolism. 2014;19:373-379. DOI: 10.1016/j.cmet.2014.01.001

[27] Neuhaus P, Klupp J, Langrehr JM. mTOR inhibitors: An overview. Liver Transplantation. 2001;7:473-484. DOI: 10.1053/jlts.2001.24645

[28] Chi H. Regulation and function of mTOR signalling in T cell fate decision. Nature reviews Immunology. 2012;12:325-338. DOI: 10.1038/nri3198

[29] Imrali A, Mao X, Yeste-Velasco M, et al. Rapamycin inhibits prostate cancer

cell growth through cyclin D1 and enhances the cytotoxic efficacy of cisplatin. American Journal of Cancer Research. 2016;6:1772-1784.

[30] Wagner AJ, Ravi V, Riedel RF, et al. Long-term follow-up for duration of response (DoR) after weekly nab-sirolimus in patients with advanced malignant perivascular epithelioid cell tumors (PEComa): Results from a registrational open-label phase II trial, AMPECT. Journal of Clinical Oncology. 2020;38:11516-11516. DOI: 10.1200/JCO.2020.38.15_suppl.11516

[31] Inhibrx, Inc. An Open-Label, Multicenter, First-in-Human, Dose-Escalation Phase 1 Study of INBRX-109 in Subjects With Locally Advanced or Metastatic Solid Tumors Including Sarcomas. Clinical Trial Registration NCT03715933, clinicaltrials.gov, https://clinicaltrials.gov/ct2/show/NCT03715933 (30 September 2020, accessed 11 January 2021)

[32] Sun S-Y. Understanding the role of the death receptor 5/FADD/caspase-8 death signaling in cancer metastasis. Molecular and Cellular Pharmacology. 2011;3:31-34.

[33] Walczak H, Miller RE, Ariail K, et al. Tumoricidal activity of tumor necrosis factor–related apoptosis–inducing ligand in vivo. Nature Medicine. 1999;5:157-163. DOI: 10.1038/5517

[34] Yuan X, Gajan A, Chu Q, et al. Developing TRAIL/TRAIL-death receptor-based cancer therapies. Cancer Metastasis Reviews. 2018;37:733-748. DOI: 10.1007/s10555-018-9728-y

[35] Elevar Therapeutics. An Open-Labeled, Phase I Study to Evaluate the Safety and Tolerability of Apatinib With Nivolumab in Patients With Unresectable or Metastatic Cancer. Clinical Trial Registration NCT03396211, clinicaltrials.gov, https://clinicaltrials.gov/ct2/show/NCT03396211 (22 June 2020, accessed 11 January 2021)

[36] Qin S, Li A, Yi M, et al. Recent advances on anti-angiogenesis receptor tyrosine kinase inhibitors in cancer therapy. Journal of Hematology & Oncology. 2019;12:27. DOI: 10.1186/s13045-019-0718-5

[37] Yi M, Jiao D, Qin S, et al. Synergistic effect of immune checkpoint blockade and anti-angiogenesis in cancer treatment. Molecular Cancer. 2019;18:60. DOI: 10.1186/s12943-019-0974-6

[38] NKMax America, Inc. Phase 1, Open-Label, Safety Study of Escalating Doses of Ex Vivo Expanded, Autologous Natural Killer Cells in Patients With Pathologically Confirmed Cancer Refractory to Conventional Therapy. Clinical Trial Registration NCT03941262, clinicaltrials.gov, https://clinicaltrials.gov/ct2/show/NCT03941262 (30 November 2020, accessed 11 January 2021)

[39] Yoo SH, Keam B, Ock C-Y, et al. Prognostic value of the association between MHC class I downregulation and PD-L1 upregulation in head and neck squamous cell carcinoma patients. Scientific Reports. 2019;9:7680. DOI: 10.1038/s41598-019-44206-2

[40] Axelrod ML, Cook RS, Johnson DB, et al. Biological consequences of MHC-II expression by tumor cells in cancer. Clinical Cancer Research. 2019;25:2392-2402. DOI: 10.1158/1078-0432.CCR-18-3200

[41] Knorr D, Bachanova V, Verneris MR, et al. Clinical utility of natural killer cells in cancer therapy and transplantation. Seminars in Immunology. 2014;26:161-172. DOI: 10.1016/j.smim.2014.02.002

[42] NKMax America, Inc. Phase 1, Open Label, Safety Study of Escalating Doses of Ex Vivo Expanded, Autologous Natural Killer Cells in Patients with Pathologically Confirmed Cancer Refractory to Conventional Therapy (Study SuperNK-01 Clinical Protocol).

[43] Immune Design. A Randomized, Open-Label, Phase 2 Trial of CMB305 (Sequentially Administered LV305 and G305) and Atezolizumab in Patients With Locally Advanced, Relapsed, or Metastatic Sarcoma Expressing NY-ESO-1. Clinical Trial Registration NCT02609984, clinicaltrials.gov, https://clinicaltrials.gov/ct2/show/NCT02609984 (26 June 2020, accessed 11 January 2021)

[44] Singh N, Kulikovskaya I, Barrett DM, et al. T cells targeting NY-ESO-1 demonstrate efficacy against disseminated neuroblastoma. Oncoimmunology. 2015;5:e1040216. DOI: 10.1080/2162402X.2015.1040216

[45] Lai J-P, Rosenberg AZ, Miettinen MM, et al. NY-ESO-1 expression in sarcomas. Oncoimmunology. 2012;1:1409-1410. DOI: 10.4161/onci.21059

[46] Robbins PF, Morgan RA, Feldman SA, et al. Tumor regression in patients with metastatic synovial cell sarcoma and melanoma using genetically engineered lymphocytes reactive with NY-ESO-1. Journal of Clinical Oncology. 2011;29:917-924. DOI: 10.1200/JCO.2010.32.2537

[47] Somaiah N, Chawla SP, Block MS, et al. A phase 1b study evaluating the safety, tolerability, and immunogenicity of CMB305, a lentiviral-based prime-boost vaccine regimen, in patients with locally advanced, relapsed, or metastatic cancer expressing NY-ESO-1. Oncoimmunology. 2020;9:e1847846. DOI: 10.1080/2162402X.2020.1847846

[48] Immune Design Halts Phase III Trial of Lead Candidate CMB305, Ramps Up G100 Development. GEN - Genetic Engineering and Biotechnology News, https://www.genengnews.com/news/immune-design-halts-phase-iii-trial-of-lead-candidate-cmb305-ramps-up-g100-development/ (2018, accessed 7 January 2021)

[49] Epeius Biotechnologies. Phase I/II Evaluation of Safety and Efficacy of Rexin-G for Recurrent or Metastatic Pancreatic Cancer. Clinical Trial Registration NCT00504998, clinicaltrials.gov, https://clinicaltrials.gov/ct2/show/NCT00504998 (9 June 2011, accessed 11 January 2021)

[50] Rawla P, Sunkara T, Gaduputi V. Epidemiology of pancreatic cancer: Global trends, etiology and risk factors. World Journal of Oncology. 2019;10:10-27. DOI: 10.14740/wjon1166

[51] Oda K, Matsuoka Y, Funahashi A, et al. A comprehensive pathway map of epidermal growth factor receptor signaling. Molecular Systems Biology. 2005;1:2005.0010. DOI: 10.1038/msb4100014

[52] Liu X, Wang P, Zhang C, et al. Epidermal growth factor receptor (EGFR): A rising star in the era of precision medicine of lung cancer. Oncotarget. 2017;8:50209-50220. DOI: 10.18632/oncotarget.16854

[53] Syendahl Dy P, Chawla SP, Hall F, et al. Immune cell trafficking in the tumor microenvironment of human cyclin G1 (CCNG1) inhibitor-treated tumors. British Journal of Cancer Research. 2018;1:202-207. DOI: 10.31488/bjcr.117

[54] Liu S, Chawla S, Bruckner H, et al. Reporting long term survival following precision tumor-targeted gene delivery to advanced chemotherapy-resistant malignancies: an academic milestone.

[55] Kitamura T, Qian B-Z, Pollard JW. Immune cell promotion of metastasis. Nature Reviews Immunology. 2015;15:73-86. DOI: 10.1038/nri3789

[56] Yaguchi T, Kawakami Y. Cancer-induced heterogeneous immunosuppressive tumor microenvironments and their personalized modulation. International Immunology. 2016;28:393-399. DOI: 10.1093/intimm/dxw030

[57] Ignacio J, San-Juan F, Manalo R, et al. The Genevieve Protocol: Phase I/II Evaluation of a Dual Targeted Approach to Cancer Gene Therapy/ Immunotherapy. Clinics in Oncology; 3, http://www.remedypublications.com/clinics-in-oncology-abstract.php?aid=1693 (2018, accessed 16 January 2021)

[58] Rothlin CV, Ghosh S. Lifting the innate immune barriers to antitumor immunity. Journal for Immunotherapy of Cancer. 2020;8:e000695. DOI: 10.1136/jitc-2020-000695

[59] Chew HY, Chan V, Simpson F, et al. Will Next-Generation immunotherapy overcome the intrinsic diversity and low immunogenicity of sarcomas to improve clinical benefit? Cancers (Basel). 2020;12:3392. DOI: 10.3390/cancers12113392

[60] Gordon EM, Ravicz JR, Liu S, et al. Cell cycle checkpoint control: The cyclin G1/Mdm2/p53 axis emerges as a strategic target for broad-spectrum cancer gene therapy - A review of molecular mechanisms for oncologists. Molecular and Clinical Oncology. 2018;9:115-134. DOI: 10.3892/mco.2018.1657

Chapter 2

Evolving Dynamic Biomarkers for Prediction of Immune Responses to Checkpoint Inhibitors in Cancer

Afsheen Raza, Maysaloun Merhi, Allan Relecom, Queenie Fernandes, Varghese Inchakalody, Abdul Rahman Zar Gul, Shahab Uddin, Mohammed Ussama Al Homsi and Said Dermime

Abstract

Immune checkpoint inhibitors (ICIs) have been approved as first or second line therapy in a large group of cancers. However, the observation of potentially long-lasting responses was restricted to limited subset of patients. Efforts have been made to identify predictive factors of response to ICIs in order to select eligible patients and to avoid exposing non-responding patients to treatment side effects. Although several biomarkers have been identified, their predictive potential remains unsatisfactory. One promising emerging approach is to focus on dynamic biomarkers to directly characterize the response and, more importantly, to identify those patients presenting an immune response failure. Several studies have shown a strong correlation between specific circulating immune cell subsets and tumor immune infiltrates. Moreover, liquid biomarkers including soluble immune checkpoint molecules have potential in predicting the modulation of the immune response under immune checkpoint blockade. In this chapter, we will discuss current advances in the study of circulatory and intra-tumoral dynamic biomarkers as predictors of responses to ICIs therapy in cancer.

Keywords: dynamic biomarkers, serum soluble biomarkers, cellular immune response, immune checkpoint inhibitors, CTLA-4, PD-1, tumor control

1. Introduction

The immune checkpoint cell surface proteins like programmed death-ligand 1 (PD-L1), programmed death 1 (PD-1) and cytotoxic T-lymphocyte-associated protein 4 (CLTA-4) represent important pathways of cancer immune evasion. Immune checkpoint inhibitors (ICIs) are identified as potent key players in providing therapeutic benefit in a range of solid cancers as well as in a subgroup of hematological malignancies. However, the response rates to these immune-modulatory molecules are sub-optimal and predictive biomarkers allowing to select for responsive cancer patients are lacking. The study of the dynamics of the immune system and of the tumors under immune checkpoint blockade has greatly improved knowledge on the mechanisms of action of ICIs, allowing the identification of a number of novel candidate dynamic biomarkers predictive of ICI treatment response meriting further exploration in validation trials.

Tumor biopsy of tissue from primary or metastatic site is a major mainstay of treatment decisions as the molecular features and histology can reveal the complex cancer landscape. However, tissue biopsy has various limitations such as high heterogeneity, invasive nature of tissue sampling and skilled expertise/techniques required for analyzing and reporting making it a difficult specimen especially for treatment monitoring purpose [1]. Therefore, emphasis on utility of liquid biopsies as prognostic and predictive soluble biomarkers especially in cancer immunotherapy is gaining a lot of attention. The main advantages of blood-based specimens are that these are easy to extract and analyze with limited skilled expertise or techniques. Furthermore, biomarkers in the blood can represent dynamic alterations of the evolving cancer in response to treatment and can help in longitudinal monitoring. In addition to this, these can also be utilized for risk prediction of immune-related adverse events (irAE) which is an important and critical monitoring parameter [2].

In this chapter, we attempt to discuss in relevant details the purpose and role of immune modulatory molecules and of the different serum soluble biomarkers in various human and animal models with an aim to show insight on to their mechanisms of action and resistance, thus conveying information predictive of therapeutic response.

2. Effect of immune checkpoint blockade on effector T cells

2.1 Effect of PD-1 blockade on effector T cells

PD-1 is an important immune checkpoint expressed on activated T cells and known to regulate their functional activity. By binding to its ligands, PD-L1 or PD-L2, which are expressed on tumor cells and a variety of immune cells [3], PD-1 is able to inhibit downstream signaling of the T cells receptor (TCR) [4]. Hence, ICIs targeting the PD-1/PD-L1 axis are developed to modulate this negative feedback loop and restore T cells activity. Indeed, response to anti PD-1 drugs is characterized by the upregulation of genes associated with activation of effector T cells [5–7]. Moreover, the blocking of PD-1 has been linked to an expansion of CD8+ effector T cells within the tumor. Interestingly, this CD8+ T cells expansion was found to follow a specific gradient that decreases from the margins of the tumor into its center [5, 8, 9]. In addition, the noted expansion in CD8+ T cells was also found to coincide with an increase in CD8+ T cell clonality in the tumor microenvironment (TME) [8]. This is clearly indicative of the fact that CD8+ T cells expanded in the tumor upon blocking PD-1 are indeed tumor-reactive and stand as a consistent correlate of treatment benefit.

Another interesting aspect is the heterogeneity noted in the tumor infiltrating CD8+ T cells depending on their different phenotypes and functional states. One such subset is known to express high levels of PD-1 and co-express the following immune modulating proteins: the T-cell immunoglobulin and mucin-domain containing-3 (TIM-3), the lymphocyte-activation gene-3 (LAG-3), the T cell immunoreceptor with Ig and ITIM domains (TIGIT) and CD39, which are all linked to T cells exhaustion [Tex] [10, 11]. Exhausted CD8+ T cells represent a dysfunctional cell state that develops due to chronic antigen exposition. However, exhausted CD8+ T cells in the TME have a higher potential for tumor antigens recognition and a higher clonal distribution than any other CD8+ T cells subset in the TME [12, 13].

Further, the Tex phenotype also defines an impaired capacity of producing effector cytokines such as IL-2, TNF-α and IFN-γ [12]. The inhibition of the PD-1/PD-L1 axis was initially suggested to reinvigorate the anti-tumoral immune response by reversing the state of these terminally exhausted tumor-reactive T cells. However, this function is challenged by the fact that this state of terminal exhaustion is characterized by a distinct epigenetic profile which limits its reversibility [14–16]. In support of this, recent evidence has shown that anti-PD-1 therapy can engage progenitor Tex subsets that co-express PD-1 and the lineage-determining transcription factor 1 (tcf-1), instead of terminally exhausted subsets [17, 18]. Similarly, certain studies on animal models also show that blocking PD-1 leads to the engaging of $PD-1^+/tcf-1^+/CD8^+$ T cells inducing their self-regeneration or differentiation into effector $tcf-1^-$ cells that eventually develop functional states of exhaustion [19, 20]. Interestingly, it has been shown that Tex subsets might promote the recruitment of other immune cells into the TME and consequently support the anti-tumoral immune response [12]. In addition, anti-PD-1 treatment was shown to engage memory-precursor like CD8+ T cell subsets, leading to their accumulation in the TME [21] and to a subsequent enhanced cytotoxicity towards cancer cells [22]. The on-treatment increase in memory CD8+ T cells was suggested to correlate with response to anti-PD-1 therapy in both preclinical models and clinical studies [9, 23].

blocking of PD-1 is known to cause an increase in the proliferation of CD8+ T cells very early during the course of treatment [24, 25]. This proliferative response can be observed in the periphery, where it peaks as early as 7 days following the introduction of anti-PD-1 therapy [24, 26]. In one of our studies on a gastric cancer patient undergoing anti-PD-1 therapy, we observed that the frequency of peripheral cytotoxic T cells $CD8^+/CD107^+$ specific for the NY-ESO-1 cancer testis antigen closely correlated with the patient clinical outcome [27]. Another study has reported that the proliferative response of peripheral $CD8^+/PD-1^+$ T cells could be predictive of durable clinical benefit in patients with solid tumors receiving anti-PD-1 therapy [26]. Thus, these studies support the fact that the systemic CD8+ effector T cells response plays a key role in tumor management under anti-PD-1 treatment and suggest their importance as a predictive biomarker of response to PD-1 blockade. In **Figure 1** we illustrate the dynamics of intra-tumoral effector T cells that are shown to correlate with anti-PD-1 treatment outcome.

2.2 Effect of CTLA-4 blockade on effector T cells

When T cells are engaged in an active immune response, the expression of the surface protein CTLA-4, a homolog of CD28 with high affinity to B7–1 and 2 ligands, will be upregulated. CTLA-4: B7–1/2 binding acts as a co-inhibitor of the TCR signal [28]. Thus, the primary role of the CTLA-4 checkpoint is to negatively regulate T cell activation especially during the priming phase upon binding to the B7 ligands expressed by antigen presenting cells (APC). In accordance with this, a major aspect of anti-CTLA-4 therapy is its ability to reinvigorate T cell proliferation and activation. Indeed, the effects of anti-CTLA-4 therapy are evident in several studies on mouse models. For example, CTLA-4 deficient mice were found to display rapidly lethal lymphoproliferation [29]. On the other hand, anti-CTLA-4 therapy led to the expansion of both $CD4^+$ and $CD8^+$ effector T cells in the tumor [30]. Although both T cells subsets are necessary in mediating tumor immune control [31], the increase in $CD4^+$ T cells appeared to be of a greater importance than that of $CD8^+$ T cells [30].

In few studies, $CD8^+$ T cells expansion has been shown to translate into an effective response to immune checkpoint blockade therapy [7, 32]. However, a study on advanced melanoma patients undergoing treatment with the anti-CTLA-4 antibody tremelimumab, reports no association between the expansion of $CD8^+$ effector

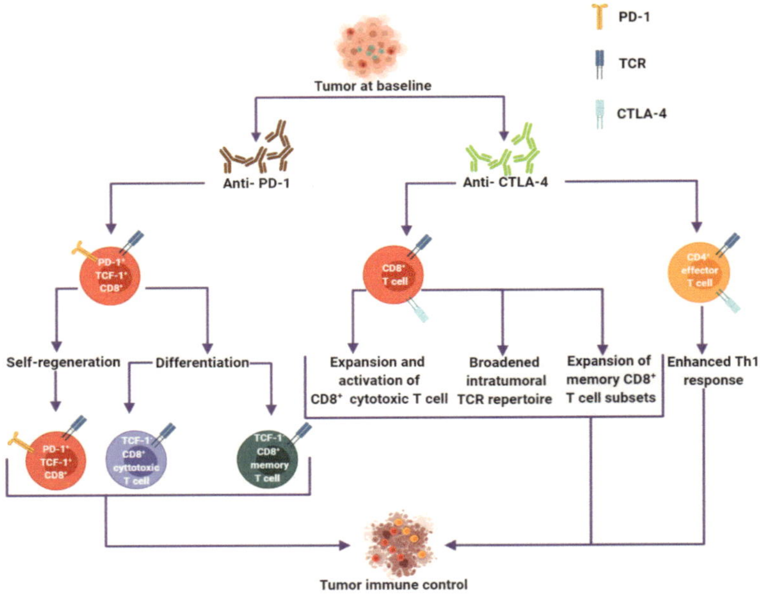

Figure 1.
Effect of immune checkpoint inhibition on effector T cells.

T cells and successful anti-tumor response [33] despite similar $CD8^+$ T cells activation profiles observed in lesions that responded to anti-CTLA-4 therapy and those that did not respond to this therapy [33]. These findings, possibly explained by the action of immunosuppressive elements in the TME, highlight that adequate $CD8^+$ effector T cells function is necessary but not sufficient for complete suppression of tumor growth under immunotherapy [34]. Another interesting effect noted upon CTLA-4 blockade is the enhanced expansion of memory $CD8^+$ T cell [35] which will help to promote long-term tumor control post-therapy. Moreover, this expansion of memory $CD8^+$ T cells is considered as an indicator of treatment benefit in a few clinical studies [36, 37].

$CD4^+$ T cells expanding in the tumors of mouse models under anti-CTLA-4 treatment are found to exhibit a Th1-like effector phenotype with a noticeable expression of ICOS, a known marker of follicular T helper cells [30]. Interestingly, this phenotype of $CD4^+$ T cell was observed in mice after genetic knock-down of negative co-inhibitory molecules such as CTLA-4 [38]. Moreover, ICOS-deficient mice showed an impaired anti-tumor T cell response to anti-CTLA-4 therapy [39]. In addition, a tumor microenvironment that is rich in $CD4^+$ Th1 effector T cells infiltration was shown to be critical to develop response to anti-CTLA-4 therapy in castration resistant prostate cancer [40]. Furthermore, a higher expression of Th1 associated genes was observed in melanoma tumors of patients responding to ipilimumab compared to non-responders, supporting the functional relevance of a Th1- response in CTLA-4 inhibitor treatment benefit [41]. Interestingly, while the presence of $CD4^+$ Th1 cells is predictive of response to anti-CTLA-4, a peripheral blood profile rich in Th17 cells was reported to be rather predictive of autoimmune toxicity under anti-CTLA-4 therapy [42]. Moreover, several clinical studies have reported an increase of $ICOS^+/CD4^+$ T cells in the tumor and peripheral blood of patients treated with anti-CTLA-4 [43–49]. Additionally, an increased proliferation of both peripheral $CD4^+$ and $CD8^+$ T cells is observed as early as 3 weeks after the first dose of anti-CTLA-4 treatment [50–52]. Such a response may partly be due to the bulk expansion in the periphery of specific T cells against known tumor antigens in anti-CTLA-4 treated patients [53–55]. Of note, an increase in absolute lymphocyte count (ALC) was shown to correlate with enhanced overall survival and response to ipilimumab in several studies [56–59].

The distribution of the TCR repertoire may be described by different metrics. For example, TCR richness invoke the number of unique T cell clones while its evenness refers to the frequency of their distribution. Some studies reported an increase in the richness of the TCR repertoire under anti-CTLA-4 therapy [60, 61]. On the contrary, the evenness of the TCR repertoire under anti-CTLA-4 therapy is comparatively less impacted [60, 62, 63]. This increase in richness of the TCR repertoire under the effect of anti-CTLA-4 therapy is indicative of unleashed T-cell priming possibly allowing for enhanced tumor immune control through the promotion of new anti-tumor T cells responses [64]. However, in a study on metastatic melanoma and prostate cancer, it has been shown that enhanced clinical outcomes under CTLA-4 blockade are associated with less clonotype loss and on-treatment stability of existing high-frequency TCR clonotypes [61]. These findings suggest that response to anti-CTLA-4 treatment occurs despite the remodeling of the peripheral TCR repertoire rather than as a result of it. In **Figure 1** we illustrate the dynamics of intra-tumoral effector T cells that are shown to correlate with anti-CTLA-4 treatment outcome.

3. Effect of immune checkpoint blockade on immune suppressive T cells

3.1 Effect of PD-1 blockade on immune suppressive T cells

Regulatory T cells (Tregs), an immunosuppressive subset of T cells, are known to be closely involved in the regulation of the immune responses to cancer [65–67]. The tumor-infiltrating subsets of Tregs are characterized by their high surface expression of PD-1 [68–70] and the PD-1/PD-L1 axis is known to modulate Tregs function via cell-intrinsic pathways. For example, the blocking of PD-1 in animal models reduced the immunosuppressive function of Tregs and declined their expression in the TME [71, 72]. Moreover, studies on murine models have shown that PD-1/PD-L1 pathway mediates the conversion of $CD4^+$ Th1 effector T cells into induced $Foxp3^+$ Tregs (iTregs) [73, 74]. Conversely, certain preclinical studies show that anti-PD-1 therapy is associated with an increase rather than a decrease in Tregs infiltration in the TME [24, 75]. The proliferation of Tregs under anti-PD-1 therapy could be explained by a treatment-induced reversal of the exhausted state of PD-1^{Hi} in the TME [76, 77]. The expansion of Tregs upon blockade of PD-1/PD-L1 axis has been observed at the tumor level as well as in the peripheral blood. One particular study showed that patients with gastric adenocarcinoma responding to anti-PD-1 displayed an on-treatment decrease in intra-tumoral Tregs, whereas non-responders had post-treatment tumor biopsies exhibiting an infiltration of highly proliferative effector Tregs (Foxp-3^{hi}/$CD45^-$ $CD4^+$) [78]. This suggests that on-treatment changes in intra-tumoral T reg infiltration could be a relevant dynamic parameter to account for in predicting anti-PD-1/PD-L1 treatment response. The predictive insight provided by the on-treatment dynamics of circulating Tregs under PD-1/PD-L1 blockade has also been investigated. In a study conducted on melanoma patients exposed to nivolumab, an expansion of circulating Tregs under therapy was shown to positively correlate with treatment benefit [79]. These observations suggest that Tregs dynamics under anti-Pd-1 therapy may contribute predictive insight into treatment benefit when monitored both in the TME and in the periphery.

Interestingly, another immunosuppressive $CD4^+$ T cell subset found to be regulated by anti-PD-1 therapy has been recently identified. These cells known as 4PD-1^{Hi} express high levels of PD-1 while lacking Foxp-3 expression [80]. Also, these 4PD-1^{Hi} cells were shown to accumulate in the tumor and to inhibit T cells effector function. Therefore, $4PD1^{Hi}$ cells are considered as a marker of tumor progression. Anti-PD-1 treatment was shown to reduce the proliferation of $4PD\text{-}1^{Hi}$ cells, whereas anti-CTLA-4 treatment showed an exactly opposite effect on these cells. In line with this interesting observation, the downregulation of $4PD\text{-}1^{Hi}$ cells under anti-PD-1 treatment was further documented as a biomarker of treatment response under anti-PD-1 pembrolizumab antibody in a melanoma patient cohort. In addition, some preclinical studies support the fact that anti-PD-1 therapy can induce the expansion of specific $CD8^+$ T cells immunosuppressive subsets [30]. Indeed, a recent study showed that PD-1 blockade in sub-optimally primed T cell conditions supported the proliferation of dysfunctional immunosuppressive $CD8^+$ T cells expressing PD-1 and high levels of CD38 and this effect was associated with treatment failure and tumor resistance in cancer patients [81]. The dynamics of these T cell subsets under treatment may therefore provide valuable predictive information, pending the validation of these candidate biomarkers in larger scale studies. The proposed mechanisms of anti-PD-1 action on Tregs subsets are summarized in **Figure 2**.

3.2 Effect of CTLA-4 blockade on regulatory T cells

Several observations suggest the action of anti-CTLA-4 on Tregs to be key in mediating treatment effects on the tumor. Indeed, some studies involving murine tumor models reported anti-CTLA-4 treatment to simultaneously induce an increased expansion of peripheral Tregs and a decreased expansion of intra-tumoral Tregs [82–84]. This dual action of anti-CTLA-4 on Tregs proliferation could be due to the higher expression of CTLA-4 on exhausted tumor-infiltrating Tregs, where their decline under treatment is suggested to be mediated by a distinct Fc-gamma receptor dependent mechanism of anti-body-mediated cell-mediated cytotoxicity (ADCC)

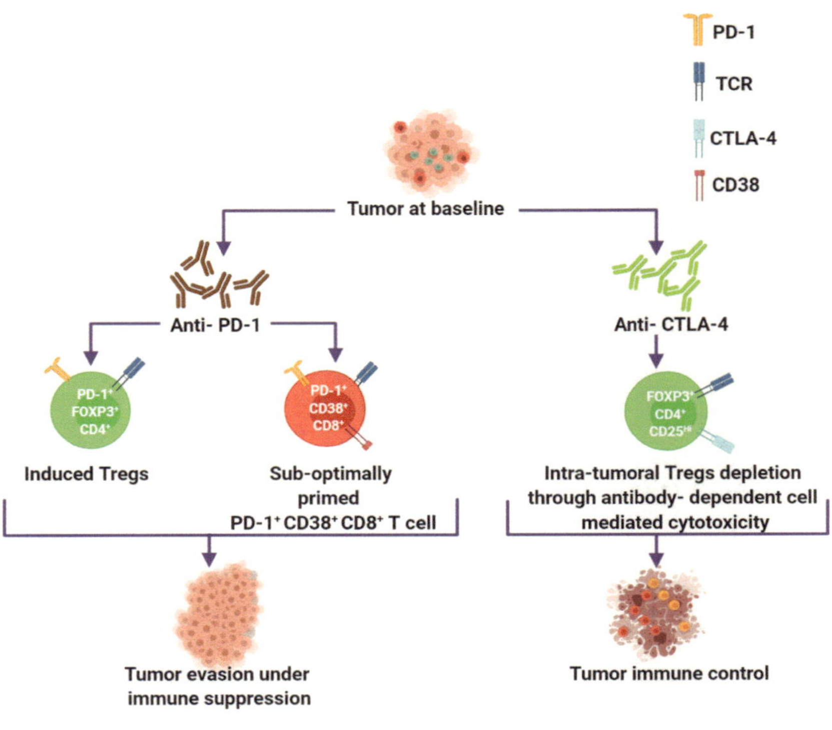

Figure 2.
Effect of immune checkpoint inhibition on immune suppressive T cells.

[85]. This feature was suggested to play a key role in tumor control under CTLA-4 blockade since it has been demonstrated that an on-treatment increase in intra-tumoral Teffs: Tregs ratio stands as the correlate of an optimal treatment response [82, 83, 86, 87]. Moreover, in another study in different murine models, the therapeutic activity of ipilimumab was found to essentially rely on this Fc-dependent Tregs depletion and not on the checkpoint inhibitor action of the drug [88]. However, there is noticeable inconsistencies in observed Tregs dynamics under CTLA-4 blockade in humans. Indeed, certain studies document a remarkable expansion of Tregs in the peripheral blood of patients treated with anti-CTLA-4 [51, 89–91], while other studies report a declined or unchanging frequency of peripheral Tregs during this therapy [37, 49, 92]. In addition, the ability of the peripheral Tregs dynamics to predict a treatment response to anti-CTLA-4 treatment is also quite unclear. For example, their change in frequency is found to correlate both negatively [93] and positively [90] with anti-CTLA-4 treatment benefit. Yet some other studies show no correlation at all between the change in Tregs frequency and a treatment response to anti-CTLA-4 therapy [56, 94, 95]. Observations of the intra-tumoral Tregs dynamics under anti-CTLA-4 is also inconclusive. A contradictory effect is put forth by a cohort on regionally advanced melanoma patients treated with 2 neoadjuvant doses of ipilimumab. This study reported a reversed association between the change in intra-tumoral Tregs frequency and treatment benefit [90]. Similarly, another study reported a marked decline in intra-tumoral Tregs levels in melanoma patients responding to ipilimumab compared to non-responding ones [96]. On the contrary, two other studies report increasing frequencies of Tregs in biopsies of patients undergoing anti-CTLA-4 therapy [13, 32]. It is interesting to note that the accumulation of Tregs within the tumors upon CTLA-4 blockade may be induced by a feedback loop triggered by a successful cytotoxic T cell response [97]. This may account for the positive correlation between the intra-tumoral levels of Tregs and patient long-term survival as reported by some studies involving solid tumors [98, 99]. These observations nonetheless suggest that Tregs dynamics under CTLA-4 treatment, in the TME and possibly in the periphery, should be accounted for when monitoring for treatment effects. The depletion of intra-tumoral Tregs under CTLA-4 blockade is illustrated in **Figure 2**.

3.3 Effect of PD-1 and CTLA-4 blockade on myeloid cell compartment

Monocytes, macrophages and dendritic cells are involved in antigen presentation and T cells priming and thereby serve as a bridge between the innate and adaptive immune response. However, chronic inflammation arising due to cancer disturbs the myeloid cell line maturation process, leading to the generation of myeloid derived suppressor cells [MDSCs] and tumor-associated macrophages [TAMs], that are both suppressors of the anti-tumor immune response [100]. These tumor associated monocytes and macrophages are known to display a wide variety of phenotypes with both pro-inflammatory [M1] and immunosuppressive [M2] functions [101]. Likewise, several studies on animal models have found that treatment with ICIs has the ability of bringing about a spectacular transformation of the intra-tumoral myeloid cell compartment from an immunosuppressive configuration to a more pro-inflammatory one [102, 103]. It has been suggested that the increased INF-γ secretion by renewed T cells would possibly indirectly mediate this myeloid cell reprogramming in the TME under immune checkpoint therapy [102]. Also, it was observed that dual PD-1 and CTLA-4 blockade induces an increase in intra-tumoral pro-inflammatory macrophages, as shown in animal models [104]. In addition, potential direct mechanisms of regulation of MDSCs by anti-PD-1 or anti-CTLA-4 treatment were also identified. As an example, an induced expression of CTLA-4 on monocyte-derived dendritic cells [mDCs] acts as a negative regulator of mDCs-associated cytokine secretion and antigen-specific CD4$^+$ T cell proliferation [105]. Moreover, subsets of intra-tumoral MDSCs that express PD-1 and CTLA-4 are found to display decreased arginase 1 expression and activity upon anti-CTLA-4 or anti-PD-1 treatment in mice [106]. In murine models, it has been shown that arginase 1 impairs T cells functions and contributes to immune evasion [107]. Furthermore, it has been recently reported that anti-PD-1 therapy was able to prevent the block in myeloid cell lineage maturation, thereby allowing the myeloid precursors to maturate into effector macrophages and dendritic cells contributing favorably to the anti-tumoral immune response [108].

A decline in circulating MDSCs under anti-CTLA-4 is found to correlate with patient outcome in several studies [37, 90, 109, 110], although this association is not universally reported [111]. Moreover, these studies showed discordant observations regarding the dynamics and predictive value of the major MDSCs subsets (monocytic MDSCs (mo-MDSCs) and polymorphonuclear MDSCs (PMN-MDSCs) subsets) [112]. In addition, several studies showed that anti-PD-1 treatment had no effect on the level of circulating mo-MDSC and PMN-MDSC subsets [9, 113, 114]. Yet a particular study revealed a prominent restructuration of the myeloid compartment after initiation of anti-PD-1 therapy in metastatic melanoma patients when studied

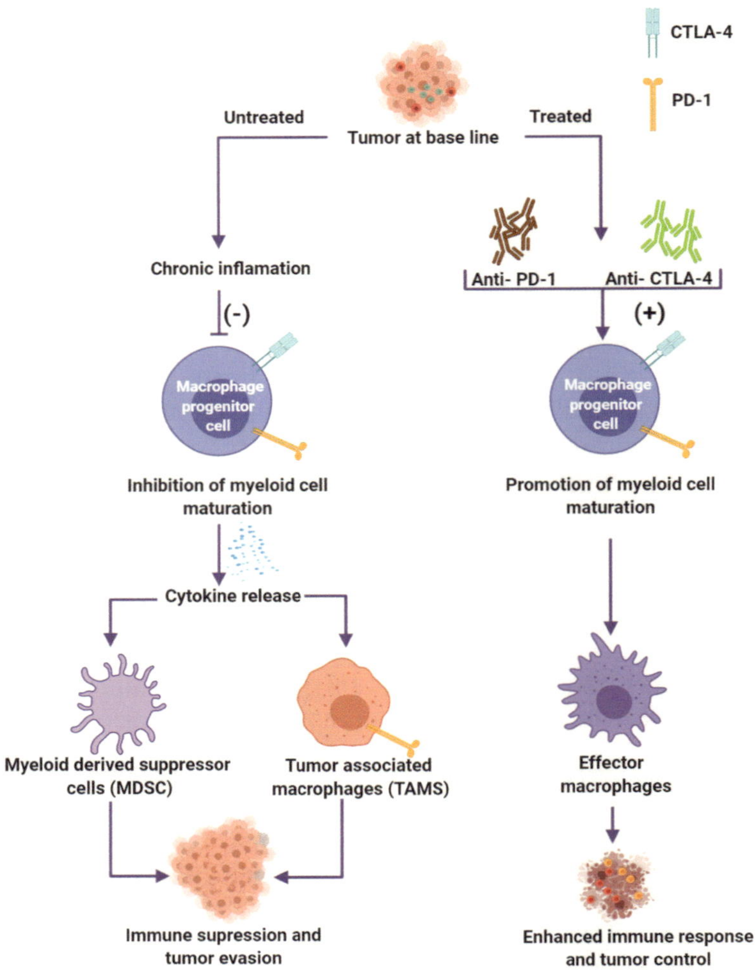

Figure 3.
Effect of PD-1 and CTLA-4 blockade on myeloid cells.

under the lens of high dimensional single cell analysis platforms [113]. Therefore, the ability to monitor the evolution of myeloid cells under immune checkpoint blockade appears to be of great predictive value, considering the important role that this cell compartment possibly plays in the modulation of the anti-tumoral immune response by either promoting or preventing the effector T cells response observed upon these therapies. One example of the described mechanisms of anti-PD-1 and anti-CTLA-4 effect on myeloid cells compartment is illustrated in **Figure 3**.

4. Dynamic predictive and prognostic soluble biomarkers in cancer immunotherapy

In the subsections below, we will focus on blood-based candidate biomarkers that can be utilized as predictive or prognostic markers in cancer immunotherapy.

4.1 Blood cell counts/ratios, C-reactive protein and lactate dehydrogenase

Changes in the blood cell counts and their ratios including neutrophils, lymphocytes, neutrophil to lymphocyte ratio as well as C-Reactive Protein (CRP) and Lactate Dehydrogenase (LDH) have been reported as prognostic/predictive outcome markers for immunotherapy [2]. Several studies have shown that low neutrophils and high lymphocytes are associated with overall survival (OS) in cancer patients [58, 115, 116]. For example, melanoma patients on nivolumab treatment having absolute lymphocyte counts of >1000/μL and absolute neutrophil count of <4000/μL were observed to have better overall survival [115]. On the other hand, pre-treatment neutrophil-to-lymphocyte ratio (NLR) and derived NLR (dNLR) can also serve as an index of the systemic inflammatory response and therefore considered as useful indicators of response in immunotherapy. Pre-treatment NLR/dNLR levels and survival association studies in advanced cancers including melanoma, non-small-cell lung cancer (NSCLC) and genitourinary have reported that high pre-treatment NLR and dNLR levels are associated with poor progression free survival (PFS)/OS with increased risks of death in immunotherapy treated patients indicating their usefulness as predictive and prognostic biomarkers [117–120].

CRP is an inflammatory marker that induces the expression of acute-phase proteins such as neutrophils and has been correlated with poor prognosis in several cancers [121, 122]. With regards to immunotherapy, post treatment increased CRP levels have been associated with inflammation, disease progression and in some cases immune-related adverse events. On the other hand, low CRP levels post immunotherapies have been associated with better antitumor response/survival [93, 123].

LDH is a final enzyme in the glycolysis pathway that catalyzes the interconversion of pyruvate and lactate. In cancers, high levels of LDH leads to increased utilization of glycolysis as their energy requirement in the microenvironment [124]. Studies have confirmed that LDH is a significant negative prognostic factor for immunotherapy treated stage 4 melanoma patients [125]. Elevated baseline LDH in melanoma and lung cancer patients treated with pembrolizumab/nivolumab is associated with poor OS and higher risk of death [126–128]. Similar results have been reported for advanced esophageal squamous cell carcinoma patients treated with the anti-PD-1 immune checkpoint inhibitor camrelizumab where elevated LDH levels were found to correlate with poor OS [129].

The fact that blood cell counts/ratios, CRP and LDH tests are performed as part of a routine diagnosis and also are highly assessable/measurable at various treatment timelines in patients making them attractive dynamic biomarkers.

4.2 Soluble immune checkpoint inhibitors

Soluble forms of immune checkpoints (sICs) are shed in the plasma/serum and have been associated with modulation of the immune system by affecting the binding capacity of immunotherapeutic drugs and thus influencing the efficiency of immune system. Studies have demonstrated that sICs can serve as markers for prognosis, response to treatment and overall response rate (ORR) in immunotherapy treated patients [130]. In addition to this, these markers can also be important for prediction of immune related adverse events which is an area poorly explored with respect to these biomarkers. Here, in this sub-section, we will discuss sICs evidenced in literature as prognostic and predictive markers in ICIs treatment.

4.2.1 Soluble immune inhibitory markers

4.2.1.1 Soluble PD-1, PDL-1 and PDL-2

sPD-1 has been documented to inhibit all three PD-L1/PD-1 interactions: PD-L1/CD80, PD-L1/PD-1, and PDL2/PD-1 [131]. Researchers have demonstrated that expressed sPD-1 blocks PD-L1/PD-1 interactions that can lead to inhibition of tumor growth via various mechanisms including blockade of PD-L1 on tumor cells, upregulation of $CD8^+$ T cells, reduction in the expression of IL-10, increased production of inducible nitric oxide synthase, TNF-α and IFN-γ and enhancement of the immune response through interaction with immune cells [132–134]. sPD-1 has been reported as a modulator of immune response during ICIs treatment in serum of cancer patients. A study on 22 NSCLC patients observed that sPD-1 decreased significantly in clinically responding patients during Nivolumab treatment. In addition to this, patients with performance status of 0 had a decreased sPD-1 during treatment and these patients were found to have better immune fitness with low levels of immunosuppression [135]. Similarly, a study on 177 unresectable metastatic melanoma patients treated with anti-PD-1 showed interesting results. High pre-treatment serum concentrations of PD-1 and PD-L1 were correlated with poor prognosis and survival. The authors postulated that circulating serum PD-1 molecules might be directly targeted by therapeutic anti-PD-1 antibodies and this interaction might impair the effectiveness of anti-PD-1 therapy via neutralization. It is possible that this is a tumor escape mechanism that facilitates poor outcome. Thus, quantification of circulating PD-1 and PD-L1 molecules can translate into prognostic and predictive factors in immunotherapy treated patients [136].

sPD-L1 is produced by tumor cells/activated mature DCs and is known to have structural similarities to mPD-L1 [137]. It has been postulated that sPD-L1 has the capability to exert a competing effect against anti-PD-L1 drugs. A study by *Gong et al.* reported that NSCLC patients who were refractory to ICIs treatment secreted a sPD-L1 variant (without the transmembrane domain) in serum and this variant competed, bound and then inhibited the activity of immunotherapeutic drug in such patients [138]. This is a critical finding as it gives evidence on the dynamic role of sPD-L1 and its utility as a biomarker of response in immunotherapy. Furthermore, studies on various cancers have also reported on this aspect. For example, a study on ipilimumab treated melanoma patients showed that patients with high pre-treatment sPD-L1 levels showed poor prognosis and disease progression [139]. This is an interesting observation and sheds light on the dynamic nature of this biomarker. Similarly, two studies on NSCLC have documented that high levels of sPD-L1 correlated with poor prognosis, OS, and abdominal metastasis [140, 141]. However, to date no correlation of sPD-L1 with tissue PD-L1expression has been reported indicating the dynamic nature of secreted PD-L1 that is distinct from tissue PD-L1.

Several published studies evidence consistent data on its utility as a monitoring tool to test the efficacy of ICIs as a prognostic biomarker. Further studies with systematic uniform methodologies may allow better understanding of sPD-L1 as an effective tool for patient stratification with regards to anti-PD-1 therapy benefit.

sPD-L2 is a splice variant protein product that lacks transmembrane domain and is secreted into the blood. Distinct expression pattern of PD-L2 variants in leukocytes of distinct cellular status have been observed suggesting that modulation of sPD-L2 expression may have an influence on the outcome of the immune response [142]. However, limited data on sPD-L2 as an immune related biomarker is available. A study by *Zizari et al.*, on NSCLC patients treated with Nivolumab showed that sPD-L2 was dynamically modulated during ICIs treatment. The concentrations of sPD-L2 were found to be significantly lower in responding patients. In addition to this, soluble mediators including low PD-L1, CD137, Tim-3 and BTLA-4 in combination with low sPD-L2 are associated with favorable clinical response indicating that sPD-L2 works in synergy with other molecules to modulate the immune response. This allows understanding on the dynamic interaction of soluble immune modulators as useful biomarkers of response [135]. In addition to response prediction, a study on NSCLC patients treated with Nivolumab reported interesting results with respect to immune related adverse events. Low sPD-L2 concentration at diagnosis as well as in pre-treatment samples was found to be associated with occurrence of immune grade 3–4 toxicity indicating that sPD-L2 can also serve as potential predictive biomarker for immune related adverse events in ICIs treated patients [143].

4.2.1.2 Soluble CTLA-4, TIM-3 and LAG-3

The major source of sCTLA-4 is Tregs, monocytes and immature DCs [144]. sCTLA-4 has been reported in several studies as a plausible marker for response in ICIs treatment. For example, in melanoma patients treated with ipilimumab, high pre-treatment expression of sCTLA-4 was associated with response to treatment and longer OS [145]. Another study on metastatic melanoma patients treated with ipilimumab showed similar results with high levels of sCTLA-4 at baseline associated with disease responsiveness and survival. Interestingly, the study observed that in responding patients, sCTLA-4 concentration increased with subsequent treatment cycles while in progressing patients, sCTLA-4 decreased subsequently indicating that sCTLA-4 can serve as a valuable dynamic marker for treatment monitoring. In addition to this, it was also observed that patients with high pre-treatment sCTLA-4 were at a higher risk of developing immune related adverse events providing further insight into its utility as a biomarker of response/adverse event monitoring [146]. However, in different cancers, its utility may be distinct based on its interaction with other molecules and subsequent immune modulation. For example, a recent study on NSCLC patients treated with nivolumab showed that lower concentration of sCTLA-4 at 3 months of clinical evaluation was associated with response. In addition to this, patients with performance status of 0 consistently maintained a lower expression of sCTLA-4 from the time of treatment initiation until 3 months of clinical evaluation indicating that sCTLA-4 can be an indicator of immune fitness in ICIs treated patients [135]. It is postulated that during ICIs treatment, sCTLA-4 might be involved in enhancing the ability of host cytotoxic T cells to attack tumor cells and thereby enhancing the antitumor effect of immunotherapy.

sTIM-3 secreted in blood lacks mucin and transmembrane domains. It is postulated that sTIM-3 is shed from the cell surface due to metalloproteinase-dependent cleavage and may serve as a decoy receptor for TIM-3 ligands thereby interfering with the inhibitory function of TIM-3 [147]. However, the exact function of sTIM-3 is still unknown. A study on plasma levels of sTIM-3 in ICIs treated patients observed that NSCLC patients treated with nivolumab had a lower level of sTIM-3 at three months of clinical evaluation and this correlated with the response and longer survival of the patient [135]. Though, the study does give an indication of sTIM-3 as biomarker of response, further studies are needed to understand its dynamic nature in ICIs treatment.

sLAG-3 plays a role in immune pathways and has been associated as a Th1 activity marker in serum. sLAG-3 has been reported to bind to MHC class II and induce maturation of dendritic cells thereby facilitating attack on tumor cells [148, 149]. This makes sLAG-3 an attractive biomarker in ICIs treatment. Though several studies on LAG-3 and cellular response has been documented, there is paucity of data on the utility of sLAG-3 in serum of ICIs treated patients. A study on nivolumab treated NSCLC patients reported that sLAG-3 was significantly increased during treatment and this increase was retained in non-responding patients. In addition to sLAG-3, other soluble mediators including sPD-1 and sPDL-2 were also increased in these patients indicating the dynamic interactive nature of LAG-3 and its role as predictive marker [135].

4.2.1.3 Soluble IDO, CD163 and NKG2DL

Indoleamine 2,3-dioxygenase (IDO) is an enzyme that acts as an immune checkpoint and inhibits T-cell proliferation by starving the cells from tryptophan (trp) in order to sensitize them to apoptosis [150]. IDO facilitates tumor immune escape and several preclinical studies have associated IDO activity with immunotherapeutic resistance [151]. A study on nivolumab treated NSCLC patients found that lower baseline level of IDO activity in serum was significantly associated with better PFS/OS while higher levels were associated with early progression indicating that high serum levels can serve as early marker of response/indicator of resistance to anti-PD-1 treatment [152]. On the other hand, a larger study on 27 NSCLC patients treated with nivolumab indicated the dynamic nature of sIDO at baseline, 2 months and at disease progression. The study aimed to evaluate the dynamic nature of IDO as a predictor of response. Interestingly, the authors observed that at baseline, IDO activity was higher in responding patients than non-responding patients. However, in patients who did not benefit from immunotherapy, a statistically significant increase was observed between baseline sample and sample taken at the time to disease progression indicating the potential utility of IDO as therapeutic resistance marker to anti-PD-1 treatment [153].

CD163 is the hemoglobin/haptoglobin complex scavenger receptor expressed exclusively on circulating monocytes/tissue macrophages. It is involved in anti-inflammatory functions associated with macrophages and therefore plays an important role in suppressing anti-tumor immune responses [154]. sCD163 is secreted in plasma via proteolytic shedding and is considered a specific marker for TAM. To demonstrate the utility of sCD163 as a marker of response in immunotherapy, *Fujimura et al.* conducted a study on 59 cases of advanced cutaneous melanoma and 16 cases of advanced mucosal melanoma treated with nivolumab. It was observed that in advanced cutaneous melanoma group, sCD163 was significantly increased at 6 weeks of treatment in the response group as compared to non-response group indicating that sCD163 is an early marker of response in nivolumab treated patients [155]. On the other hand, another study by the same group determined the utility of sCD163 as predictor of immune related adverse events (irAE) in nivolumab treated advanced melanoma patients. It was observed that at day 42 of treatment, the absolute value of sCD163 significantly increased in patients with adverse nivolumab-induced, immune-related events indicating that sCD163 can also serve as a valuable predictor of irAEs in immunotherapy [155]. However, due to limited published data, further studies will provide a better understanding on this marker.

NKG2D is an activating immunoreceptor of cytotoxic lymphocytes and is expressed on T, NK, and NKT cells. NKG2D has eight ligands including MIC (MICA and MICB) or ULBP (ULBP1, ULBP2, ULBP3, ULBP4, RAET1G, and RAET1L) family. These NKG2D ligands are absent on normal cells but are usually overexpressed on tumor cells. Soluble NKG2D ligands (sNKG2DLs) are generated by proteolytic shedding of tumor cells which boosts tumor immune escape by binding and subsequent endocytosis/degradation of NKG2D receptor on NK/T cells thus suppressing antitumor immune responses [156, 157]. Various sNKG2DLs have been studied as predictive biomarkers of response in immunotherapy. A study in melanoma patients by *Maccalli et al.,* showed that absence of soluble sMICB, sULBP-1 and sULBP-2 in baseline serum of anti-PD-1 treated patients correlated with improved survival while detectable levels of these molecules was correlated with poor survival [158]. Similarly, another study by the same group on melanoma patients showed that elevated sULBP2 in early-stage patients on ICIs treatment was a strong indicator of poor prognosis indicating the clinical usefulness of sULBP2 as a distinguishing marker for classifying prognosis in early- and late-stage melanoma patients on treatment [156].

4.2.2 Soluble immune stimulatory markers

4.2.2.1 Soluble CD27 and CD28

CD27 is expressed in lymphocytes and is activated by its ligand, CD70, which is a member of the tumor necrosis factor receptor superfamily. Upon binding of CD70 to CD27, soluble CD27 (sCD27) is cleaved off by metalloproteinases and is secreted in serum, plasma, and urine samples. Studies have suggested that changes in sCD27 levels reflect the activity of systemic immunity [159]. In various hematological malignancies increased levels of sCD27 have been reported to correlate with poor prognosis [160]. A study on 16 advanced lung cancer patients on anti-PD-1 treatment were tested for their pretreatment sCD27 levels and correlated with their response patterns. It was observed that a sCD27 level was higher in patients with longer survival and in such patients the duration of treatment was shorter. The authors suggested that sCD27 levels can serve as prognostic marker for predicting effectiveness of ICIs in advanced lung cancer [161].

CD28 is a second messenger of T cell activation and is a critical immune checkpoint for recognition of dendritic cells by T cells. Previous studies have suggested that PD-1 antibodies rely on the activation of the CD28/B7 pathway to rescue the depletion $CD8^+$ T cells and then achieve anti-tumor effects [162]. Soluble sCD28 has been reported as a modulator of T cells for proliferation and is therefore considered an attractive biomarker of response to ICIs treatment [163]. Recently, a study on 44 patients with various cancers (lung, tongue, esophageal and nasopharyngeal, colorectal, cholangiocarcinoma, gastric, duodenal adenocarcinoma, renal cell carcinoma, hepatocellular carcinoma, and malignant melanoma) on anti-PD-1 treatment were tested for serum CD28 along with other soluble markers. It was observed that patients with higher baseline sCD28 expression had a longer PFS and responded better to treatment than non-responsive patients [164]. This dynamic change in sCD28 during treatment gives a credible index in terms of its predictive efficiency as a promising response marker. However, larger studies on this aspect are needed to understand the role of this marker.

5. Conclusion

Using ICIs have shown promising effect in treating cancers. However, only small group of patients are responsive to this treatment strategy. Tumor resistance to the immune response can be mediated by the involvement of several immunological pathways. In this chapter, we reviewed the different immunological pathways that can be modulated by immune checkpoint blockade and more specifically PD-1 and CTLA-4 inhibitors. We have summarized all the findings obtained in pre-clinical and clinical trials reporting an impact of anti-PD-1 and anti-CTLA-4 on intra-tumoral and peripheral immune response. Interestingly, the study of the dynamics of the immune system under CTLA-4 and PD-1 inhibitors shows a noticeable distinction in their regulatory mode of action on the anti-tumoral and peripheral immune response. Moreover, the findings discussed in this chapter show that CTLA-4 and PD-1 inhibitors do not only restore intra-tumoral effector T cells activity upon exhaustion but are also able to induce a consequential remodeling of the tumor microenvironment as well as the systemic immune response. Indeed, the field of immunological liquid biomarkers is fast evolving with many novel predictive and prognostics markers gaining attention. Though, liquid biopsies have many advantages including minimal invasiveness, longitudinal monitoring and simultaneous parallel testing with highly sensitive/specific high throughput applications. Although several studies state the utility of soluble ICIs markers, it is observed that the characteristic feature of these markers is to modulate the immune response in synergy with each other. This makes them attractive candidates as up and down regulation of a combination of markers can allow better understanding of the immune modulatory and dynamic nature of soluble immune molecules involved in ICIs treatment. However, there are several limitations that need to be addressed for these markers. Mainly, standardization of sampling/measurement techniques as well as larger validation studies are required to verify the utility of these markers as promising tools to guide and monitor treatment decisions in ICIs treated patients. Finally, identification of dynamic biomarkers for prediction of ICIs tumor control and for monitoring of patient response under treatment is gaining considerable knowledge through recent technologies including proteomics and transcriptomics. Progress along this approach is critical to build reasoning for novel therapeutic combinations and to set forth a more personalized cancer immunotherapeutic strategy.

Acronyms and abbreviations

ICI	immune checkpoint inhibitors
PD-L1	programmed death-ligand 1
PD-1	programmed death- 1
CTLA-4	cytotoxic T-lymphocyte-associated protein 4
TCR	T cell receptor
TME	tumor microenvironment
TIM-3	T-cell immunoglobulin and mucin-domain containing-3
LAG-3	lymphocyte-activation gene-3
TIGIT	T cell immunoreceptor with Ig and ITIM domains
Tex	exhausted T cells
Teff	effector T cells
ALC	absolute lymphocyte count
MDSCs	myeloid derived suppressor cells
TAM	tumor-associated macrophages
irAE	immune-related adverse events
CRP	C-reactive protein
LDH	lactate dehydrogenase
OS	overall survival
NLR	neutrophil-to-lymphocyte ratio
dNLR	derived Neutrophil-to-lymphocyte ratio
NSCLC	non-small-cell lung cancer
PFS	progression free survival

sICs	soluble forms of immune checkpoints
ICI	immune checkpoint inhibitors
ORR	overall response rate
sPD-1	soluble programmed cell death protein 1
sPDL-1	soluble programmed death-ligand 1
sPDL-2	soluble programmed cell death 1 ligand 2
sCTLA-4	soluble cytotoxic T-lymphocyte-associated protein 4
sTIM-3	soluble T-cell immunoglobulin and mucin domain-3
sLAG-3	soluble lymphocyte-activation gene 3
sIDO	soluble indoleamine 2,3-dioxygenase
sCD163	soluble cluster of differentiation 163
NKG2D	natural killer group 2D
sNKG2DL	soluble natural killer group 2D ligands
MICA	major histocompatibility complex class I-related chain A
MICB	major histocompatibility complex class I-related chain B
NK	natural killer
NKT	natural killer T cells
ULBP 1,2,3,4	UL-16-binding proteins 1,2,3,4
RAET1G	retinoic acid early transcript 1G
RAET1L	retinoic acid early transcript 1 L
sCD27	soluble cluster of differentiation 27
sCD28	soluble cluster of differentiation 28

Author details

Afsheen Raza[1,2†], Maysaloun Merhi[1,2†], Allan Relecom[3†], Queenie Fernandes[1,5†], Varghese Inchakalody[1,2†], Abdul Rahman Zar Gul[2], Shahab Uddin[4], Mohammed Ussama Al Homsi[2] and Said Dermime[1,2*]

1 Translational Cancer Research Facility and Clinical Trial Unit, Interim Translational Research Institute, Hamad Medical Corporation, Doha, Qatar

2 National Center for Cancer Care and Research, Hamad Medical Corporation, Doha, Qatar

3 Department of Oncology, Geneva University Hospitals, Geneva, Switzerland

4 Translational Research Institute, Academic Health System, Hamad Medical Corporation, Doha, Qatar

5 College of Medicine, Qatar University, Doha, Qatar

*Address all correspondence to: sdermime@hamad.qa

† These authors equally contributed in writing this book chapter.

References

[1] Arora, S., et al., *Existing and Emerging Biomarkers for Immune Checkpoint Immunotherapy in Solid Tumors.* Adv Ther, 2019. **36**(10): p. 2638-2678.

[2] Shindo, Y., et al., *Novel Biomarkers for Personalized Cancer Immunotherapy.* Cancers (Basel), 2019. **11**(9).

[3] Latchman, Y., et al., *PD-L2 is a second ligand for PD-1 and inhibits T cell activation.* Nat Immunol, 2001. **2**(3): p. 261-8.

[4] Topalian, S.L., C.G. Drake, and D.M. Pardoll, *Targeting the PD-1/B7-H1(PD-L1) pathway to activate anti-tumor immunity.* Curr Opin Immunol, 2012. **24**(2): p. 207-12.

[5] Herbst, R.S., et al., *Predictive correlates of response to the anti-PD-L1 antibody MPDL3280A in cancer patients.* Nature, 2014. **515**(7528): p. 563-7.

[6] Riaz, N., et al., *Tumor and Microenvironment Evolution during Immunotherapy with Nivolumab.* Cell, 2017. **171**(4): p. 934-949 e16.

[7] Chen, P.L., et al., *Analysis of Immune Signatures in Longitudinal Tumor Samples Yields Insight into Biomarkers of Response and Mechanisms of Resistance to Immune Checkpoint Blockade.* Cancer Discov, 2016. **6**(8): p. 827-37.

[8] Tumeh, P.C., et al., *PD-1 blockade induces responses by inhibiting adaptive immune resistance.* Nature, 2014. **515**(7528): p. 568-71.

[9] Ribas, A., et al., *PD-1 Blockade Expands Intratumoral Memory T Cells.* Cancer Immunol Res, 2016. **4**(3): p. 194-203.

[10] Paley, M.A., et al., *Progenitor and terminal subsets of CD8+ T cells cooperate to contain chronic viral infection.* Science, 2012. **338**(6111): p. 1220-5.

[11] Blackburn, S.D., et al., *Coregulation of CD8+ T cell exhaustion by multiple inhibitory receptors during chronic viral infection.* Nat Immunol, 2009. **10**(1): p. 29-37.

[12] Thommen, D.S., et al., *A transcriptionally and functionally distinct PD-1(+) CD8(+) T cell pool with predictive potential in non-small-cell lung cancer treated with PD-1 blockade.* Nat Med, 2018. **24**(7): p. 994-1004.

[13] Sharma, A., et al., *Anti-CTLA-4 Immunotherapy Does Not Deplete FOXP3(+) Regulatory T Cells (Tregs) in Human Cancers-Response.* Clin Cancer Res, 2019. **25**(11): p. 3469-3470.

[14] Pauken, K.E., et al., *Epigenetic stability of exhausted T cells limits durability of reinvigoration by PD-1 blockade.* Science, 2016. **354**(6316): p. 1160-1165.

[15] Philip, M., et al., *Chromatin states define tumour-specific T cell dysfunction and reprogramming.* Nature, 2017. **545**(7655): p. 452-456.

[16] Ghoneim, H.E., et al., *De Novo Epigenetic Programs Inhibit PD-1 Blockade-Mediated T Cell Rejuvenation.* Cell, 2017. **170**(1): p. 142-157 e19.

[17] Im, S.J., et al., *Defining CD8+ T cells that provide the proliferative burst after PD-1 therapy.* Nature, 2016. **537**(7620): p. 417-421.

[18] Jadhav, R.R., et al., *Epigenetic signature of PD-1+ TCF1+ CD8 T cells that act as resource cells during chronic viral infection and respond to PD-1 blockade.* Proc Natl Acad Sci U S A, 2019. **116**(28): p. 14113-14118.

[19] Siddiqui, I., et al., *Intratumoral Tcf1(+)PD-1(+)CD8(+) T Cells with Stem-like Properties Promote Tumor Control in Response to Vaccination and*

Checkpoint Blockade Immunotherapy. Immunity, 2019. **50**(1): p. 195-211 e10.

[20] Miller, B.C., et al., *Subsets of exhausted CD8(+) T cells differentially mediate tumor control and respond to checkpoint blockade.* Nat Immunol, 2019. **20**(3): p. 326-336.

[21] Kurtulus, S., et al., *Checkpoint Blockade Immunotherapy Induces Dynamic Changes in PD-1(-)CD8(+) Tumor-Infiltrating T Cells.* Immunity, 2019. **50**(1): p. 181-194 e6.

[22] Ganesan, A.P., et al., *Tissue-resident memory features are linked to the magnitude of cytotoxic T cell responses in human lung cancer.* Nat Immunol, 2017. **18**(8): p. 940-950.

[23] Spitzer, M.H., et al., *Systemic Immunity Is Required for Effective Cancer Immunotherapy.* Cell, 2017. **168**(3): p. 487-502 e15.

[24] Huang, A.C., et al., *A single dose of neoadjuvant PD-1 blockade predicts clinical outcomes in resectable melanoma.* Nat Med, 2019. **25**(3): p. 454-461.

[25] Huang, A.C., et al., *T-cell invigoration to tumour burden ratio associated with anti-PD-1 response.* Nature, 2017. **545**(7652): p. 60-65.

[26] Kim, K.H., et al., *The First-week Proliferative Response of Peripheral Blood PD-1(+)CD8(+) T Cells Predicts the Response to Anti-PD-1 Therapy in Solid Tumors.* Clin Cancer Res, 2019. **25**(7): p. 2144-2154.

[27] Merhi, M., et al., *Persistent anti-NY-ESO-1-specific T cells and expression of differential biomarkers in a patient with metastatic gastric cancer benefiting from combined radioimmunotherapy treatment: a case report.* J Immunother Cancer, 2020. **8**(2).

[28] Walunas, T.L., et al., *CTLA-4 can function as a negative regulator of T cell activation.* Immunity, 1994. **1**(5): p. 405-13.

[29] Waterhouse, P., et al., *Lymphoproliferative disorders with early lethality in mice deficient in Ctla-4.* Science, 1995. **270**(5238): p. 985-8.

[30] Wei, S.C., et al., *Distinct Cellular Mechanisms Underlie Anti-CTLA-4 and Anti-PD-1 Checkpoint Blockade.* Cell, 2017. **170**(6): p. 1120-1133 e17.

[31] Gubin, M.M., et al., *Checkpoint blockade cancer immunotherapy targets tumour-specific mutant antigens.* Nature, 2014. **515**(7528): p. 577-81.

[32] Ribas, A., et al., *Intratumoral immune cell infiltrates, FoxP3, and indoleamine 2,3-dioxygenase in patients with melanoma undergoing CTLA4 blockade.* Clin Cancer Res, 2009. **15**(1): p. 390-9.

[33] Huang, R.R., et al., *CTLA4 blockade induces frequent tumor infiltration by activated lymphocytes regardless of clinical responses in humans.* Clin Cancer Res, 2011. **17**(12): p. 4101-9.

[34] Hosoi, A., et al., *Increased diversity with reduced "diversity evenness" of tumor infiltrating T-cells for the successful cancer immunotherapy.* Sci Rep, 2018. **8**(1): p. 1058.

[35] Pedicord, V.A., et al., *Single dose of anti-CTLA-4 enhances CD8+ T-cell memory formation, function, and maintenance.* Proc Natl Acad Sci U S A, 2011. **108**(1): p. 266-71.

[36] Felix, J., et al., *Ipilimumab reshapes T cell memory subsets in melanoma patients with clinical response.* Oncoimmunology, 2016. **5**(7): p. 1136045.

[37] de Coana, Y.P., et al., *Ipilimumab treatment decreases monocytic MDSCs and increases CD8 effector memory T cells in long-term survivors with advanced melanoma.* Oncotarget, 2017. **8**(13): p. 21539-21553.

[38] Wei, S.C., et al., *Negative Co-stimulation Constrains T Cell Differentiation by Imposing Boundaries on Possible Cell States.* Immunity, 2019. **50**(4): p. 1084-1098 e10.

[39] Fu, T., Q. He, and P. Sharma, *The ICOS/ICOSL pathway is required for optimal antitumor responses mediated by anti-CTLA-4 therapy.* Cancer Res, 2011. **71**(16): p. 5445-54.

[40] Jiao, S., et al., *Differences in Tumor Microenvironment Dictate T Helper Lineage Polarization and Response to Immune Checkpoint Therapy.* Cell, 2019. **179**(5): p. 1177-1190 e13.

[41] Ji, R.R., et al., *An immune-active tumor microenvironment favors clinical response to ipilimumab.* Cancer Immunol Immunother, 2012. **61**(7): p. 1019-31.

[42] von Euw, E., et al., *CTLA4 blockade increases Th17 cells in patients with metastatic melanoma.* J Transl Med, 2009. 7: p. 35.

[43] Chen, H., et al., *Anti-CTLA-4 therapy results in higher CD4+ICOShi T cell frequency and IFN-gamma levels in both nonmalignant and malignant prostate tissues.* Proc Natl Acad Sci U S A, 2009. **106**(8): p. 2729-34.

[44] Liakou, C.I., et al., *CTLA-4 blockade increases IFNgamma-producing CD4+ICOShi cells to shift the ratio of effector to regulatory T cells in cancer patients.* Proc Natl Acad Sci U S A, 2008. **105**(39): p. 14987-92.

[45] Carthon, B.C., et al., *Preoperative CTLA-4 blockade: tolerability and immune monitoring in the setting of a presurgical clinical trial.* Clin Cancer Res, 2010. **16**(10): p. 2861-71.

[46] Ng Tang, D., et al., *Increased frequency of ICOS+ CD4 T cells as a pharmacodynamic biomarker for anti-CTLA-4 therapy.* Cancer Immunol Res, 2013. **1**(4): p. 229-34.

[47] Weber, J.S., et al., *Ipilimumab increases activated T cells and enhances humoral immunity in patients with advanced melanoma.* J Immunother, 2012. **35**(1): p. 89-97.

[48] Kitano, S., et al., *Enhancement of tumor-reactive cytotoxic CD4+ T cell responses after ipilimumab treatment in four advanced melanoma patients.* Cancer Immunol Res, 2013. **1**(4): p. 235-44.

[49] Vonderheide, R.H., et al., *Tremelimumab in combination with exemestane in patients with advanced breast cancer and treatment-associated modulation of inducible costimulator expression on patient T cells.* Clin Cancer Res, 2010. **16**(13): p. 3485-94.

[50] Das, R., et al., *Combination therapy with anti-CTLA-4 and anti-PD-1 leads to distinct immunologic changes in vivo.* J Immunol, 2015. **194**(3): p. 950-9.

[51] Kavanagh, B., et al., *CTLA4 blockade expands FoxP3+ regulatory and activated effector CD4+ T cells in a dose-dependent fashion.* Blood, 2008. **112**(4): p. 1175-83.

[52] Wang, W., et al., *Biomarkers on melanoma patient T cells associated with ipilimumab treatment.* J Transl Med, 2012. **10**: p. 146.

[53] Klein, O., et al., *Melan-A-specific cytotoxic T cells are associated with tumor regression and autoimmunity following treatment with anti-CTLA-4.* Clin Cancer Res, 2009. **15**(7): p. 2507-13.

[54] Yuan, J., et al., *CTLA-4 blockade enhances polyfunctional NY-ESO-1 specific T cell responses in metastatic melanoma patients with clinical benefit.* Proc Natl Acad Sci U S A, 2008. **105**(51): p. 20410-5.

[55] Hodi, F.S., et al., *Immunologic and clinical effects of antibody blockade of cytotoxic T lymphocyte-associated antigen 4 in previously vaccinated cancer patients.* Proc Natl Acad Sci U S A, 2008. **105**(8): p. 3005-10.

[56] Martens, A., et al., *Increases in Absolute Lymphocytes and Circulating CD4+ and CD8+ T Cells Are Associated with Positive Clinical Outcome of Melanoma Patients Treated with Ipilimumab.* Clin Cancer Res, 2016. **22**(19): p. 4848-4858.

[57] Kelderman, S., et al., *Lactate dehydrogenase as a selection criterion for ipilimumab treatment in metastatic melanoma.* Cancer Immunol Immunother, 2014. **63**(5): p. 449-58.

[58] Ku, G.Y., et al., *Single-institution experience with ipilimumab in advanced melanoma patients in the compassionate use setting: lymphocyte count after 2 doses correlates with survival.* Cancer, 2010. **116**(7): p. 1767-75.

[59] Delyon, J., et al., *Experience in daily practice with ipilimumab for the treatment of patients with metastatic melanoma: an early increase in lymphocyte and eosinophil counts is associated with improved survival.* Ann Oncol, 2013. **24**(6): p. 1697-703.

[60] Robert, L., et al., *CTLA4 blockade broadens the peripheral T-cell receptor repertoire.* Clin Cancer Res, 2014. **20**(9): p. 2424-32.

[61] Cha, E., et al., *Improved survival with T cell clonotype stability after anti-CTLA-4 treatment in cancer patients.* Sci Transl Med, 2014. **6**(238): p. 238ra70.

[62] Oh, D.Y., et al., *Immune Toxicities Elicted by CTLA-4 Blockade in Cancer Patients Are Associated with Early Diversification of the T-cell Repertoire.* Cancer Res, 2017. **77**(6): p. 1322-1330.

[63] Arakawa, A., et al., *Clonality of CD4(+) Blood T Cells Predicts Longer Survival With CTLA4 or PD-1 Checkpoint Inhibition in Advanced Melanoma.* Front Immunol, 2019. **10**: p. 1336.

[64] Messaoudi, I., et al., *Direct link between mhc polymorphism, T cell avidity, and diversity in immune defense.* Science, 2002. **298**(5599): p. 1797-800.

[65] Facciabene, A., G.T. Motz, and G. Coukos, *T-regulatory cells: key players in tumor immune escape and angiogenesis.* Cancer Res, 2012. **72**(9): p. 2162-71.

[66] Mougiakakos, D., et al., *Regulatory T cells in cancer.* Adv Cancer Res, 2010. **107**: p. 57-117.

[67] Wei, T., W. Zhong, and Q. Li, *Role of heterogeneous regulatory T cells in the tumor microenvironment.* Pharmacol Res, 2020. **153**: p. 104659.

[68] Sakaguchi, S., et al., *FOXP3+ regulatory T cells in the human immune system.* Nat Rev Immunol, 2010. **10**(7): p. 490-500.

[69] Lowther, D.E., et al., *PD-1 marks dysfunctional regulatory T cells in malignant gliomas.* JCI Insight, 2016. **1**(5).

[70] Togashi, Y., K. Shitara, and H. Nishikawa, *Regulatory T cells in cancer immunosuppression - implications for anticancer therapy.* Nat Rev Clin Oncol, 2019. **16**(6): p. 356-371.

[71] Duraiswamy, J., et al., *Dual blockade of PD-1 and CTLA-4 combined with tumor vaccine effectively restores T-cell rejection function in tumors.* Cancer Res, 2013. **73**(12): p. 3591-603.

[72] Yoshida, K., et al., *Anti-PD-1 antibody decreases tumour-infiltrating regulatory T cells.* BMC Cancer, 2020. **20**(1): p. 25.

[73] Amarnath, S., et al., *The PDL1-PD1 axis converts human TH1 cells into regulatory T cells.* Sci Transl Med, 2011. **3**(111): p. 111ra120.

[74] Francisco, L.M., et al., *PD-L1 regulates the development, maintenance, and function of induced regulatory T cells.* J Exp Med, 2009. **206**(13): p. 3015-29.

[75] Dodagatta-Marri, E., et al., *alpha-PD-1 therapy elevates Treg/Th balance and increases tumor cell pSmad3 that are both targeted by alpha-TGFbeta antibody to promote durable rejection and immunity in squamous cell carcinomas.* J Immunother Cancer, 2019. **7**(1): p. 62.

[76] Franceschini, D., et al., *PD-L1 negatively regulates CD4+CD25+Foxp3+ Tregs by limiting STAT-5 phosphorylation in patients chronically infected with HCV.* J Clin Invest, 2009. **119**(3): p. 551-64.

[77] Penaloza-MacMaster, P., et al., *CD4 T Cell Depletion Substantially Augments the Rescue Potential of PD-L1 Blockade for Deeply Exhausted CD8 T Cells.* J Immunol, 2015. **195**(3): p. 1054-63.

[78] Kamada, T., et al., *PD-1(+) regulatory T cells amplified by PD-1 blockade promote hyperprogression of cancer.* Proc Natl Acad Sci U S A, 2019. **116**(20): p. 9999-10008.

[79] Woods, D.M., et al., *Decreased Suppression and Increased Phosphorylated STAT3 in Regulatory T Cells are Associated with Benefit from Adjuvant PD-1 Blockade in Resected Metastatic Melanoma.* Clin Cancer Res, 2018. **24**(24): p. 6236-6247.

[80] Zappasodi, R., et al., *Non-conventional Inhibitory CD4(+)Foxp3(-) PD-1(hi) T Cells as a Biomarker of Immune Checkpoint Blockade Activity.* Cancer Cell, 2018. **34**(4): p. 691.

[81] Verma, V., et al., *PD-1 blockade in subprimed CD8 cells induces dysfunctional PD-1(+)CD38(hi) cells and anti-PD-1 resistance.* Nat Immunol, 2019. **20**(9): p. 1231-1243.

[82] Peggs, K.S., et al., *Blockade of CTLA-4 on both effector and regulatory T cell compartments contributes to the antitumor activity of anti-CTLA-4 antibodies.* J Exp Med, 2009. **206**(8): p. 1717-25.

[83] Selby, M.J., et al., *Anti-CTLA-4 antibodies of IgG2a isotype enhance antitumor activity through reduction of intratumoral regulatory T cells.* Cancer Immunol Res, 2013. **1**(1): p. 32-42.

[84] Tang, F., et al., *Anti-CTLA-4 antibodies in cancer immunotherapy: selective depletion of intratumoral regulatory T cells or checkpoint blockade?* Cell Biosci, 2018. **8**: p. 30.

[85] Saito, T., et al., *Two FOXP3(+) CD4(+) T cell subpopulations distinctly control the prognosis of colorectal cancers.* Nat Med, 2016. **22**(6): p. 679-84.

[86] Quezada, S.A., et al., *CTLA4 blockade and GM-CSF combination immunotherapy alters the intratumor balance of effector and regulatory T cells.* J Clin Invest, 2006. **116**(7): p. 1935-45.

[87] Simpson, T.R., et al., *Fc-dependent depletion of tumor-infiltrating regulatory T cells co-defines the efficacy of anti-CTLA-4 therapy against melanoma.* J Exp Med, 2013. **210**(9): p. 1695-710.

[88] Du, X., et al., *A reappraisal of CTLA-4 checkpoint blockade in cancer immunotherapy.* Cell Res, 2018. **28**(4): p. 416-432.

[89] Bjoern, J., et al., *Immunological correlates of treatment and response in stage IV malignant melanoma patients treated with Ipilimumab.* Oncoimmunology, 2016. **5**(4): p. e1100788.

[90] Tarhini, A.A., et al., *Immune monitoring of the circulation and the tumor microenvironment in patients with regionally advanced melanoma receiving neoadjuvant ipilimumab.* PLoS One, 2014. **9**(2): p. e87705.

[91] Khan, S., et al., *Tremelimumab (anti-CTLA4) mediates immune responses mainly by direct activation of T effector cells rather than by affecting T regulatory*

cells. Clin Immunol, 2011. **138**(1): p. 85-96.

[92] Phan, G.Q., et al., *Cancer regression and autoimmunity induced by cytotoxic T lymphocyte-associated antigen 4 blockade in patients with metastatic melanoma.* Proc Natl Acad Sci U S A, 2003. **100**(14): p. 8372-7.

[93] Simeone, E., et al., *Immunological and biological changes during ipilimumab treatment and their potential correlation with clinical response and survival in patients with advanced melanoma.* Cancer Immunol Immunother, 2014. **63**(7): p. 675-83.

[94] Sarnaik, A.A., et al., *Extended dose ipilimumab with a peptide vaccine: immune correlates associated with clinical benefit in patients with resected high-risk stage IIIc/IV melanoma.* Clin Cancer Res, 2011. **17**(4): p. 896-906.

[95] Maker, A.V., P. Attia, and S.A. Rosenberg, *Analysis of the cellular mechanism of antitumor responses and autoimmunity in patients treated with CTLA-4 blockade.* J Immunol, 2005. **175**(11): p. 7746-54.

[96] Romano, E., et al., *Ipilimumab-dependent cell-mediated cytotoxicity of regulatory T cells ex vivo by nonclassical monocytes in melanoma patients.* Proc Natl Acad Sci U S A, 2015. **112**(19): p. 6140-5.

[97] Spranger, S., et al., *Up-regulation of PD-L1, IDO, and T(regs) in the melanoma tumor microenvironment is driven by CD8(+) T cells.* Sci Transl Med, 2013. **5**(200): p. 200ra116.

[98] Fridman, W.H., et al., *The immune contexture in cancer prognosis and treatment.* Nat Rev Clin Oncol, 2017. **14**(12): p. 717-734.

[99] Pages, F., et al., *International validation of the consensus Immunoscore for the classification of colon cancer: a prognostic and accuracy study.* Lancet, 2018. **391**(10135): p. 2128-2139.

[100] Nakamura, K. and M.J. Smyth, *Myeloid immunosuppression and immune checkpoints in the tumor microenvironment.* Cell Mol Immunol, 2020. **17**(1): p. 1-12.

[101] Martinez, F.O. and S. Gordon, *The M1 and M2 paradigm of macrophage activation: time for reassessment.* F1000Prime Rep, 2014. **6**: p. 13.

[102] Gubin, M.M., et al., *High-Dimensional Analysis Delineates Myeloid and Lymphoid Compartment Remodeling during Successful Immune-Checkpoint Cancer Therapy.* Cell, 2018. **175**(5): p. 1443.

[103] Xiong, H., et al., *Anti-PD-L1 Treatment Results in Functional Remodeling of the Macrophage Compartment.* Cancer Res, 2019. **79**(7): p. 1493-1506.

[104] Beavis, P.A., et al., *Dual PD-1 and CTLA-4 Checkpoint Blockade Promotes Antitumor Immune Responses through CD4(+)Foxp3(-) Cell-Mediated Modulation of CD103(+) Dendritic Cells.* Cancer Immunol Res, 2018. **6**(9): p. 1069-1081.

[105] Laurent, S., et al., *CTLA-4 is expressed by human monocyte-derived dendritic cells and regulates their functions.* Hum Immunol, 2010. **71**(10): p. 934-41.

[106] Liu, Y., et al., *Regulation of arginase I activity and expression by both PD-1 and CTLA-4 on the myeloid-derived suppressor cells.* Cancer Immunol Immunother, 2009. **58**(5): p. 687-97.

[107] Rodriguez, P.C., et al., *Arginase I production in the tumor microenvironment by mature myeloid cells inhibits T-cell receptor expression and*

antigen-specific T-cell responses. Cancer Res, 2004. **64**(16): p. 5839-49.

[108] Strauss, L., et al., *Targeted deletion of PD-1 in myeloid cells induces antitumor immunity.* Sci Immunol, 2020. 5(43).

[109] Pico de Coana, Y., et al., *Ipilimumab treatment results in an early decrease in the frequency of circulating granulocytic myeloid-derived suppressor cells as well as their Arginase1 production.* Cancer Immunol Res, 2013. **1**(3): p. 158-62.

[110] Gebhardt, C., et al., *Myeloid Cells and Related Chronic Inflammatory Factors as Novel Predictive Markers in Melanoma Treatment with Ipilimumab.* Clin Cancer Res, 2015. **21**(24): p. 5453-9.

[111] Meyer, C., et al., *Frequencies of circulating MDSC correlate with clinical outcome of melanoma patients treated with ipilimumab.* Cancer Immunol Immunother, 2014. **63**(3): p. 247-57.

[112] Gabrilovich, D.I. and S. Nagaraj, *Myeloid-derived suppressor cells as regulators of the immune system.* Nat Rev Immunol, 2009. **9**(3): p. 162-74.

[113] Krieg, C., et al., *High-dimensional single-cell analysis predicts response to anti-PD-1 immunotherapy.* Nat Med, 2018. **24**(2): p. 144-153.

[114] Bonomi, M., et al., *Circulating immune biomarkers as predictors of the response to pembrolizumab and weekly low dose carboplatin and paclitaxel in NSCLC and poor PS: An interim analysis.* Oncol Lett, 2019. **17**(1): p. 1349-1356.

[115] Nakamura, Y., et al., *Nivolumab for advanced melanoma: pretreatment prognostic factors and early outcome markers during therapy.* Oncotarget, 2016. 7(47): p. 77404-77415.

[116] Valpione, S., et al., *Personalised medicine: Development and external validation of a prognostic model for metastatic melanoma patients treated with ipilimumab.* Eur J Cancer, 2015. **51**(14): p. 2086-94.

[117] Ferrucci, P.F., et al., *Baseline neutrophils and derived neutrophil-to-lymphocyte ratio: prognostic relevance in metastatic melanoma patients receiving ipilimumab.* Ann Oncol, 2016. **27**(4): p. 732-8.

[118] Jin, J., et al., *Association of the neutrophil to lymphocyte ratio and clinical outcomes in patients with lung cancer receiving immunotherapy: a meta-analysis.* BMJ Open, 2020. **10**(6): p. e035031.

[119] Maymani, H., et al., *Predicting outcomes in patients with advanced non-small cell lung cancer enrolled in early phase immunotherapy trials.* Lung Cancer, 2018. **120**: p. 137-141.

[120] Shindo, Y., et al., *Predictive biomarkers for the efficacy of peptide vaccine treatment: based on the results of a phase II study on advanced pancreatic cancer.* J Exp Clin Cancer Res, 2017. **36**(1): p. 36.

[121] Akamine, T., et al., *Association of preoperative serum CRP with PD-L1 expression in 508 patients with non-small cell lung cancer: A comprehensive analysis of systemic inflammatory markers.* Surg Oncol, 2018. **27**(1): p. 88-94.

[122] Shrotriya, S., et al., *C-Reactive Protein Is an Important Biomarker for Prognosis Tumor Recurrence and Treatment Response in Adult Solid Tumors: A Systematic Review.* PLoS One, 2015. **10**(12): p. e0143080.

[123] Nakamura, Y., *Biomarkers for Immune Checkpoint Inhibitor-Mediated Tumor Response and Adverse Events.* Front Med (Lausanne), 2019. **6**: p. 119.

[124] Wong, N., J. De Melo, and D. Tang, *PKM2, a Central Point of Regulation in Cancer Metabolism.* Int J Cell Biol, 2013. **2013**: p. 242513.

[125] Balch, C.M., et al., *Final version of 2009 AJCC melanoma staging and classification.* J Clin Oncol, 2009. **27**(36): p. 6199-206.

[126] Deng, T., et al., *Higher pretreatment lactate dehydrogenase concentration predicts worse overall survival in patients with lung cancer.* Medicine (Baltimore), 2018. **97**(38): p. e12524.

[127] Diem, S., et al., *Serum lactate dehydrogenase as an early marker for outcome in patients treated with anti-PD-1 therapy in metastatic melanoma.* Br J Cancer, 2016. **114**(3): p. 256-61.

[128] Wagner, N.B., et al., *S100B and LDH as early prognostic markers for response and overall survival in melanoma patients treated with anti-PD-1 or combined anti-PD-1 plus anti-CTLA-4 antibodies.* Br J Cancer, 2018. **119**(3): p. 339-346.

[129] Wang, X., et al., *Lactate dehydrogenase and baseline markers associated with clinical outcomes of advanced esophageal squamous cell carcinoma patients treated with camrelizumab (SHR-1210), a novel anti-PD-1 antibody.* Thorac Cancer, 2019. **10**(6): p. 1395-1401.

[130] Gu, D., et al., *Soluble immune checkpoints in cancer: production, function and biological significance.* J Immunother Cancer, 2018. **6**(1): p. 132.

[131] Song, M.Y., et al., *Enhancement of vaccine-induced primary and memory CD8(+) T-cell responses by soluble PD-1.* J Immunother, 2011. **34**(3): p. 297-306.

[132] Geng, H., et al., *HSP70 vaccine in combination with gene therapy with plasmid DNA encoding sPD-1 overcomes immune resistance and suppresses the progression of pulmonary metastatic melanoma.* Int J Cancer, 2006. **118**(11): p. 2657-64.

[133] Qiu, H., et al., *Regulating immunity and inhibiting tumor growth by the recombinant peptide sPD-1-CH50.* Anticancer Res, 2009. **29**(12): p. 5089-94.

[134] Shin, S.P., et al., *Adenovirus expressing both thymidine kinase and soluble PD1 enhances antitumor immunity by strengthening CD8 T-cell response.* Mol Ther, 2013. **21**(3): p. 688-95.

[135] Zizzari, I.G., et al., *Soluble Immune Checkpoints, Gut Metabolites and Performance Status as Parameters of Response to Nivolumab Treatment in NSCLC Patients.* J Pers Med, 2020. **10**(4).

[136] Ugurel, S., et al., *Elevated baseline serum PD-1 or PD-L1 predicts poor outcome of PD-1 inhibition therapy in metastatic melanoma.* Ann Oncol, 2020. **31**(1): p. 144-152.

[137] Frigola, X., et al., *Soluble B7-H1: differences in production between dendritic cells and T cells.* Immunol Lett, 2012. **142**(1-2): p. 78-82.

[138] Gong, B., et al., *Secreted PD-L1 variants mediate resistance to PD-L1 blockade therapy in non-small cell lung cancer.* J Exp Med, 2019. **216**(4): p. 982-1000.

[139] Zhu, X. and J. Lang, *Soluble PD-1 and PD-L1: predictive and prognostic significance in cancer.* Oncotarget, 2017. **8**(57): p. 97671-97682.

[140] Vecchiarelli, S., et al., *Circulating programmed death ligand-1 (cPD-L1) in non-small-cell lung cancer (NSCLC).* Oncotarget, 2018. **9**(25): p. 17554-17563.

[141] Zhang, J., et al., *Circulating PD-L1 in NSCLC patients and the correlation between the level of PD-L1 expression and the clinical characteristics.* Thorac Cancer, 2015. **6**(4): p. 534-8.

[142] He, X.H., et al., *Cloning and identification of two novel splice variants of human PD-L2.* Acta Biochim Biophys Sin (Shanghai), 2004. **36**(4): p. 284-9.

[143] Costantini, A., et al., *Predictive role of plasmatic biomarkers in advanced non-small cell lung cancer treated by nivolumab.* Oncoimmunology, 2018. 7(8): p. e1452581.

[144] Ward, F.J., et al., *The soluble isoform of CTLA-4 as a regulator of T-cell responses.* Eur J Immunol, 2013. **43**(5): p. 1274-85.

[145] Leung, A.M., et al., *Clinical Benefit from Ipilimumab Therapy in Melanoma Patients may be Associated with Serum CTLA4 Levels.* Front Oncol, 2014. **4**: p. 110.

[146] Pistillo, M.P., et al., *Soluble CTLA-4 as a favorable predictive biomarker in metastatic melanoma patients treated with ipilimumab: an Italian melanoma intergroup study.* Cancer Immunol Immunother, 2019. **68**(1): p. 97-107.

[147] Wolf, Y., A.C. Anderson, and V.K. Kuchroo, *TIM3 comes of age as an inhibitory receptor.* Nat Rev Immunol, 2020. **20**(3): p. 173-185.

[148] El Mir, S. and F. Triebel, *A soluble lymphocyte activation gene-3 molecule used as a vaccine adjuvant elicits greater humoral and cellular immune responses to both particulate and soluble antigens.* J Immunol, 2000. **164**(11): p. 5583-9.

[149] Huard, B., et al., *CD4/major histocompatibility complex class II interaction analyzed with CD4- and lymphocyte activation gene-3 (LAG-3)-Ig fusion proteins.* Eur J Immunol, 1995. **25**(9): p. 2718-21.

[150] Hwu, P., et al., *Indoleamine 2,3-dioxygenase production by human dendritic cells results in the inhibition of T cell proliferation.* J Immunol, 2000. **164**(7): p. 3596-9.

[151] Holmgaard, R.B., et al., *Indoleamine 2,3-dioxygenase is a critical resistance mechanism in antitumor T cell immunotherapy targeting CTLA-4.* J Exp Med, 2013. **210**(7): p. 1389-402.

[152] Botticelli, A., et al., *Can IDO activity predict primary resistance to anti-PD-1 treatment in NSCLC?* J Transl Med, 2018. **16**(1): p. 219.

[153] Agullo-Ortuno, M.T., et al., *Blood Predictive Biomarkers for Patients With Non-small-cell Lung Cancer Associated With Clinical Response to Nivolumab.* Clin Lung Cancer, 2020. **21**(1): p. 75-85.

[154] Jensen, T.O., et al., *Macrophage markers in serum and tumor have prognostic impact in American Joint Committee on Cancer stage I/II melanoma.* J Clin Oncol, 2009. **27**(20): p. 3330-7.

[155] Fujimura, T., et al., *Serum Level of Soluble CD163 May Be a Predictive Marker of the Effectiveness of Nivolumab in Patients With Advanced Cutaneous Melanoma.* Front Oncol, 2018. **8**: p. 530.

[156] Paschen, A., et al., *Differential clinical significance of individual NKG2D ligands in melanoma: soluble ULBP2 as an indicator of poor prognosis superior to S100B.* Clin Cancer Res, 2009. **15**(16): p. 5208-15.

[157] Raulet, D.H., *Roles of the NKG2D immunoreceptor and its ligands.* Nat Rev Immunol, 2003. **3**(10): p. 781-90.

[158] Maccalli, C., et al., *Soluble NKG2D ligands are biomarkers associated with the clinical outcome to immune checkpoint blockade therapy of metastatic melanoma patients.* Oncoimmunology, 2017. **6**(7): p. e1323618.

[159] Hintzen, R.Q., et al., *A soluble form of the human T cell differentiation antigen CD27 is released after triggering of the TCR/CD3 complex.* J Immunol, 1991. **147**(1): p. 29-35.

[160] Kok, M., et al., *Serum soluble CD27, but not thymidine kinase, is an*

independent prognostic factor for outcome in indolent non-Hodgkin's lymphoma. Tumour Biol, 2003. **24**(1): p. 53-60.

[161] Kashima, J., et al., *High Serum Soluble CD27 Level Correlates with Poor Performance Status and Reduced Survival in Patients with Advanced Lung Cancer.* Oncology, 2019. **97**(6): p. 365-372.

[162] Hui, E., et al., *T cell costimulatory receptor CD28 is a primary target for PD-1-mediated inhibition.* Science, 2017. **355**(6332): p. 1428-1433.

[163] Hebbar, M., et al., *Detection of circulating soluble CD28 in patients with systemic lupus erythematosus, primary Sjogren's syndrome and systemic sclerosis.* Clin Exp Immunol, 2004. **136**(2): p. 388-92.

[164] Zhang, C., et al., *Anti-PD-1 Therapy Response Predicted by the Combination of Exosomal PD-L1 and CD28.* Front Oncol, 2020. **10**: p. 760.

Chapter 3

The Endocrinological Side Effects of Immunotherapies

Anush Patel, Haisam Abid and Amrat Kumar

Abstract

The use of immunotherapies is gaining importance in the treatment of advanced malignancies. There are many checkpoints in the immune system which prevents T-cells from attacking one's own body cells. The cancer cells can camouflage from the T-cells and the immune system is unable to mount an effective anti-tumor response. The immunotherapies, mainly monoclonal antibodies anti-cytotoxic T-lymphocyte antigen 4 (CTLA-4), anti-programmed cell death protein-1 (PD-1) and anti-PD-1 ligand molecules (PD-L1 and L2) reactivate the immune system to act against cancerous cells but they can also cause T-cells to attack healthy cells causing various autoimmune diseases, which are known as immune related adverse events (irAEs). Current clinical data shows increased incidence of pituitary disorders with CTLA4 inhibitors and thyroid dysfunction in patients with PD-1/PD L-1 1 blockade. There have also been association of type 1 diabetes mellitus and primary adrenal insufficiency in patients with immune check point inhibitors. In this chapter we will discuss the incidence, characteristic findings, diagnosis and management of various endocrinological side effects due to targeted immunotherapies used in various malignancies.

Keywords: cancer immunotherapy, immune check point inhibitors, endocrine side effects, thyroid dysfunction, hypophysitis, primary adrenal insufficiency, Type 1 diabetes mellitus

1. Introduction

Immune system detects and destroys abnormal cells through immune surveillance and as a part of this prevents growth of many impending cancers. Immunotherapies work by either activating or suppressing the immune system and have emerged as important part of how we treat different types of cancers in last few decades [1].

Immune inhibitor pathway plays an important role in maintenance of self-tolerance, and cancer cells evade immune mediated destruction by upregulation of immune inhibitory pathways. Immunotherapy can be used to suppress these immune checkpoints resulting in antitumor activity. Immune check point inhibitors have significantly improved prognosis for patients with various advanced malignancies like melanoma, non-small cell lung carcinoma, Hodgkin lymphoma, urothelial carcinoma, renal cell carcinoma and head and neck cancer. As medical oncology treatments are changing from anatomical sites to molecular sites – immunotherapies have established role in certain molecular patterns as well (i.e. MSI high, TMB high metastatic tumors).

Immunotherapies include wide array of drugs with different mechanisms including monoclonal antibodies, immunomodulators, cytokines, checkpoint

IntechOpen

inhibitors, chimeric antigen receptor T cell therapy, cancer vaccines and oncolytic viruses while many other new approaches are being investigated.

Targeting the immune inhibitory pathways for cancer treatment can lead to immunologic self-tolerance imbalance, resulting in immune-related adverse events (irAEs) which can virtually affect all the organ systems; including eye and brain which are usually unaffected by immune system [2–4]. Different immunotherapies usually affect different organs, as Anti-CTLA-4 mAbs are likely to affect colon and pituitary gland, while anti-PD-1 (L1) mAbs affect thyroid gland.

Among Anti-CTLA-4 mAbs, Ipilimumab has been approved for melanoma, kidney cancer and now NSCLC, and has significantly changed the natural history of advanced tumor. Another immunotherapeutic drug tremelimumab is under development. Common side effects associated with anti-CTAL-4 mAbs include pruritis, diarrhea, rash and fatigue with severe to life-threatening adverse events occurring in less than 5% cases. Anti PD-1 and PD-L1 mABs have similar toxicity profile [5]. Nivolumab, pembrolizumab, and cemiplimab are anti PD-1 mABs, while atezolizumab, avelumab, and durvalumab target PD-L1. In general, anti-PD-1 mAbs are associated with far fewer irAEs than Anti-CTLA-4 mAbs. Common side effects associated with Anti PD-1 (L1) mAbs fatigue, rash, pruritus and idea with severe to life-threatening adverse events occurring in 2–3% of cases. The combination of Anti-CTLA-4 and Anti PD-1 (L-1) antibodies have shown better antitumor results but however they have been associated with higher incidence of immune therapy related adverse event than monotherapy [6, 7].

Usually these irAEs arise within 3–6 months of starting the immunotherapy but it may take few years and thus needs close monitoring for years after completion of therapy. These side effects can be graded from mild to moderate as Grade 1–2 and severe to life threatening as Grade 3–4 [2, 8].

In general, mild Grade 1 side effects usually requires symptom management and does not require immunotherapy discontinuation. Grade 2 or moderate side effects usually managed with temporary discontinuation of checkpoint inhibitor. For severe to life-threatening Grade 3 and 4 side effects immunotherapy is permanently discontinued and these patient usually require high dose of corticosteroids.

Some studies have shown association of irAEs with better antitumor efficacy, the data remains conflicting and needs further research confirm whether occurrence of irAEs predicts better outcome [9–13].

2. Endocrinological adverse effects of immunotherapy

Immunotherapy can cause wide array of endocrine side effects. More common irAEs are hypophysitis leading to hypopituitarism, primary or secondary thyroid dysfunction, primary or secondary adrenal insufficiency, autoimmune diabetes mellitus leading to diabetic ketoacidosis.

3. Pituitary dysfunction

3.1 Incidence

3.1.1 Anti-CTLA-4 mAbs

Hypophysitis is one of the more common immunotherapies induced endocrinopathies and is more common after anti CTLA–4 therapy, reaching around 13% after treatment with ipilimumab [14, 15]. Ipilimumab induced hypophysitis (IH) occurs more frequently in males and in older age when compared to lymphocytic autoimmune hypophysitis even when adjusted for melanoma incidence for age and sex [15–17].

IH is a type II hypersensitivity reaction in which CTLA-4 antibodies bind to antigen expressed on pituitary cells resulting in compliment activation and gland destruction [18, 19]. Some studies have suggested that IH development may be associated with better antitumor outcomes in terms of morbidity and mortality [14]. The data on whether other agents and radiotherapy can alter the risks of hypophysitis is limited.

In the reported studies the average time to IH diagnosis is about 9 weeks; though time to endocrine abnormalities development has not been routinely reported in trials.

The radiographic changes seen on MRI including heterogenous pituitary enlargement with thickening of stalk are the sensitive and specific indicator of hypophysitis and may be the first signs of pituitary dysfunction occurring before hormonal disturbances or development of symptoms [1, 20]. The degree of pituitary enlargement can be mild in the patient's with IH and resolves quickly after glucocorticoids treatment [14].

Most common laboratory abnormalities observed at the time of diagnosis includes central hypothyroidism with reduction of TSH and secondary adrenal insufficiency. Hyponatremia secondary to adrenal insufficiency and hypothyroidism is frequently noted but central diabetes insipidus is rare with IH. Also growth hormone or prolactin axis disturbances occur less compared to other hormonal deficiencies. Usually, other hormonal deficiencies improved with treatment except for adrenal insufficiency which requires lifelong with steroid treatment [14, 21, 22].

3.1.2 Anti-PD-1 and anti PD-L1 mAbs

Multiple studies have shown that incidence of Anti-PD-1 and anti PD-L1 mAbs associated hypophysitis is less compared to Anti-CTLA-4 antibodies. Average incidence of hypophysitis was 0.6% in patients treated with pembrolizumab and novilumab, <0.1% in durvalumab and 0.2% with atezolizumab [23–26].

3.2 Diagnosis and treatment

3.2.1 Monitoring

Patients receiving immunotherapy treatments should have baseline pituitary function test done. Routine thyroid function test monitoring with monthly TSH and free T4 level checks is recommended during the treatment and when patient develops symptoms suggestive of hypophysitis. Those patients who receives anti-CTLA-4 agents routine monitoring of ACTH and cortisol level should be done.

3.2.2 Diagnosis

A clinician must have high index of suspicion for the hypophysitis diagnosis as patient may present with vague symptoms or use of exogenous glucocorticoids may mask their presentation so regular monitoring is critical. When suspected, MRI should be performed to assess pituitary and rule out other causes of pituitary dysfunction along with hormone profile evaluation including TSH and free T4, ACTH, cortisol, LH, FSH, prolactin, estradiol and females and distress return in males. It is recommended to investigate for diabetes insipidus only if patient is presenting with symptoms such as polyuria or polydipsia.

3.2.3 Treatment

High dose glucocorticoids course is given when hypophysitis is suspected which may reverse inflammatory process and prevent the need for longer term hormone replacement in some cases. However, in most patient's long-term hormonal supplementation for affected hormones is required with thyroid hormone replacement for central hypothyroidism or steroid replacement for secondary adrenal insufficiency. In premenopausal female estradiol replacement and in men testosterone placement should be considered.

4. Thyroid dysfunction

Immunotherapy related thyroid dysfunction can range from painless thyroiditis with transient thyrotoxicosis, transient or long-standing hypothyroidism, thyroid associated orbitopathy, and occasionally thyroid storm [27–29].

4.1 Incidence

Thyroid disorder can present with nonspecific symptoms such as fatigue and weakness. It is important to distinguish between primary versus secondary hypothyroidism, as former is more likely with anti-PD-1 and anti-PD-L1 mAbs with incidence ranging from 4–19.5%; and later is more suggestive from hypophysitis induced by anti-CTLA-4 mAbs [30].

For patients treated with nivolumab and pembrolizumab, the incidence rates of hypothyroidism were similar at 6.5% and 7.9% respectively. Incidence rate for hypothyroidism with ipilimumab, nivolumab or pembrolizumab, atezolizumab, and the combination of ipilimumab plus nivolumab were 3.8, 7.0, 3.9, and 13.2 percent, respectively [31].

Primary hyperthyroidism is seen less frequently with immunotherapy with incidence rates for hyperthyroidism with ipilimumab, nivolumab or pembrolizumab, atezolizumab, and the combination of ipilimumab plus nivolumab were 1.7, 3.2, 0.6, and 8 percent, respectively [31].

4.2 Monitoring

Baseline thyroid function test should be obtained before initiation of immunotherapy and after that regular monitoring of thyroid hormone levels including TSH and free T4 is recommended before each treatment and also when symptoms arise.

4.3 Diagnosis

High TSH with low free T4 indicates primary hypothyroidism and a low TSH and low free T4 indicates hypophysitis. In thyroiditis with transient thyrotoxicosis low TSH and high free T4 may be followed by more long-standing hypothyroidism high TSH and low free T4.

4.4 Treatment

While asymptomatic patients with mildly elevated TSH level < 10 can be observed, thyroid hormone replacement remains the mainstay of treatment in hypothyroidism. Dosage adjustment should be done every 4–6 weeks based on TSH level. Patients with thyroiditis and transient thyrotoxicosis can be managed symptomatically with beta blockers. Immunotherapy can be continued except and case of severe thyrotoxicosis when drug might need to be paused until symptoms resolve. Many patients may have subclinical hypothyroidism (TSH >20 mIU/L and normal T4) with symptoms, and in our experience, this should be treated with close monitoring for clinical improvement.

5. Primary adrenal insufficiency

5.1 Incidence

The adrenal insufficiency with immunotherapy is rare [32], there have been case reports which showed the association of immunotherapies and adrenal insufficiency. Data shows that there is a risk of 0.8–1.6% of adrenal insufficiency with ipilimumab either as a monotherapy or combination with anti-PDL 1 therapy. There is a 1% risk of primary adrenal insufficiency with nivolumab and median time of onset is around 4.5 months. Data suggests that there is 0.5% risk of primary adrenal insufficiency with avelumab and 0.4% risk of adrenal insufficiency in patients with atezolizumab.

There have been reports of subclinical form of adrenalitis with immune check point inhibitors, with normal endocrine function but radiographic evidence of inflammation of adrenal glands known as adrenalitis-symmetrically enlarged and smooth adrenal glands [33].

5.2 Characteristic findings

It is very rare to have primary adrenal insufficiency associated with adrenal crisis. Characteristic findings may include weight loss, fatigue, anorexia, nausea, vomiting, abdominal pain, orthostatic hypotension, hypoglycemia, eosinophilia, hyperpigmentation, hyponatremia, hyperkalemia or hypercalcemia.

5.3 Diagnosis

Low or suppressed morning serum cortisol with high ACTH levels will be seen in patients with adrenal insufficiency.

5.4 Treatment

Adrenal crisis is one of the most serious and life-threatening endocrinological side effect of immunotherapy, which requires prompt diagnosis and treatment. If there is high clinical suspicion of adrenal crisis, after obtaining serum cortisol and ACTH levels, treatment should be started without waiting for the results to come back. Patients should be given stress doses of steroids, IV hydrocortisone 100 mg every six to eight hours and aggressive fluid resuscitation should be made as there is high risk of hypovolemic shock. Endocrinologist consult is highly recommended as well.

6. Type 1 diabetes mellitus

6.1 Incidence

Type 1 diabetes mellitus is also a rare a side effect in patients treated with immunotherapy. Type 1 DM has been observed in around 1% of patients treated with nivolumab and in 0.2% of patients treated with pembrolizumab. The median time of onset from starting immunotherapy is around 4.5 months.

6.2 Diagnosis

Type 1 DM is rare but when present, ketoacidosis must be investigated and treated [34]. Anti-GAD65 can be performed to look for autoimmunity.

6.3 Mechanism

The most likely mechanism of developing insulin dependent diabetes mellitus is inappropriate activation of T cells which cause destruction of pancreatic islet cells [35].

6.4 Treatment

Patients with immune mediated type 1 diabetes mellitus should be referred to endocrinology and treated with basal-bolus insulin regimen.

7. Conclusion

With the widespread use of immunotherapies in cancer, the incidence of side effects of immune check point inhibitors is also increasing. Physicians should be aware of different immune related adverse events (irAE).

Hypophysitis and thyroid dysfunction are the most common endocrinological side effects of immune check point inhibitors. Patients who receive anti-CTLA-4 therapy, the pituitary hormones should be regularly monitored and if there is concern for central adrenal or thyroid dysfunction, treatment should be instituted as soon as possible, and immunotherapy should be held.

Primary thyroid dysfunction is more common in patients who receive anti-PD1 and anti-PD-L1 antibodies. Patients may develop hyper or hypothyroidism. Hyperthyroidism is mainly transient, which can lead to hypothyroidism requiring life-long thyroid hormone treatment.

Most of the endocrine side effects of immune check point inhibitors can be adequately treated, clinicians should regularly monitor hormone levels so that it can be promptly diagnosed and treated. In patients with mild to moderate endocrinopathies, immunotherapy can be continued with careful monitoring.

Physicians should be aware that irAEs can occur during and after the treatment with immunotherapies and a multidisciplinary approach should be used in managing it. Patient's education is also very important, and physicians should guide them about the symptoms and signs to look for and notify the physicians.

Author details

Anush Patel[1]*, Haisam Abid[2] and Amrat Kumar[3]

1 Hematology/Oncology, Bassett Medical Center, Cooperstown, NY, USA

2 Internal Medicine, Medical College of Wisconsin, Milwaukee, WI, USA

3 Internal Medicine, Bassett Medical Center, Cooperstown, NY, USA

*Address all correspondence to: anushpatel@gmail.com

References

[1] Horvat, Troy Z., et al. "Immune-related adverse events, need for systemic immunosuppression, and effects on survival and time to treatment failure in patients with melanoma treated with ipilimumab at Memorial Sloan Kettering Cancer Center." Journal of Clinical Oncology 33.28 (2015): 3193.

[2] Michot, J. M., et al. "Immune-related adverse events with immune checkpoint blockade: a comprehensive review." European journal of cancer 54 (2016): 139-148.

[3] Crews, Jonathan, et al. "Ipilimumab-associated retinopathy." Ophthalmic Surgery, Lasers and Imaging Retina 46.6 (2015): 658-660.

[4] Bossart, Simon, et al. "Case report: encephalitis, with brainstem involvement, following checkpoint inhibitor therapy in metastatic melanoma." The Oncologist 22.6 (2017): 749.

[5] Pillai, Rathi Narayana, et al. "Evaluation of toxicity profile of PD-1 versus PD-L1 inhibitors in non-small cell lung cancer (NSCLC)." (2016): 9035-9035.

[6] Hodi, F. Stephen, et al. "Clinical response, progression-free survival (PFS), and safety in patients (pts) with advanced melanoma (MEL) receiving nivolumab (NIVO) combined with ipilimumab (IPI) vs IPI monotherapy in CheckMate 069 study." (2015): 9004-9004.

[7] Larkin, James, et al. "Combined nivolumab and ipilimumab or monotherapy in untreated melanoma." New England journal of medicine 373.1 (2015): 23-34.

[8] Friedman, Claire F., Tracy A. Proverbs-Singh, and Michael A. Postow. "Treatment of the immune-related adverse effects of immune checkpoint inhibitors: a review." JAMA oncology 2.10 (2016): 1346-1353.

[9] Weber, Jeffrey S., et al. "Safety profile of nivolumab monotherapy: a pooled analysis of patients with advanced melanoma." (2017).

[10] Maher, V. Ellen, et al. "Analysis of the association between adverse events and outcome in patients receiving a programmed death protein 1 or programmed death ligand 1 antibody." Journal of Clinical Oncology 37.30 (2019): 2730-2737.

[11] Eggermont, Alexander MM, et al. "Association between immune-related adverse events and recurrence-free survival among patients with stage III melanoma randomized to receive pembrolizumab or placebo: a secondary analysis of a randomized clinical trial." JAMA oncology 6.4 (2020): 519-527.

[12] Lo, Jennifer A., David E. Fisher, and Keith T. Flaherty. "Prognostic significance of cutaneous adverse events associated with pembrolizumab therapy." JAMA oncology 1.9 (2015): 1340-1341.

[13] Teulings, Hansje-Eva, et al. "Vitiligo-like depigmentation in patients with stage III-IV melanoma receiving immunotherapy and its association with survival: a systematic review and meta-analysis." J Clin Oncol 33.7 (2015): 773-781.

[14] Faje, Alexander T., et al. "Ipilimumab-induced hypophysitis: a detailed longitudinal analysis in a large cohort of patients with metastatic melanoma." The Journal of Clinical Endocrinology & Metabolism 99.11 (2014): 4078-4085.

[15] Faje, Alexander. "Immunotherapy and hypophysitis: clinical presentation, treatment, and biologic insights." Pituitary 19.1 (2016): 82-92.

[16] Corsello, Salvatore Maria, et al. "Endocrine side effects induced by immune checkpoint inhibitors." The Journal of Clinical Endocrinology & Metabolism 98.4 (2013): 1361-1375.

[17] Min, Le, et al. "Systemic high-dose corticosteroid treatment does not improve the outcome of ipilimumab-related hypophysitis: a retrospective cohort study." Clinical Cancer Research 21.4 (2015): 749-755.

[18] Laurent, Stefania, et al. "The engagement of CTLA-4 on primary melanoma cell lines induces antibody-dependent cellular cytotoxicity and TNF-α production." Journal of translational medicine 11.1 (2013): 108.

[19] Iwama, Shintaro, et al. "Pituitary expression of CTLA-4 mediates hypophysitis secondary to administration of CTLA-4 blocking antibody." Science translational medicine 6.230 (2014): 230ra45-230ra45.

[20] Van der Hiel, Bernies, et al. "Detection of early onset of hypophysitis by (18) F-FDG PET-CT in a patient with advanced stage melanoma treated with ipilimumab." Clinical nuclear medicine 38.4 (2013): e182-4.

[21] Blansfield, Joseph A., et al. "Cytotoxic T-lymphocyte–associated antigen-4 blockage can induce autoimmune hypophysitis in patients with metastatic melanoma and renal cancer." Journal of immunotherapy (Hagerstown, Md.: 1997) 28.6 (2005): 593.

[22] Albarel, Frédérique, et al. "Long-term follow-up of ipilimumab-induced hypophysitis, a common adverse event of the anti-CTLA-4 antibody in melanoma." European Journal of Endocrinology 172.2 (2015): 195-204.

[23] Weber, Jeffrey S., et al. "Nivolumab versus chemotherapy in patients with advanced melanoma who progressed after anti-CTLA-4 treatment (CheckMate 037): a randomised, controlled, open-label, phase 3 trial." The lancet oncology 16.4 (2015): 375-384.

[24] Ribas, Antoni, et al. "Association of pembrolizumab with tumor response and survival among patients with advanced melanoma." Jama 315.15 (2016): 1600-1609.

[25] Rizvi, Naiyer A., et al. "Safety and clinical activity of MEDI4736, an anti-programmed cell death-ligand 1 (PD-L1) antibody, in patients with non-small cell lung cancer (NSCLC)." (2015): 8032-8032.

[26] Rosenberg, Jonathan E., et al. "Atezolizumab in patients with locally advanced and metastatic urothelial carcinoma who have progressed following treatment with platinum-based chemotherapy: a single-arm, multicentre, phase 2 trial." The Lancet 387.10031 (2016): 1909-1920.

[27] Borodic, Gary, David M. Hinkle, and Yihong Cia. "Drug-induced graves disease from CTLA-4 receptor suppression." Ophthalmic Plastic & Reconstructive Surgery 27.4 (2011): e87-e88.

[28] Hamnvik, Ole-Petter Riksfjord, P. Reed Larsen, and Ellen Marqusee. "Thyroid dysfunction from antineoplastic agents." Journal of the National Cancer Institute 103.21 (2011): 1572-1587.

[29] Orlov, Steven, et al. "Induction of painless thyroiditis in patients receiving programmed death 1 receptor immunotherapy for metastatic malignancies." The Journal of Clinical Endocrinology & Metabolism 100.5 (2015): 1738-1741.

[30] Cukier, Priscilla, et al. "Endocrine side effects of cancer immunotherapy."

Endocrine-related cancer 24.12 (2017): T331-T347.

[31] Barroso-Sousa, Romualdo, et al. "Incidence of endocrine dysfunction following the use of different immune checkpoint inhibitor regimens: a systematic review and meta-analysis." JAMA oncology 4.2 (2018): 173-182.

[32] Brahmer, Julie, et al. "Nivolumab versus docetaxel in advanced squamous-cell non–small-cell lung cancer." New England Journal of Medicine 373.2 (2015): 123-135.

[33] Bacanovic, Sara, et al. "Ipilimumab-induced adrenalitis: a possible pitfall in 18F-FDG-PET/CT." Clinical nuclear medicine 40.11 (2015): e518-e519.

[34] Kitabchi, Abbas E., et al. "Hyperglycemic crises in adult patients with diabetes." Diabetes care 32.7 (2009): 1335-1343.

[35] Abid, Haisam, Kanramon Watthanasuntorn, and Rosana Gnanajothy. "SUN-LB036 Diabetic Ketoacidosis: A Rare Side Effect of Nivolumab Induced Insulin Dependent Diabetes Mellitus." Journal of the Endocrine Society 3.Supplement_1 (2019): SUN-LB036.

Chapter 4

Immunotherapy in Malignant Pleural Mesothelioma

Asako Matsuda and Nobukazu Fujimoto

Abstract

Malignant pleural mesothelioma (MPM) is an extremely aggressive plural malignancy mainly caused by asbestos exposure. Basic research about the immune suppressive tumor microenvironment in MPM has suggested that MPM might be a good candidate for immune therapy. Immunocheckpoint inhibitors have shown some promising results. A phase Ib trial with pembrolizumab, an antibody specific for the programmed cell death 1 protein (anti-PD-1), showed efficacy in patients with programmed death-ligand 1 (PD-L1)-positive MPM. Among 25 patients tested, 5 patients (20%) achieved a partial response. A Japanese group evaluated the efficacy and safety of nivolumab, an anti-PD-L1 antibody, for patients with advanced MPM in a phase II study. Ten (29%) patients showed an objective response. Based on those results, nivolumab was approved in Japan for unresectable recurrent MPM. A phase III randomized study was conducted to compare nivolumab plus ipilimumab to platinum doublet chemotherapy as a first-line therapy in unresectable MPM. The primary endpoint, overall survival (OS), was significantly improved in the nivolumab plus ipilimumab group. Cellular therapies and cancer vaccines are limited by many challenges; therefore, improvements to overcome these difficulties are urgently warranted. Further research is needed, including large-scale clinical trials, to clarify the utility and safety of immunotherapy in MPM.

Keywords: asbestos, ipilimumab, nivolumab, mesothelioma, pembrolizumab

1. Introduction

Malignant pleural mesothelioma (MPM) is an extremely aggressive plural malignancy, which is mainly caused by asbestos exposure [1]. The benefit of surgical resection is controversial, because only a minority of patients with MPM meets the criteria for surgery, and it is unrealistic to assume that surgery will achieve a complete tumor resection without a micro residual tumor. Systemic chemotherapy with platinum plus pemetrexed is the recommended first-line systemic therapy for advanced MPM. However, the median overall survival (OS) is only approximately 12 months [2]. For patients that fail first-line chemotherapy, a standard second-line chemotherapy has not been defined [3]. Hence, it is critically essential to develop a new treatment option.

Recently, immunocheckpoint inhibitors (ICIs) have achieved great success in treating several cancer types [4–7]. Basic research about the immune-suppressive tumor microenvironment in MPM has suggested that MPM might be a good candidate for immune therapy [8, 9]. CD8+ tumor-infiltrating lymphocytes were reported to predict a favorable prognosis after a resection of MPM [10]. In fact, recently, ICIs have shown promising results for patients with MPM.

In this chapter, we summarize recent studies on immunotherapy for MPM.

2. Anti-cytotoxic T-lymphocyte antigen 4 antibody

Anti-cytotoxic T-lymphoctye antigen 4 (CTLA-4) antibody was the first reported ICI for treating MPM. To date, three clinical trials have tested anti CTLA 4 antibody monotherapy for MPM.

In the first phase II trial (MESOT-TREM-2008), the anti-CTLA-4 monoclonal antibody, tremelimumab (15 mg/kg) was administered intravenously once every 90 days to patients with MPM [11]. Twenty-nine patients with MPM that had failed a first-line platinum-based regimen were enrolled. Of these, no patients achieved a complete response, 2 patients achieved a partial response, and 7 others achieved durable disease control. The median progression-free survival (PFS) was 6.2 months, and the median OS was 10.7 months. The second phase II trial (MESOT-TREM-2012), enrolled 29 patients with MPM that were treated with 10 mg/kg tremelimumab, initially every 4 weeks for 6 doses, then every 12 weeks [12]. The disease control rate was slightly improved after this regimen modification; one patient achieved a partial response, and 11 patients achieved disease control.

Based on these two trials, a large scale, randomized trial (DETERMINE) was conducted [13] with 571 patients with MPM. Of these, 382 patients were assigned to tremelimumab and 189 patients were assigned to placebo. However, there was no significant difference in PFS or OS between these two groups. After the DETERMINE trial, anti-CTLA-4 antibodies were investigated only in combination with an anti-programmed cell death protein 1 (anti-PD-1) antibody or anti-programmed death ligand 1 (PD-L1) antibody.

3. Anti-PD-L1 antibody

Mansfield et al. reported that PD-L1 was expressed in approximately 42 of 106 MPM specimens, and that PD-L1 expression was significantly correlated with poor survival (OS: 5 months in a PD-L1-positive group vs. 14.5 months in a PD-L1-negative group) [14]. Cedrés et al. also reported that PD-L1 expression was a negative prognostic factor in patients with MPM [15]. These results supported the notion that PD-L1 might serve as a potential target for immunotherapy in MPM.

Avelumab is a human IgG1 monoclonal antibody that binds to PD-L1 [16]. Hassan et al. described a phase I trial (JAVELIN Solid Tumor) that enrolled 53 patients with unresectable MPM. Those patients had failed first-line chemotherapy with platinum and pemetrexed. When they were treated with avelumab, the objective response rate was 9% (one complete response and four partial responses) [17]. Responses were durable (median, 15.2 months), and they were observed both in patients with PD-L1-positive tumors (objective response rate [ORR]: 19%) and in those with PD-L1-negative tumors (ORR: 7%). The median PFS was 4.1 months, and median OS was 10.7 months.

Another anti-PD-L1 antibody, durvalumab, was recently evaluated for efficacy in 54 patients with MPM that were not treated previously. Durvalumab was combined with cisplatin and pemetrexed as a first-line chemotherapy (DREAM trial) [18]. The ORR was 48%, and, 31/54 (57%) patients were progression-free at 6 months. Based on the phase II trial results, a phase III trial is currently planned.

4. Anti-PD-1 antibody

4.1 Pembrolizumab

Pembrolizumab is an antibody against PD-1. Pembrolizumab was tested for efficacy in 25 patients with PD-L1-positive MPM in a non-randomized, phase Ib trial [19]. Five patients (20%) achieved a partial response, and 72% of patients achieved disease control. The median OS was 18 months.

A phase II trial of pembrolizumab monotherapy was conducted in 65 patients with MPM that had been treated previously [20]. Among those patients, 19% achieved a partial response to pembrolizumab. The median PFS and OS were 4.5 and 11.5 months, respectively.

Based on these two trials, pembrolizumab was administered, off-label, to 93 patients with MPM in Switzerland and Australia [21]. The ORR was 18%, and the median PFS and OS were 3.1 months and 7.2 months, respectively. Patients with high PD-L1 expression showed improved ORR (44%) and PFS (6.2 months). Recently, a retrospective study from Australia analyzed data from patients with MPM that received pembrolizumab as the first-, second-, or subsequent-line treatment. They found an ORR of 18%, and a disease control rate of 56%. The median PFS was 4.8 months, and the median OS was 9.5 months [22].

4.2 Nivolumab

Nivolumab is a fully humanized monoclonal anti-PD-1 antibody. It was first tested in 34 patients with recurrent MPM in the Netherlands [23]. In that single-center trial, patients with MPM received 3 mg/kg intravenous nivolumab every 2 weeks. Among 34 patients, 8 patients (24%) achieved a partial response, and another 8 patients (24%) displayed stable disease at 12 weeks.

A Japanese group also evaluated the efficacy and safety of nivolumab in 34 patients with advanced MPM. That study tested nivolumab as a salvage therapy in a single-arm phase II study (MERIT study) [24]. Patients received 240 mg nivolumab intravenously every 2 weeks. Ten (29%) patients showed an objective response. The median duration of the response was 11.1 months, and the disease control rate was 68%. The median PFS and OS were 6.1 and 17.3 months, respectively. Among patients with PD-L1-positive tumors ($\geq$1% expression), the ORR was 40%. Based on those results, nivolumab was approved in Japan for unresectable recurrent MPM.

5. Combination therapy with ICIs

Based on the favorable results obtained with ICI monotherapy, recent investigations tested combination treatments, with an anti-PD-1 or anti-PD-L1 antibody combined with an anti-CTLA-4 antibody. This combination was expected to maximize T-cell activation.

NIBIT-MESO-1 was open-label, non-randomized, phase II trial, in which 40 patients with MPM received at least one dose each of tremelimumab and durvalumab [25]. Eleven patients (28%) displayed an objective response. The median PFS was 5.7 months and the median OS was 16.6 months.

IFCT-1501 MAPS2 was a multicenter, open-label, randomized, phase II trial, in which 108 patients with MPM were randomly assigned to receive intravenous nivolumab or intravenous nivolumab plus ipilimumab. In the intention-to-treat population, 12-week disease control (primary endpoint) was achieved by 25/63

Agent	Year	N	ORR (%)	mPFS (mo)	mOS (mo)	Study type	Reference
Anti-CTLA4							
Tremelimumab	2013	29	7	6.2	10.7	2	Calabro et al. [11]
Tremelimumab	2015	20	3	6.2	11.3	2	Calabro et al. [12]
Tremelimumab	2017	571	5	2.8	7.7	2b	Maio et al. [13]
Anti-PD-L1							
Avelumab	2019	53	9	4.1	10.7	1b	Hassen et al. [17]
Anti-PD-1							
Pembrolizumab	2017	25	20	5.4	18	1b	Alley et al. [19]
Pembrolizumab	2018	65	19	4.5	11.5	2	Desai et al. [20]
Nivolumab	2018	34	24	2.6	11.8	2	Quispel-Janssen et al. [23]
Nivolumab	2018	34	29	6.1	17.3	2	Okada et al. [24]
Combination therapy							
Tremelimumab/Durvalumab	2018	40	28	5.7	16.6	2	Calabro et al. [25]
Nivolumab/Ipilimumab	2019	62	28	5.6	15.9	2	Scherpereel et al. [26]
Nivolumab		63	19	4	11.9		
Nivolumab/Ipilimumab	2019	34	29	6.2	NR	2	Disselhorst et al. [27]
Nivolumab/Ipilimumab	2020	303	40	6.8	18.1	3	Baas et al. [28]

ORR: objective response rate; mPFS: median progression free survival; mo: months; mOS: median overall survival; CTLA: cytotoxic T-lymphocyte antigen; PD-L1: programmed death ligand 1; PD-1: programmed cell death protein 1.

Table 1.
Overview of clinical trials that tested immunocheckpoint inhibitors for malignant pleural mesothelioma.

(40%) patients in the nivolumab group and 32/62 (52%) patients in the combination group [26]. The INITIATE study also evaluated the efficacy of nivolumab combined with ipilimumab in patients with MPM. In that study, among 34 patients included in the efficacy assessment, ten (29%) patients achieved a partial response, and 23 patients (68%) achieved 12 weeks of disease control [27]. Based on these favorable results, a phase III randomized study was conducted to compare nivolumab plus ipilimumab to platinum doublet chemotherapy as a first-line therapy in unresectable MPM. In that study, 303 patients were randomized to nivolumab plus ipilimumab and 302 patients were randomized to platinum doublet chemotherapy. With a minimum follow-up of 22 months, the primary endpoint, OS, was significantly improved with nivolumab plus ipilimumab compared to chemotherapy (median, 18.1 vs. 14.1 months; hazard ratio, 0.74; 95% confidence interval, 0.61–0.89; P = 0.002) [28].

Overview of clinical trials of that tested ICIs for MPM was summarized in **Table 1**.

6. Vaccine

Cancer vaccines have been tested for various cancer types. These vaccines have included tumor lysate, attenuated bacteria, and single or multiple peptides. Wilms tumor 1 (WT-1) is one of the most well investigated cancer antigens. WT-1 was expressed in tumors in 97% of patients with MPM [29]. Galinpepimut-S, a multivalent vaccine against the WT 1 peptide, can activate both CD4+ and CD8+ T-cells [30]. The efficacy and safety of galinpepimut-S was investigated in a phase II trial. The pilot study demonstrated that the median PFS was 7.4 months in the placebo group and 10.1 months in the vaccine group. The median OS was 18.3 months in the placebo group and 22.8 months in the vaccine group. Based on th0se findings, a clinical trial is currently ongoing to investigate a combination treatment of galinpepimut-S plus nivolumab in patients with MPM (with WT-1-positive tumors). Combining cancer vaccines with ICIs might improve the clinical outcome and open a new avenue of therapeutic strategies for MPM.

7. Dendritic cell therapy

Vaccination strategies have been developed that involve dendritic cells (DCs), which are antigen-presenting cells for T-cell activation. The DCs are pulsed with tumor lysate to overcome the shortcomings of autologous DCs. These strategies have shown remarkable anti-tumor activity, with low toxicity, in several cancer types. In the area of MPM, 9 patients received three vaccinations of autologous mature DCs loaded with autologous tumor cell lysate [31]. Among these patients, 3 showed a partial response in the first 8 weeks after the DC vaccination. However, two of those three patients had received chemotherapy before the DC vaccination, which might have influenced the anti-tumor effect. In the next step of treatment, they added cyclophosphamide to increase the anti-tumor activity by inhibiting regulatory T cells [32]. Ten patients with MPM received cyclophosphamide and a vaccination of autologous mature DCs loaded with autologous tumor cell lysate. Of those ten patients, seven lived longer than 24 months, and the mean OS was 37 months.

Obtaining autologous tumor cell lysate is time consuming, because patients have to undergo multiple tumor biopsies. In one study, allogeneic tumor lysate obtained from a tumor cell line was applied to autologous DCs [33]. Nine patients with MPM were treated with DC vaccinations (autologous DCs pulsed with tumor lysate from five mesothelioma cell lines). Of these, two patients experienced a partial response and all nine patients established disease control. The median OS was longer than 22.8 months. Based on those promising results, an ongoing phase II/III study is currently testing DCs loaded with allogeneic tumor cell lysate as a maintenance therapy after chemotherapy (DENIM trial) [34].

8. Chimeric antigen receptor T-cell therapy

Chimeric antigen receptor (CAR) T-cells can be used to target specific tumor antigens directly. CAR T-cell therapy has shown clinical efficacy for hematological malignancies, and it was approved by the United States Food and Drug Administration for B cell acute leukemia and diffuse large B-cell lymphoma. Several clinical trials are ongoing to test CAR T-cell therapy on both hematological malignancies and solid tumors [35]. CAR T-cells that targeted WT-1, fibroblast activation protein (FAP), or mesothelin (MSLN) were tested in a clinical trial on MPM. Hass et al. reported the results of a clinical trial for testing CAR T-cells that targeted MSLN on 15 patients with MPM. The CAR T-cells were applied as a monotherapy or in combination with low-dose cyclophosphamide, for solid tumors [36]. The best overall response was stable disease (11 of 15 patients). Currently, several phase I trials are ongoing to examine the efficacy of CAR T-cell therapy in solid tumors, including MPM.

9. Conclusion

The prognosis of MPM remains poor. A PD-1/PD-L1 blockade is an effective treatment option for MPM. The combination of nivolumab (anti-PD-1 antibody) and ipilimumab (anti-CTLA-4 antibody) could be a standard first-line treatment. Additionally, the combination of an ICI with conventional chemotherapy might be a promising treatment option. Cellular therapies and cancer vaccines must overcome many challenges, such as T-cell migration to the tumor and infiltration into the tumor. Improvements in cancer therapies are urgently needed to overcome these difficulties. Further research with large-scale clinical trials are needed to clarify the utility and safety of these immunotherapies in MPM. In addition, in this new era of precision medicine, we need to develop biomarkers to identify which patients would benefit from ICI-ICI combinations, ICI plus chemotherapy, or cellular therapy.

Acknowledgements

This study was supported by grants-in-aid from the Ministry of Health, Labor, and Welfare, Japan.

Conflict of interest

Dr. Fujimoto received consultancy fees from Boehringer Ingelheim, Ono, Bristol-Myers Squibb, Kyorin, and Kissei. Dr. Fujimoto also received honoraria or research funding from Hisamitsu, Chugai, Ono, Taiho, Boehringer Ingelheim, Bristol-Myers Squibb, Novartis, GlaxoSmithKline, and MSD.

Author details

Asako Matsuda and Nobukazu Fujimoto*
Department of Medical Oncology, Okayama Rosai Hospital, Okayama, Japan

*Address all correspondence to: nobufujimot@gmail.com

References

[1] Carbone M, Adusumilli PS, Alexander HR, Jr., Baas P, Bardelli F, Bononi A, Bueno R, Felley-Bosco E, Galateau-Salle F, Jablons D, Mansfield AS, Minaai M, de Perrot M, Pesavento P, Rusch V, Severson DT, Taioli E, Tsao A, Woodard G, Yang H, Zauderer MG, Pass HI. Mesothelioma: Scientific clues for prevention, diagnosis, and therapy. CA Cancer J Clin. 2019;69:402-429. doi: 10.3322/caac.21572.

[2] Vogelzang NJ, Rusthoven JJ, Symanowski J, Denham C, Kaukel E, Ruffie P, Gatzemeier U, Boyer M, Emri S, Manegold C, Niyikiza C, Paoletti P. Phase III study of pemetrexed in combination with cisplatin versus cisplatin alone in patients with malignant pleural mesothelioma. J Clin Oncol. 2003;21:2636-2644. DOI: 10.1016/S1525-7304(11)70322-9.

[3] Buikhuisen WA, Hiddinga BI, Baas P, van Meerbeeck JP. Second line therapy in malignant pleural mesothelioma: A systematic review. Lung Cancer. 2015;89:223-231. doi: 10.1016/j.lungcan.2015.06.018.

[4] Ferris RL, Blumenschein G, Jr., Fayette J, Guigay J, Colevas AD, Licitra L, Harrington K, Kasper S, Vokes EE, Even C, Worden F, Saba NF, Iglesias Docampo LC, Haddad R, Rordorf T, Kiyota N, Tahara M, Monga M, Lynch M, Geese WJ, Kopit J, Shaw JW, Gillison ML. Nivolumab for Recurrent Squamous-Cell Carcinoma of the Head and Neck. N Engl J Med. 2016;375:1856-1867. DOI: 10.1016/S1470-2045(17)30421-7.

[5] Jelinek T, Mihalyova J, Kascak M, Duras J, Hajek R. PD-1/PD-L1 inhibitors in haematological malignancies: update 2017. Immunology. 2017;152:357-371. doi: 10.1111/imm.12788.

[6] Le DT, Durham JN, Smith KN, Wang H, Bartlett BR, Aulakh LK, Lu S, Kemberling H, Wilt C, Luber BS, Wong F, Azad NS, Rucki AA, Laheru D, Donehower R, Zaheer A, Fisher GA, Crocenzi TS, Lee JJ, Greten TF, Duffy AG, Ciombor KK, Eyring AD, Lam BH, Joe A, Kang SP, Holdhoff M, Danilova L, Cope L, Meyer C, Zhou S, Goldberg RM, Armstrong DK, Bever KM, Fader AN, Taube J, Housseau F, Spetzler D, Xiao N, Pardoll DM, Papadopoulos N, Kinzler KW, Eshleman JR, Vogelstein B, Anders RA, Diaz LA Jr. Mismatch repair deficiency predicts response of solid tumors to PD-1 blockade. Science. 2017;357:409-413. DOI: 10.1126/science.aan6733.

[7] Topalian SL, Hodi FS, Brahmer JR, Gettinger SN, Smith DC, McDermott DF, Powderly JD, Carvajal RD, Sosman JA, Atkins MB, Leming PD, Spigel DR, Antonia SJ, Horn L, Drake CG, Pardoll DM, Chen L, Sharfman WH, Anders RA, Taube JM, McMiller TL, Xu H, Korman AJ, Jure-Kunkel M, Agrawal S, McDonald D, Kollia GD, Gupta A, Wigginton JM, Sznol M. Safety, activity, and immune correlates of anti-PD-1 antibody in cancer. N Engl J Med. 2012;366:2443-2454. DOI: 10.1056/NEJMoa1200694.

[8] Hegmans JP, Hemmes A, Hammad H, Boon L, Hoogsteden HC, Lambrecht BN. Mesothelioma environment comprises cytokines and T-regulatory cells that suppress immune responses. Eur Respir J. 2006;27:1086-1095. DOI: 10.1183/09031936.06.00135305

[9] Bograd AJ, Suzuki K, Vertes E, Colovos C, Morales EA, Sadelain M, Adusumilli PS. Immune responses and immunotherapeutic interventions in malignant pleural mesothelioma. Cancer Immunol Immunother. 2011;60:1509-1527. DOI: 10.1007/s00262-011-1103-6

[10] Yamada N, Oizumi S, Kikuchi E, Shinagawa N, Konishi-Sakakibara J, Ishimine A, Aoe K, Gemba K,

Kishimoto T, Torigoe T, Nishimura M. CD8+ tumor-infiltrating lymphocytes predict favorable prognosis in malignant pleural mesothelioma after resection. Cancer Immunol Immunother. 2010;59:1543-1549. DOI: 10.1007/s00262-010-0881-6.

[11] Calabrò L, Morra A, Fonsatti E, Cutaia O, Amato G, Giannarelli D, Di Giacomo AM, Danielli R, Altomonte M, Mutti L, Maio M. Tremelimumab for patients with chemotherapy-resistant advanced malignant mesothelioma: an open-label, single-arm, phase 2 trial. Lancet Oncol. 2013;14:1104-1111. DOI: 10.1016/S1470-2045(13)70381-4.

[12] Calabro L, Morra A, Fonsatti E, Cutaia O, Fazio C, Annesi D, Lenoci M, Amato G, Danielli R, Altomonte M, Giannarelli D, Di Giacomo AM, Maio M. Efficacy and safety of an intensified schedule of tremelimumab for chemotherapy-resistant malignant mesothelioma: an open-label, single-arm, phase 2 study. The Lancet Respir Med. 2015;3:301-309. DOI: 10.1016/S2213-2600(15)00092-2.

[13] Maio M, Scherpereel A, Calabrò L, Aerts J, Perez SC, Bearz A, Nackaerts K, Fennell DA, Kowalski D, Tsao AS, Taylor P, Grosso F, Antonia SJ, Nowak AK, Taboada M, Puglisi M, Stockman PK, Kindler HL. Tremelimumab as second-line or third-line treatment in relapsed malignant mesothelioma (DETERMINE): a multicentre, international, randomised, double-blind, placebo-controlled phase 2b trial. Lancet Oncol. 2017;18:1261-1273. DOI: 10.1016/S1470-2045(17)30446-1.

[14] Mansfield AS, Roden AC, Peikert T, Sheinin YM, Harrington SM, Krco CJ, Dong H, Kwon ED. B7-H1 expression in malignant pleural mesothelioma is associated with sarcomatoid histology and poor prognosis. J Thorac Oncol. 2014;9:1036-1040. DOI: 10.1097/JTO.0000000000000177.

[15] Cedrés S, Ponce-Aix S, Zugazagoitia J, Sansano I, Enguita A, Navarro-Mendivil A, Martinez-Marti A, Martinez P, Felip E. Analysis of expression of programmed cell death 1 ligand 1 (PD-L1) in malignant pleural mesothelioma (MPM). PLoS One. 2015;10:e0121071. DOI: 10.1371/journal.pone.0121071.

[16] Heery CR, O'Sullivan-Coyne G, Madan RA, Cordes L, Rajan A, Rauckhorst M, Lamping E, Oyelakin I, Marte JL, Lepone LM, Donahue RN, Grenga I, Cuillerot JM, Neuteboom B, Heydebreck AV, Chin K, Schlom J, Gulley JL. Avelumab for metastatic or locally advanced previously treated solid tumours (JAVELIN Solid Tumor): a phase 1a, multicohort, dose-escalation trial. Lancet Oncol. 2017;18:587-598. DOI: 10.1016/S1470-2045(17)30239-5.

[17] Hassan R, Thomas A, Nemunaitis JJ, Patel MR, Bennouna J, Chen FL, Delord JP, Dowlati A, Kochuparambil ST, Taylor MH, Powderly JD, Vaishampayan UN, Verschraegen C, Grote HJ, von Heydebreck A, Chin K, Gulley JL. Efficacy and safety of avelumab treatment in patients with advanced unresectable mesothelioma: Phase 1b results from the JAVELIN Solid Tumor Trial. JAMA Oncol. 2019;5:351-357. DOI: 10.1001/jamaoncol.2018.5428.

[18] Nowak AK, Lesterhuis WJ, Kok PS, Brown C, Hughes BG, Karikios DJ, John T, Kao SC, Leslie C, Cook AM, Pavlakis N, Briscoe K, O'Byrne KJ, Karapetis CS, Lam WS, Langford A, Yip S, Stockler MR. Durvalumab with first-line chemotherapy in previously untreated malignant pleural mesothelioma (DREAM): a multicentre, single-arm, phase 2 trial with a safety run-in. The Lancet Oncology. 2020;21:1213-1223. DOI: 10.1016/S1470-2045(20)30462-9.

[19] Alley EW, Lopez J, Santoro A, Morosky A, Saraf S, Piperdi B, van

Brummelen E. Clinical safety and activity of pembrolizumab in patients with malignant pleural mesothelioma (KEYNOTE-028): preliminary results from a non-randomised, open-label, phase 1b trial. Lancet Oncol. 2017;18:623-630. DOI: 10.1016/S1470-2045(17)30169-9.

[20] Desai A KT, Rose B, Tan Y, Hill B, Pemberton E, Straus C, Seiwert T, Kindler HL. Phase II trial of pembrolizumab (NCT02399371) in previously-treated malignant mesothelioma: Final analysis. J Thorac Oncol. 2018;13:S339. DOI:https://doi.org/10.1016/j.jtho.2018.08.277

[21] Metaxas Y, Rivalland G, Mauti LA, Klingbiel D, Kao S, Schmid S, Nowak AK, Gautschi O, Bartnick T, Hughes BG, Bouchaab H, Rothschild SI, Pavlakis N, Wolleb S, Petrausch U, O'Byrne K, Froesch P, Loffler-Baumann M, Pratsch-Peter S, Russell P, Mingrone W, Savic S, Thapa B, Fruh M, Pless M, von Moos R, John T. Pembrolizumab as Palliative Immunotherapy in Malignant Pleural Mesothelioma. J Thorac Oncol. 2018;13:1784-1791. DOI: 10.1016/j.jtho.2018.08.007

[22] Ahmadzada T, Cooper WA, Holmes M, Mahar A, Westman H, Gill AJ, Nordman I, Yip PY, Pal A, Zielinski R, Pavlakis HN, Nagrial A, Daneshvar D, Brungs D, Karikios D, Aleksova V, Burn J, Asher R, Grau GE, Hosseini-Beheshti E, Reid G, Clarke S, Kao S. Retrospective Evaluation of the Use of Pembrolizumab in Malignant Mesothelioma in a Real-World Australian Population. J Thorac Oncol Clin Res Rep. 2020;1(4):100075. DOI:https://doi.org/10.1016/j.jtocrr.2020.100075

[23] Quispel-Janssen J, van der Noort V, de Vries JF, Zimmerman M, Lalezari F, Thunnissen E, Monkhorst K, Schouten R, Schunselaar L, Disselhorst M, Klomp H, Hartemink K, Burgers S, Buikhuisen W, Baas P. Programmed Death 1 Blockade With Nivolumab in Patients With Recurrent Malignant Pleural Mesothelioma. J Thorac Oncol. 2018;13:1569-1576. DOI: 10.1016/j.jtho.2018.05.038

[24] Okada M, Kijima T, Aoe K, Kato T, Fujimoto N, Nakagawa K, Takeda Y, Hida T, Kanai K, Imamura F, Oizumi S, Takahashi T, Takenoyama M, Tanaka H, Hirano J, Namba Y, Ohe Y. Clinical Efficacy and Safety of Nivolumab: Results of a Multicenter, Open-label, Single-arm, Japanese Phase II study in Malignant Pleural Mesothelioma (MERIT). Clin Can Res. 2019;25:5485-5492. DOI:10.1158/1078-0432.CCR-19-0103

[25] Calabrò L, Morra A, Giannarelli D, Amato G, D'Incecco A, Covre A, Lewis A, Rebelatto MC, Danielli R, Altomonte M, Di Giacomo AM, Maio M. Tremelimumab combined with durvalumab in patients with mesothelioma (NIBIT-MESO-1): an open-label, non-randomised, phase 2 study. Lancet Respir Med. 2018;6:451-460. DOI: 10.1016/S2213-2600(18)30151-6

[26] Scherpereel A, Mazieres J, Greillier L, Lantuejoul S, Dô P, Bylicki O, Monnet I, Corre R, Audigier-Valette C, Locatelli-Sanchez M, Molinier O, Guisier F, Urban T, Ligeza-Poisson C, Planchard D, Amour E, Morin F, Moro-Sibilot D, Zalcman G. Nivolumab or nivolumab plus ipilimumab in patients with relapsed malignant pleural mesothelioma (IFCT-1501 MAPS2): a multicentre, open-label, randomised, non-comparative, phase 2 trial. Lancet Oncol. 2019;20:239-253. DOI:10.1016/S1470-2045(18)30765-4

[27] Disselhorst MJ, Quispel-Janssen J, Lalezari F, Monkhorst K, de Vries JF, van der Noort V, Harms E, Burgers S, Baas P. Ipilimumab and nivolumab in the treatment of recurrent malignant pleural mesothelioma (INITIATE):

results of a prospective, single-arm, phase 2 trial. Lancet Respir Med. 2019;7:260-270. DOI: 10.1016/S2213-2600(18)30420-X

[28] Baas P, Scherpereel A, Nowak AK, Fujimoto N, Peters S, Tsao A, Mansfield A, Popat S, Jahan T, Antonia S, Oulkhouir Y, Bautista Y, Cornelissen R, Greillier L, Grossi F, Kowalski DM, Rodriguez-Cid J, Aanur P, Baudelet C, Zalcman G. First-line nivolumab + ipilimumab vs chemotherapy in unresectable malignant pleural mesothelioma: CheckMate 743. J Thorac Oncol. 2020;15(10 suppl):e42. DOI:https://doi.org/10.1016/j.jtho.2020.08.004

[29] Eguchi T, Kadota K, Mayor M, Zauderer MG, Rimner A, Rusch VW, Travis WD, Sadelain M, Adusumilli PS. Cancer antigen profiling for malignant pleural mesothelioma immunotherapy: expression and coexpression of mesothelin, cancer antigen 125, and Wilms tumor 1. Oncotarget. 2017;8:77872-77882. DOI: 10.18632/oncotarget.20845

[30] Zauderer MG, Tsao AS, Dao T, Panageas K, Lai WV, Rimner A, Rusch VW, Adusumilli PS, Ginsberg MS, Gomez D, Rice D, Mehran R, Scheinberg DA, Krug LM. A Randomized Phase II Trial of Adjuvant Galinpepimut-S, WT-1 Analogue Peptide Vaccine, After Multimodality Therapy for Patients with Malignant Pleural Mesothelioma. Clin Cancer Res. 2017;23:7483-7489. DOI: 10.1158/1078-0432.CCR-17-2169

[31] Hegmans JP, Veltman JD, Lambers ME, de Vries IJ, Figdor CG, Hendriks RW, Hoogsteden HC, Lambrecht BN, Aerts JG. Consolidative dendritic cell-based immunotherapy elicits cytotoxicity against malignant mesothelioma. Am J Respir Crit Care Med. 2010;181:1383-1390. DOI:10.1164/rccm.200909-1465OC eng.

[32] Cornelissen R, Hegmans JP, Maat AP, Kaijen-Lambers ME, Bezemer K, Hendriks RW, Hoogsteden HC, Aerts JG. Extended Tumor Control after Dendritic Cell Vaccination with Low-Dose Cyclophosphamide as Adjuvant Treatment in Patients with Malignant Pleural Mesothelioma. Am J Respir Crit Care Med. 2016;193:1023-1031. DOI: 10.1164/rccm.201508-1573OC

[33] Aerts J, de Goeje PL, Cornelissen R, Kaijen-Lambers MEH, Bezemer K, van der Leest CH, Mahaweni NM, Kunert A, Eskens F, Waasdorp C, Braakman E, van der Holt B, Vulto AG, Hendriks RW, Hegmans J, Hoogsteden HC. Autologous Dendritic Cells Pulsed with Allogeneic Tumor Cell Lysate in Mesothelioma: From Mouse to Human. Clin Cancer Res. 2018;24:766-776. DOI: 10.1158/1078-0432.CCR-17-2522

[34] Belderbos RA, Baas P, Berardi R, Cornelissen R, Fennell DA, van Meerbeeck JP, Scherpereel A, Vroman H, Aerts J. A multicenter, randomized, phase II/III study of dendritic cells loaded with allogeneic tumor cell lysate (MesoPher) in subjects with mesothelioma as maintenance therapy after chemotherapy: DENdritic cell Immunotherapy for Mesothelioma (DENIM) trial. Transl Lung Cancer Res. 2019;8:280-285. DOI: 10.21037/tlcr.2019.05.05

[35] Ma S, Li X, Wang X, Cheng L, Li Z, Zhang C, Ye Z, Qian Q. Current Progress in CAR-T Cell Therapy for Solid Tumors. Int J Biol Sci. 2019;15:2548-2560. DOI: 10.7150/ijbs.34213

[36] Haas AR, Tanyi JL, O'Hara MH, Gladney WL, Lacey SF, Torigian DA, Soulen MC, Tian L, McGarvey M, Nelson AM, Farabaugh CS, Moon E, Levine BL, Melenhorst JJ, Plesa G, June CH, Albelda SM, Beatty GL. Phase I Study of Lentiviral-Transduced Chimeric Antigen Receptor-Modified T Cells Recognizing Mesothelin in Advanced Solid Cancers. Mol Ther. 2019;27:1919-1929. DOI: 10.1016/j.ymthe.2019.07.015

Chapter 5

Targeted Cancer Therapy Using Nanoparticles and Antibody Fragments

Sankha Bhattacharya and Kapil Gore

Abstract

Cancer is caused by an uncontrolled cell division, forming a tumor capable of metastasis. Cancer is the second leading cause of death worldwide. Conventional treatments kill healthy cells, causing side effects. Recently, nanomaterials are explored due to properties such as as- nano-size, high loading, and ligands' attachment for a selective delivery. Apart from normal body cells, cancer cells express many receptors in excess, which serve as 'targets' for attacking the cells. Various ligands like proteins, peptides, polysaccharides can be attached to nanoparticles to allow proper and specific reach to the tumor. Such nanoparticles go to their desired site and stick onto the receptors, taken inside the cells by various methods. Antibodies are natural proteins that bind to foreign substances and remove them. IgG being the most explored antibody, suffers from many disadvantages such as non-specificity for required antigen, limited binding sites, low tumor penetration. Hence many researchers experimented by removing and adjusting the binding sites, using only the binding sites, enhancing the valency of naturally available IgG. It gave many benefits such as enhanced penetration, reduced immunogenicity, better delivery of drugs with fewer side effects. Continuing advancements in the field of protein engineering will help scientists to come up with better solutions. The properties allow easy surface interaction and entry, achieve better biodistribution, and reduce the amount of drug required. Targeting is based on Paul Ehrlich's 'magic bullet, 'where the therapeutic moiety has two parts-one to identify the target and the second to eliminate it. This concept is revised to incorporate a third component, a carrier. Many nanocarriers can be used to target cancer cells containing ligands to identify malignant cells. Approaches to targeting are passive, active and physical targeting. Many such nanoparticles are in clinical trials and can be a better solution to cancer therapy.

Keywords: nanoparticles, cancer immunotherapy, targeted drug delivery, cancer, targeting, nanomedicine, antibody fragments

1. Introduction

For the innovative treatment of cancer, it is necessary to boost target-based cancer therapy, ensuring that it could differentiate between normal and cancer cells while targeting cells [1]. Targeted cancer therapies are far better than the conventional method [2]. Therefore, targeted cancer therapy enjoys lesser unwanted side effects and an excellent molecular mechanism, which promotes minimum toxicity caused by chemotherapeutic drugs [3]. The rapid clearance from the body can be seen when the drug was administered in a higher tolerable dose, which ultimately leads to higher toxicity [4]. During targeted therapy, the drug could be modified to target biological transduction pathways and cellular factors. It also targets angiogenesis and apoptosis inducing molecules [5]. In recent years, several studies have been designed to investigate the effects of nanosized medicines inoperative targeting and diagnosis of cancer cells. Nanoparticles can possibly entrench drugs, theranostic agents, and genes [6]. It was also observed from the various research findings that, nanoparticular approach while drug targeting improves drug tolerability and bioavailability [7]. In formulation drug delivery, anchoring, fabricating, protection of payload from getting degradation by enzymes are possible [8]. The anchored nanoparticles can able to deliver a higher dose into tumor cells while bypassing the normal cells. The modified scaffold integration of nanoparticles facilitates biodistribution of specific drug delivery, which conjugates with ligands and eventually binds with tumor biomarkers [9]. Paul Ehrlich recently suggested a magic bullet, where two different targetings are possible with consistent therapeutic action [10]. In recent research articles and patents, it was often observed that many pharmaceutical carriers such as liposomes, micelles, polymeric nanoparticles designed from natural or synthetic sources were used to target chemotherapeutic medicaments in different cancer cells [11]. Many nanoparticles have passed phase II of the clinical trials stage. This suggests that effective active and passive targeting is possible, due to which greater specificity while selecting cancer target is achieved [12]. Nowadays, conjugation of antibodies, peptides, small chemical entities are versatile in delivering anticancer agents in the form of nanoparticle composite [13]. However, tumor targeting is not an easy job! Scientists are targeting tumors in three different mechanisms; (a) Where nanoparticles were pre-exposed with leaky vasculature of tumor cells and encountered with the reticuloendothelial system (RES) or enhanced permeability and retention (EPR) effects [14]. However, (b) active targeting is more advantageous, as inactive targeting, uncontrolled cell proliferative targeting of tumors, and pH and temperature-dependent targeting is possible. In physical targeting (c) pathological conditions such as pH and temperature play a key role. Nevertheless, targeting the tumor side also depends on the size of the nanoparticles. The nanoparticles, which are less than 7 nm, come under hydrodynamic diameters, easily passing through renal excretion [15]. The nanoparticles that are larger than 100 nm are eventually cleared from the circulation by the phagocytic system [16]. The nanoparticles' surface charge also plays a pivotal role, as the particles' cationic charge helps to facilitate internalization [17]. Sometimes surface addition of poly (sarcosine) and poly (ethylene glycol) [18] enhances the circulating half-life of the particles, on the other hand, preventing nanoparticles from getting engulfed by the reticuloendothelial system; by which accumulation of a certain amount of nanoparticles on the outer surface of the cancerous tissue is possible. To make nanoparticles more advanced, hooking ligands onto the nanoparticles' body facilitates internalization into cancer cells.

2. Molecular targets in cancer

To target cancerous cells, it is essential to target molecular aberrations. Effective nanoparticular therapy for cancer targeting relies on the ability to targets such genetic alterations to provide significant clinical benefits [19]. Nowadays, scientists are more focused on targeting p53, ALK PIK3CA, KRAS, G-NAQ, MET, BRAF, EGFR, CKIT genes, and certain pathways, i.e., PI3K/Akt/mTOR, etc. [20].

3. Ligands for cancer targeting

Ligands are a prerequisite for cancer. Recently, immunotoxin has obtained clinical approval from USFDA, and more than 100 ligand-targeted therapies are under clinical trials [21]. Newly developed phase-display techniques allow selective targeting with higher affinity. The bispecific antibodies and fusion proteins have been used for therapeutic purposes. Mostly the nanoreservior systems viz., niosomes, and polymeric nanoparticles are most suitable for ligand-based targeting [22]. However, pharmacokinetic behaviors and bio-distribution understanding of the molecules are still unknown. The principles of Ligands for cancer targeting can also be applied to the targeted delivery of gene medicines such as antisense oligonucleotides [23].

4. Attachment of ligands to carriers

Most of the nanoparticles as specially lipid-based formulations and polymeric nanoparticles are emerging as the best carrier system to deliver the molecule in cancerous tissues [24]. Monoclonal antibodies and peptides are possibly the best carriers. The surface-bound ligands specifically bind to the target cells. The various techniques viz., covalent and non-covalent techniques help in effective active targeting of cancer cells (**Figure 1**).

5. Receptor approaches of drug targeting in cancer

Receptor based targeting is being focused on ensuring the accurate delivery of carriers to their desired location [25]. It allows targeting not only to a localized tumor but also to traveling cancerous cells. This ensures precise delivery. Due to the excessive expression of receptors, targeting becomes easy. Ligands carry out the functionality through active targeting [26].

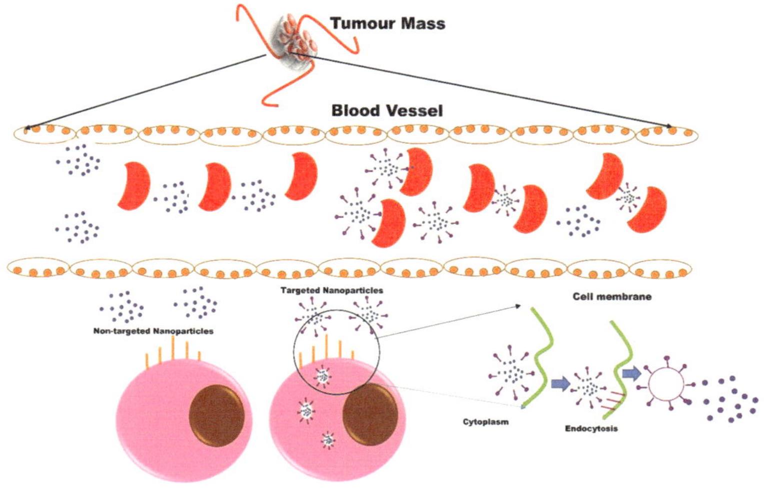

Figure 1.
Due to the active targeting, the nanoparticles are getting accumulated in the tumor site. Compered to non-targeted nanoparticles, actively targeted nanoparticles reach the tumor site with higher efficiency and through the endocytosis process, the nanocomposite triggers cancer cells death.

Receptor based targeting is being focused on ensuring the accurate delivery of carriers to their desired location [25]. It allows targeting not only to a localized tumor but also to traveling cancerous cells. This ensures precise delivery. Due to the excessive expression of receptors, targeting becomes easy. Ligands carry out the functionalization through active targeting (this has to be deleted) [27].

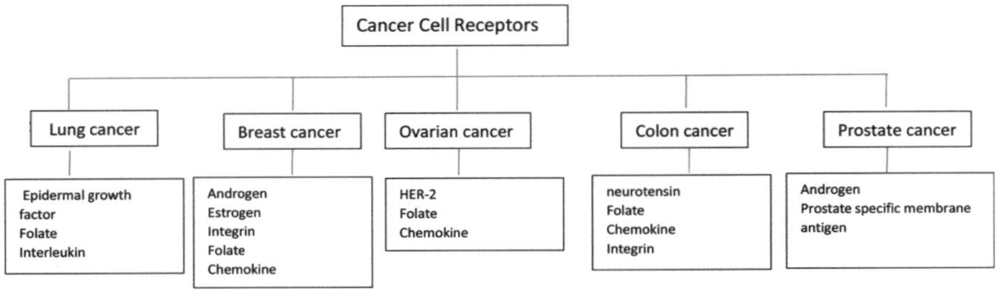

6. Receptors

6.1 EGFR

EGFR is a glycoprotein spanning across cell membranes. It is a target for Epidermal Growth Factor [28]. It initiates a signaling pathway leading to cell proliferation and mitosis. This is overexpressed in breast, colon, head and neck, ovarian tumors, and renal and glioma. The binding of antibodies against this receptor reduces cell proliferation. Many researchers prepared drug-loaded vesicles to target EFGR, which increased the drug's efficacy more than 10-fold [29]. Recently, cancer varieties like colorectal, lung, head, and neck carcinoma showed resistance to EGFR targeting due to mutations in the gene causing inhibition of activation and hence signaling.

6.2 Interleukin receptors

As interleukin receptors are majorly expressed, they are essential as a target for delivery. Among many varieties, types-3, 4, 6, 11, 13 & 16 were investigated as a target. The complex of ligand and receptor is taken inside the cell and hence helps cell growth and proliferation. But an overexpression may cause resistance to apoptosis and malignant growth (**Table 1**).

Interleukin type	Overexpressed in
IL-6	Ovarian cancer
IL-4	Glioblastoma, ovarian cancer, lung cancer, breast cancer
IL-3	Chronic Myelogenous leukemia, acute myeloid leukemia blast
IL-13	Head and neck cancer

Table 1.
Type of interleukin.

Various researchers used many ways to target IL receptors and obtained positive results such as reduced proliferation, enhanced uptake of carriers, decreased tumor volume, as well as accumulation and entry into the tumor as well as increased survival. This is not a full-proof strategy as blocking signaling of one type may be compensated with another type. And if the interleukins are blocked, it hinders the functioning of the immune system.

6.3 Folate receptors

Folate receptor is a glycoprotein present on the external cell surface. It is rich in cystine content. It has three subtypes- α, β and γ [30]. It is responsible for the entry of folic acid into cell, which is important for nucleic acid synthesis. The α subtype is overexpressed in breast, lung, colon cancer, and mesothelioma [31]. According to studies from many researchers, positive results such as a reduced tumor volume, nuclear delivery of therapeutic moieties, increased survival of cells, upregulation of cell death were observed. As folate receptors are present in the body on abundant sites, the selectivity may not always be achieved. Also, there are no animal models for therapeutic advantages or toxicity profiling.

6.4 Integrin receptors

Integrins are proteins that bind to the extracellular matrix and promote cell binding to tissues. Due to this action, this receptor is essential in the progression and metastasis of tumors. 'RGD motif' is a polypeptide chain important for binding and has been majorly exploited as a drug target [32]. Targeting the RGD motif has advantages such as improved survival, reduced tumor mass, and tumor growth inhibition. A major drawback of integrin targeting is diseases such as progressing lymphadenopathy [33].

7. Receptors to inhibit metastasis

7.1 The cluster of differentiation receptors

CD receptors initiate tumor development and can self-renew, overexpression of ABC, dormant. These features give tumor characteristics such as resistance, recurrence, and metastasis. Blocking these receptors prevents metastasis. CD subtypes 14, 22, 36, 44, 133 have been explored as drug targets for delivery. Targeting CD-44 receptors on cells allowed delivery into even the resistant tumors and showed enhanced cytotoxicity [34].

7.2 Estrogen receptors

These are nuclear receptors binding to the hormone estrogen. Estradiol acts as a transcription factor and controls cell growth. Estrogen helps in the development of sexual and reproductive functions, initiation and forming of lungs, mammary glands, and prostate gland. These receptors are excessively expressed in the majority of types of breast cancers, making it an ideal target. Initially, hormone analogs were used as ligands to target, but the binding strength was not optimal due to the modified structure of hormones. Also, another drawback was excessive RES uptake of such liposomes, which was overcome by formulating stealth liposomes. These formulations showed reduced tumor volume [35].

8. Targets for resistant tumors

8.1 Transferrin receptor

It is a receptor present on the cell membrane which is responsible for obtaining iron inside the cell. Iron binds to transferrin, and this complex binds to the receptor, which is then internalized [36]. Iron is necessary for many functions, such as DNA synthesis. This receptor can be targeted even if the tumor is Multi-drug resistant. Targeting this receptor has shown excellent results in resistant tumors such as increased formulation internalization, reduced drug required, higher cell death, and enhanced cytotoxicity [37]. This receptor's drawback is its presence at non-malignant sites such as endocrine glands may cause a loss in efficacy.

8.2 HER2

Human epidermal growth factor receptor-2 (HER-2) is a receptor spanning across the cell membrane with having a protein kinase internal subunit [38]. It is excessively expressed in gastric, lung, breast, and ovarian cancers. Overexpression of this receptor makes it challenging to forecast carcinoma. But, commercial products such as Herceptin have shown a promise targeting this receptor [39]. Targeting the HER-2 may help in cases of tumors showing resistance. This type of targeting has also demonstrated reduced cancer cell viability, enhanced cytotoxicity in resistant tumors, and increased uptake in the studies. A significant drawback is the absence of any natural ligand for the HER-2 receptor, which makes targeting difficult [39].

8.3 Antibodies for targeting cancer

Cancer cells are derived from normal body cells; hence they have a similar receptor constitution on the cell surface. Due to this lack of specialized markers, chemotherapeutic agents cannot differentiate between normal and cancer cells. Hence, they show toxicity. Keeping a low dose may result in resistance [40]. Therefore to achieve a specific targeting, antibodies specific for antigens presented by cancer cells can be targeted.

8.4 Engineering of antibodies

IgG is the majorly used antibody for targeting cancer [41]. Antibodies have 'Y' shaped structures where two arms have the sites for antigen binding. Monoclonal antibodies which are derived from a single clone of cells themselves or only the targeting fragments, can be used for cancer therapy. These agents bind the antigen and cause cell death by antibody-dependent toxicity, complement activation, or blocking signal transduction inside the cell. The antibody has a high affinity for its specific antigen and has excellent binding strength due to the presence of two binding sites. Entire antibodies may cause activation of the immune system inside the body. And due to their long half-lives, detection also becomes an issue. Using antibodies from species other than humans may cause severe allergic reactions. Hence to combat this situation, researchers have developed various molecules based on antibodies. Antibodies have been developed where binding sites from mouse have been attached to human antibody (chimeric antibody), humanized or human antibodies have also been developed. Researchers have separated the F_c fragments responsible for binding and have used them for targeting.

9. Effector mechanism of antibodies

Antibodies usually target antigens that are unique to cancer cells or which are excessively expressed on the cell surface. The majority of antibodies induce cancer cell death by binding to their target receptor, either blocking the receptor or changing the receptor's activation requirements [42]. They disturb signaling pathways responsible for cell growth and survival; hence, they end up killing the cells [43]. For example, Cetuximab is an antibody directed against EGFR. Epidermal growth factor upon binding to EFGR causes tumor growth, proliferation, and migration. EFGR is seen in many cancers. Cetuximab binds to EGFR and blocks the receptor hence preventing ligand binding and subsequent receptor dimerization. This process leads to apoptosis. Human epidermal growth factor receptor 2 is a member of the tyrosine kinase family. It is overexpressed in breast and ovarian cancers. The unique feature of this receptor is the absence of any known natural ligand. Instead, it forms dimers with other growth factor receptors and exerts its effects. Hence antibodies that are made to target this receptor prevent its dimerization with any other receptor and prevent survival.

Indirect action of antibodies involves host immune system participation and causes cytotoxicity by activation of complement system, antibody-dependent phagocytosis, and antibody-dependent cytotoxicity. Most antibodies are able to activate the complement system, which targets and destroys the cancer cell. Ofatumumab, an anti-CD20 antibody, intensifies the process of cytotoxicity through complement activation. Antibody-dependent phagocytosis occurs after a cancer cell opsonized by mAb attaches to a macrophage FcyRI glycoprotein. Then macrophage consumes such a marked cell [44].

10. Resistance to mAb

Even if mAb therapy is successful, many patients show resistance to it. The resistance may be innate or acquired after exposure to antibodies. Natural resistance is already present in mutations in cancer cells prior to the therapy, and acquired resistance is received after the exposure to therapy [45]. Another limitation is the dependency of the therapy on the overexpression of receptors. Mutations of receptors and the components in the signaling pathway may decrease the efficacy of antibody-targeted therapy. If cells express a variant of the receptor, therapy's potency may still decrease even if the binding site does not change [46].

11. Antibody fragments

Advancement in protein sciences has enabled scientists to produce antibody fragments with a smaller size but the same efficacy. The ideal characteristics of an antibody fragment are discussed in **Figure 2**.

In the beginning, proteolysis was the method of choice to produce smaller antibody fragments [47]. These fragments had a molecular weight of around 54 kDa–100 kDa (Fab, Fab_2). In the later stages, recombinant DNA technology was used to prepare univalent and bivalent fragments which had heavy and light chains of a variable section of antibody [48]. Such a structure was the smallest targeting unit to be generated. The two chains were joined with a flexible polypeptide linkage giving a 'single chain variable fragment' (scFv). It was convenient to use because of its small size and easy production.

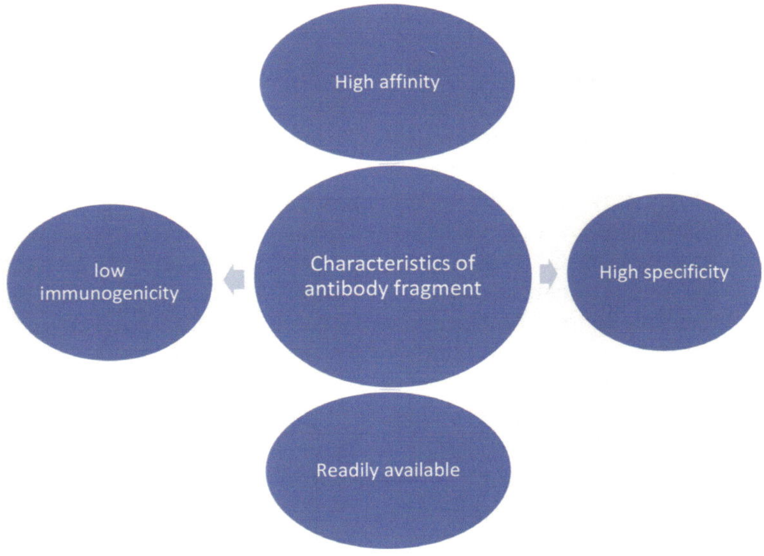
High affinity
low immunogenicity
Characteristics of antibody fragment
High specificity
Readily available

Figure 2.
Different characteristics of antibody fragments.

In the 1980s, researchers isolated and screened a heavy chain of the murine antibody for its binding to lysosomes [49]. It was called a single domain antibody' (dAb) as it contained only a heavy or light chain and had a meager molecular weight (15 kDa). However, it had drawbacks like poor solubility and aggregation, and a major issue was that the fragments did not retain the original's binding efficacy [49]. Components from animals such as camels, llamas, and fish such as sharks were used as more soluble, but they suffered from immunogenicity issues. Efforts like immunization and bioengineering to reduce agglomeration were carried out for effective use in therapy [50].

Later the above types were converted from univalent to multivalent through protein engineering, which was then used to target multiple entities at once [51]. These multivalent fragments show slower dissociation from the receptor and high functionality. One great example of multivalent fragments is a 'diabody' formed by linking light and heavy chain by a single chain variable fragment to be self-assembled into a dimer [52]. Diabodies have an advantage such as moderate molecular weight, multivalency which give them characteristics like improved penetration in tissue, rapid clearance. These diabodies bind to tumor antigen as well as to CD3 cells to kill tumors through T-cell mediated toxicity. The mini body is another type of synthesized antibody fragment, which is a pair of single chains of variable fragments interconnected by-CH_3 bonds, and a variable region specific for any antigen is attached to this pair. Minibodies are more suitable for targeted radiotherapy because they show better uptake and are cleared faster as compared to other types of fragments and are cleared rapidly. In the structure of the Mini body, the single variable region can be replaced by a cytotoxic agent, radioisotope, for its delivery.

Nanobody is the shortest antibody fragment. It is isolated from camelid heavy chains of variable antibody region. It is produced by making phage viral coat cover the desired fragment. As these antibodies do not have light chains, they are structurally different than normal antibodies. They have a concave antigen-binding region larger than other antibodies. Hydrophilic structures replace the usual hydrophobic amino acid residue. Such adjustments allow antigen-binding property even in the absence of light region. Another specific property is its ability to cross blood–brain barrier.

12. Application of fragments in imaging

12.1 Cancer imaging

Antibodies that bind to the target can be coupled with a radionuclide, fluorescent molecules to obtain images of cancer. Antibodies that have longer half-life need more time for imaging and may blur the image. These fragments have a short half-life and higher permeability, which allow easy detection. Techniques such as Positron emission tomography (PET), Computed tomography (CT), Single-photon emission computed tomography (SPECT) are now being performed where the antibody fragments are employed [53].

12.2 Nuclear imaging

Nuclear imaging is essential for the detection of cancer. Using fragments reduces nuclear exposure to radiation. The bifunctional connector connects antibody fragment and radionuclide, and such complexity easily accumulates at the tumor and gives clear visualization [54]. This method can be used to measure the absorption of drugs and the expression of receptors. One issue with the complex is increased radiation in the kidney due to complex breakdown and retention of radionuclide in the kidney [37].

12.3 Dual modality imaging

It involves non-invasive assessment of disease and fluorescence imaging of tumors during surgery. This technique shows accurate and reliable results [55]. Heterodimeric antibodies are used to target two issues at once and have a stronger affinity than homodimer.

12.4 Other imaging

Antibody fragments can be coupled with microbubbles, and it enhances the targeting efficiency [56]. Photoacoustic imaging also can be performed with antibody fragments to give high-resolution images. The laser causes expansion of tissues, and it produces sound waves, which later can be converted to images by the ultrasonic transducer.

13. Application in cancer therapy

13.1 Intrinsic therapeutic effect

The selection of antigen is most important for targeting. The target antigen is highly expressed in cancer cells but not on a normal cell. Single, as well as multiple targeting, can be achieved through the use of an engineered antibody. Multivalent antibodies not only block signaling but also overcome resistance through multiple targets [57].

13.2 Targeted drug delivery

The delivery of anti-tumor drugs using antibody fragments is a common practice of targeting medicine to the tumor [58]. Such systems ensure accurate delivery and improve the pharmacokinetics of agents. Effector molecules such as siRNA cannot target and have very low uptake. Coupling them with antibodies shows enhanced tumor uptake and reduced side effects [59]. An example is CXC chemokine receptor siRNA delivered by coupling with anti-HER2 peptide fusion protein e23sFv-9R is used to target breast cancer cells, having an excess of HER-2 receptors, which promotes apoptosis. Immunotoxins also can be targeted for effective therapy. Immunotoxins from plants and animals may show a rapid immunogenicity and have toxic side effects that may be harmful to humans. For example, an immunotoxin was synthesized by a combination of *Pseudomonas aeruginosa* exotoxin and short-chain variable fragment, which reduced tumor cells' reduced survival and improved the survival rate. An antibody fragment can also be attached to nanoparticles, which then enter the tumor cells via receptor-mediated endocytosis. An example is the anti-HER-2 short-chain variable fragment attached to the PEG-coated iron oxide particle, which shows a better targeting and improved serum half-life.

13.3 Application in immunotherapy

Tumor cells have barriers to protect them from the body's immune system, such as an impenetrable stroma and immunosuppressive cells in the tumor environment [60]. Tumor cells block antigen overexpression and increase regulatory-T cells and hence escape the immune system of the body. Immunotherapy overturns this mechanism and brings about the death of cancer cells. Bispecific antibodies can target two antigens at once, including an antigen on the cancer cell and a receptor on the cell of the immune system. Then the proteins in cell death signaling are activated by phosphorylation, which then initiates apoptosis. Bispecific antibodies link two cells hence bypassing innate as well as acquired resistance.

Chimeric antigen receptor on T cells (CAR-T) is being focused on as a target of antibodies as it helps in specific recognition of cancer cells [61]. Upon activation, it shows a high amount of cytokine release, which then kills cancer cells. This also can help to circumvent tumor resistance for killer T-cells.

For immunotherapy, a specific target is required for the immune system to attack or else; there can be severe side effects related to immunity. Also, the extent of immune response should also be considered for the efficacy of the treatment. An immune response, which is too low may not be able to kill the malignant cells, and a very strong immune response may cause cytokine storms and harm the healthy cells instead.

14. Antibody derivatives

IgG is the most explored antibody of choice for cancer targeting. Antigen binding if is the desired mechanism; only antigen-binding fragment can be separated and used. In such cases, the binding affinity and crystallization properties remain the same with smaller size and hybridization, which give enhanced tumor penetration. Also, modifications can be made to increase the specificity and valency of antibodies.

15. IgG formats

Involves changes in the structure of IgG to alter its natural properties to obtain desired attributes. The most common structural change includes changes in antibody binding region, e.g., ranibizumab. Right now, there are many fragment-based therapeutics in preclinical and clinical trials. The most advanced is otlertuzumab for treating chronic lymphocytic leukemia. Fragment-based derivatives are not able to activate the immune system without a crystallization region [62]. But they show advantages like enhanced penetration, longer circulation and increased diffusion in the tumor. Hybrids can also be made with Fc from IgG and scFv from a targeting antibody. They do not penetrate in the tumor but instead retain activities of Fc such as immunization.

16. Multivalent binders

IgG can only bind a single type of antigen. Hence it is bivalent but not bispecific. Hence, to increase the specificity, the valency of antibodies is being enhanced. Many different regions from different sources are connected together to form molecules that are multivalent and can bind to more than one type of molecules.

16.1 Bispecific

This is the most used type from multispecific modified IgG. These can bind to two different antigens at once. For e.g., blinatumomab is used for some types of acute lymphocytic leukemia. It binds to CD19 protein on the cancer cell and CD3 protein on T-cell. It causes the release of cytotoxic chemicals that kill the cancer cell. Dual affinity targeting agents are made from two separate light and heavy regions linked by disulfide bonds after translation.it can be stored for a long time and should be stable for a long time [63].

16.2 Multispecific and multivalent

A combination makes multivalent antibodies of three or more antibody domains joined sequentially or in a row. These are proteins specific for two antigens containing two pairs of light and heavy variable regions connected in a single chain forming a polypeptide. By virtue of their multivalency, tandem Abs not only target tumors but also cause infiltration and destruction of tumors by killer T-cells. These have longer storage life, better pharmacokinetics, are highly potent [64].

17. Antibody conjugates and fusion

Antibodies can be linked with other molecules such as proteins and peptides to form hybrids. Such combinations give altered biodistribution by targeting a different receptor, extend the half-life of formulation, or impart a new mechanism of action [65].

18. Antibody-drug conjugates

These hybrid molecules contain antibodies linked to a therapeutic agent. They combine the selective nature of antibodies with cytotoxicity of active agents [66]. It can reduce side effects to a minimum and shows maximum therapeutic success. Conjugates such as Mylotarg have been approved by the FDA. This has caused the emergence of many compounds that differ just by changing the method and site of conjugation. The drugs or linkers are attached to free lysine or cysteine, which gives different products based on the location of conjugation. The most recent trend involves forming a homogenous product by conjugation at particular sites only. It can be done by altering the structure of antibodies to incorporate non-natural amino acids, which act as a handle for attachment. Available tags have been discovered, such as sortase A tag, which attaches the drug to antibody at the glutamic acid site and attaches to therapeutic moiety through a polyglycine tag.

19. Antibody-fusion constructs

These are molecules synthesized using recombinant DNA technology. They combine targeting efficiency of IgG and various protein domains. This fusion affects selectivity and PK parameters extensively. Toxic proteins can be used to form immunotoxic compounds such as diphtheria toxin attached to antibodies. Dose-limiting toxicity and immunogenicity are the main challenges in the formation of such complexes. The most successful examples of protein fusion complex are

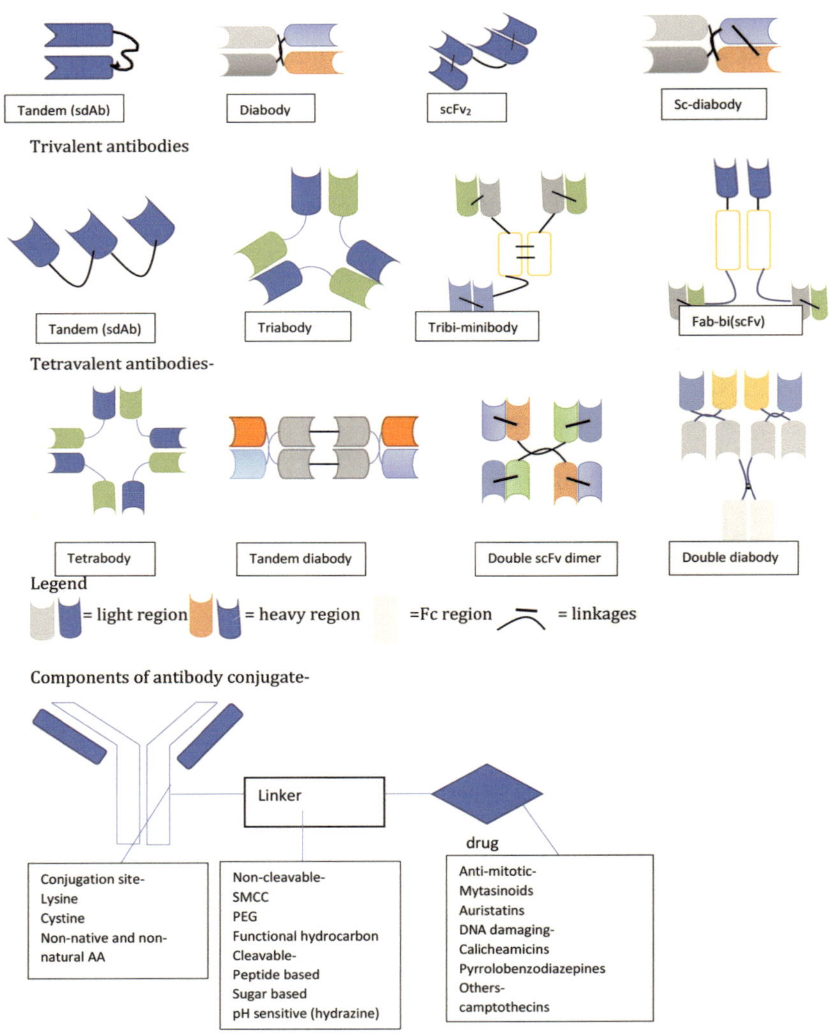

Figure 3.
Types of antibody fragments.

bioactive proteins attached to the crystallization region of IgG. Amevive and zaltrap are two such complexes approved by USFDA for release in the market. This combination shows an excellent immune response against the tumor [67].

Types of antibody fragments: Deferent type of antibody fragments are mentioned in **Figure 3**.

20. Conclusion

There is no single magic remedy that acts against all of the diseases. Antibodies are ingenious proteins targeted toward specific foreign molecules inside the body. Their therapeutic use involves their ability to disrupt signal transduction, block receptor, which further affects cell growth and cell death. They also can be used to stimulate the immune system so as to destroy any foreign or ingenious harmful materials. IgG's natural structure can be modified to remove problematic residues and add newly modified proteins for the purpose of targeting and immunostimulating. These attachments come with issues like immunogenicity, acquired resistance. But more research in field of antibody engineering is required to address this issue.

Author details

Sankha Bhattacharya* and Kapil Gore
Department of Pharmaceutics School of Pharmacy and Technology Management, SVKM'S NMIMS Deemed-to-be University, Shirpur, Maharashtra, India

*Address all correspondence to: sankhabhatt@gmail.com

References

[1] Noble, C.O., et al., *Development of ligand-targeted liposomes for cancer therapy.* 2004.**8**(4): p. 335-353.

[2] Papadopoulos, N., K.W. Kinzler, and B.J.N.b. Vogelstein, *The role of companion diagnostics in the development and use of mutation-targeted cancer therapies.* 2006. **24**(8): p. 985-995.

[3] Mattheolabakis, G., et al., *Hyaluronic acid targeting of CD44 for cancer therapy: from receptor biology to nanomedicine.* 2015. **23**(7-8): p. 605-618.

[4] Blume, K., et al., *Total body irradiation and high-dose etoposide: a new preparatory regimen for bone marrow transplantation in patients with advanced hematologic malignancies [published erratum appears in Blood 1987 Jun; 69 (6): 1789].* 1987.

[5] Sies, H. and D.P.J.N.R.M.C.B. Jones, *Reactive oxygen species (ROS) as pleiotropic physiological signalling agents.* 2020: p. 1-21.

[6] Louvel, S., *The Policies and Politics of Interdisciplinary Research: Nanomedicine in France and in the United States*. 2020: Routledge.

[7] Kumar, V., et al., *Current status and future directions of hepatocellular carcinoma-targeted nanoparticles and nanomedicine.* 2020.

[8] Lee, S.H., et al., *Strategic approaches for colon targeted drug delivery: An overview of recent advancements.* 2020. **12**(1): p. 68.

[9] Mirza, Z. and S. Karim. *Nanoparticles-based drug delivery and gene therapy for breast cancer: Recent advancements and future challenges*. in *Seminars in cancer biology*. 2019. Elsevier.

[10] Xiong, G.M., K. Venkatraman, and S.J.P.i.B.E. Venkatraman, *The magic bullet as cancer therapeutic—has nanotechnology failed to find its mark?* 2020. **2**(4): p. 042004.

[11] Sur, S., et al., *Recent developments in functionalized polymer nanoparticles for efficient drug delivery system.* 2019. **20**: p. 100397.

[12] Ahmad, A., et al., *Precision cancer nanotherapy: evolving role of multifunctional nanoparticles for cancer active targeting.* 2019. **62**(23): p. 10475-10496.

[13] Taghipour-Sabzevar, V., T. Sharifi, and M.M.J.T.d. Moghaddam, *Polymeric nanoparticles as carrier for targeted and controlled delivery of anticancer agents.* 2019. **10**(8): p. 527-550.

[14] Nomura, S., et al., *Highly reliable, targeted photothermal cancer therapy combined with thermal dosimetry using a near-infrared absorbent.* 2020. **10**(1): p. 1-7.

[15] Huang, H., et al., *Inorganic nanoparticles in clinical trials and translations.* 2020. **35**: p. 100972.

[16] Nikitin, M.P., et al., *Enhancement of the blood-circulation time and performance of nanomedicines via the forced clearance of erythrocytes.* 2020. **4**(7): p. 717-731.

[17] Kaddour, H., et al., *Electrostatic surface properties of blood and semen extracellular vesicles: Implications of sialylation and HIV-induced changes on EV internalization.* 2020. **12**(10): p. 1117.

[18] Bhattacharya, S.J.J.o.D.D.S. and Technology, *Fabrication of poly (sarcosine), poly (ethylene glycol), and poly (lactic-co-glycolic acid) polymeric nanoparticles for cancer drug delivery.* 2020: p. 102194.

[19] Yao, H.-P., et al., *MET and RON receptor tyrosine kinases in colorectal*

adenocarcinoma: molecular features as drug targets and antibody-drug conjugates for therapy. 2020. **39**(1): p. 1-18.

[20] Elsevier, A., et al., *Combined Analysis of Tumor RNAseq, Urine Proteomics and WES Profiles from Patient with Gallbladder Cancer.* 2019.

[21] Li, Y., et al., *Liposomes modified with bio-substances for cancer treatment.* 2020. **8**(23): p. 6442-6468.

[22] Khazaei-poul, Y., et al., *Monocyclic peptides: types, synthesis and applications.* 2020.

[23] de la Torre, P., et al., *Cell-Based Nanoparticles Delivery Systems for Targeted Cancer Therapy: Lessons from Anti-Angiogenesis Treatments.* 2020. **25**(3): p. 715.

[24] Duwa, R., et al., *Polymeric and lipid-based drug delivery systems for treatment of glioblastoma multiforme.* 2019. **79**: p. 261-273.

[25] Rios de la Rosa, J.M., et al., *Binding and Internalization in Receptor-Targeted Carriers: The Complex Role of CD44 in the Uptake of Hyaluronic Acid-Based Nanoparticles (siRNA Delivery).* 2019. **8**(24): p. 1901182.

[26] Harris, J.C., M.A. Scully, and E.S.J.C. Day, *Cancer cell membrane-coated nanoparticles for cancer management.* 2019. **11**(12): p. 1836.

[27] Shukla, N., et al., *Combinational Chemotherapy and Photothermal Therapy Using a Gold Nanorod Platform for Cancer Treatment.* 2020. **37**(8): p. 2000099.

[28] Heby, M., et al., *Additive clinical impact of epidermal growth factor receptor and podocalyxin-like protein expression in pancreatic and periampullary adenocarcinomas.* 2020. **10**(1): p. 1-10.

[29] Sabbah, D.A., R. Hajjo, and K.J.C.T.i.M.C. Sweidan, *Review on Epidermal Growth Factor Receptor (EGFR) Structure, Signaling Pathways, Interactions, and Recent Updates of EGFR Inhibitors.* 2020.

[30] Qu, Y., et al., *Folate and macrophage folate receptor-β in idiopathic pulmonary fibrosis disease: the potential therapeutic target?* 2020. **131**: p. 110711.

[31] Thakkar, S., et al., *Tumor microenvironment targeted nanotherapeutics for cancer therapy and diagnosis: A review.* 2020. **101**: p. 43-68.

[32] Bourgot, I., et al., *Reciprocal Interplay Between Fibrillar Collagens and Collagen-Binding Integrins: Implications in Cancer Progression and Metastasis.* 2020. **10**: p. 1488.

[33] Harjunpää, H., et al., *Cell adhesion molecules and their roles and regulation in the immune and tumor microenvironment.* 2019. **10**: p. 1078.

[34] Li, J., et al., *Facile strategy by hyaluronic acid functional carbon dot-doxorubicin nanoparticles for CD44 targeted drug delivery and enhanced breast cancer therapy.* 2020. **578**: p. 119122.

[35] Padmasree, M., et al., *Formulation, Characterization and Stability Study of Encapsulated Anticancer drug in multilayered PEGylated Tumor targeting stealth Liposomes.* 2019. **12**(10): p. 4689-4695.

[36] Kell, D.B., E.L. Heyden, and E.J.F.i.I. Pretorius, *The Biology of Lactoferrin, an Iron-Binding Protein That Can Help Defend Against Viruses and Bacteria.* 2020. **11**: p. 1221.

[37] Akhter, M.H., et al., *Receptor-based targeting of engineered nanocarrier against solid tumors: Recent progress and challenges ahead.* 2020: p. 129777.

[38] Kumar, R., et al., *HER family in cancer progression: From discovery to 2020 and beyond.* 2020. **147**: p. 109-152.

[39] Shrestha, L., *Anti-tumor Efficacy and Stability Assessment of a Peptidomimetic Targeting HER2 Receptor in Non-small Cell Lung Cancer*. 2020, University of Louisiana at Monroe.

[40] Autio, K.A., et al., *Probody therapeutics: an emerging class of therapies designed to enhance on-target effects with reduced off-tumor toxicity for use in immuno-oncology.* 2020. **26**(5): p. 984-989.

[41] Vikrant, R. and K.J.E. Geetank, *Bi-SPECIFIC ANTIBODIES: AN EMERGING IMMUNOTHERAPEUTIC AGENT.* **23**: p. 20.4.

[42] Janes, P.W., et al., *Antibody Targeting of Eph Receptors in Cancer.* 2020. **13**(5): p. 88.

[43] Zhang, F., et al., *Asparanin a from Asparagus officinalis L. Induces G0/G1 cell cycle arrest and apoptosis in human endometrial carcinoma ishikawa cells via mitochondrial and PI3K/AKT signaling pathways.* 2019. **68**(1): p. 213-224.

[44] Davis, R., *Cellular and Molecular Immunology*. 2019: Scientific e-Resources.

[45] Collins, D.M., et al., *Acquired resistance to antibody-drug conjugates.* 2019. **11**(3): p. 394.

[46] McDaid, W.J., et al., *Repurposing of Cetuximab in antibody-directed chemotherapy-loaded nanoparticles in EGFR therapy-resistant pancreatic tumours.* 2019. **11**(42): p. 20261-20273.

[47] Alfaleh, M.A., et al., *Phage display derived monoclonal antibodies: from bench to bedside.* 2020. **11**.

[48] Wozniak-Knopp, G., *Bispecific Antibodies*, in *Introduction to Antibody Engineering*. Springer. p. 161-187.

[49] Ullman, J.C., et al., *Brain delivery and activity of a lysosomal enzyme using a blood-brain barrier transport vehicle in mice.* 2020. **12**(545).

[50] Dube, T., et al., *Repurposed Drugs, Molecular Vaccines, Immune-Modulators, and Nanotherapeutics to Treat and Prevent COVID-19 Associated with SARS-CoV-2, a Deadly Nanovector.* 2020: p. 2000172.

[51] Jefferies, W.A., *CNS-targeted conjugates having modified fc regions and methods of use thereof*. 2019, Google Patents.

[52] Qi, T., et al., *The role of antibody delivery formation in cancer therapy.* 2020: p. 1-11.

[53] Pietzsch, H.-J., et al., *Single Photon Emission Computed Tomography Tracer*, in *Molecular Imaging in Oncology*. 2020, Springer. p. 227-282.

[54] Spiegel, D.A., P. McEnaney, and K. Fitzgerald, *Synthetic antibody mimetic compounds (syams) targeting cancer, especially prostate cancer*. 2019, Google Patents.

[55] Habibalahi, A., et al., *Novel automated non invasive detection of ocular surface squamous neoplasia using multispectral autofluorescence imaging.* 2019. **17**(3): p. 540-550.

[56] Punjabi, M., et al., *Ultrasound molecular imaging of atherosclerosis with nanobodies: translatable microbubble targeting murine and human VCAM (vascular cell adhesion molecule) 1.* 2019. **39**(12): p. 2520-2530.

[57] Bracken, C.J., et al., *Bi-paratopic and multivalent VH domains block ACE2 binding and neutralize SARS-CoV-2.* 2020: p. 1-9.

[58] Dougan, M. and S.K.J.N.M. Dougan, *Programmable bacteria as cancer therapy.* 2019. **25**(7): p. 1030-1031.

[59] Van Herck, S. and B.G.J.A.P.S. De Geest, *Nanomedicine-mediated alteration*

of the pharmacokinetic profile of small molecule cancer immunotherapeutics. 2020: p. 1-14.

[60] Xie, Y., et al., *Stromal modulation and treatment of metastatic pancreatic cancer with local intraperitoneal triple miRNA/siRNA nanotherapy.* 2020. **14**(1): p. 255-271.

[61] Strohl, W.R. and M.J.A. Naso, *Bispecific T-cell redirection versus chimeric antigen receptor (CAR)-T cells as approaches to kill cancer cells.* 2019. **8**(3): p. 41.

[62] Lee, C., M. Choi, and J.A.J.A.D.D.R. MacKay, *Live long and active: Polypeptide-mediated assembly of antibody variable fragments.* 2020.

[63] Leipheimer Jr, J.B., *Translational Control Promotes Oxidative Stress Resistance in the Human Fungal Pathogen Cryptococcus neoformans*. 2020, State University of New York at Buffalo.

[64] Wu, C., *Fabs-in-tandem immunoglobulin and uses thereof*. 2019, Google Patents.

[65] Datta, P., S.J.J.o.L.C. Ray, and Radiopharmaceuticals, *Nanoparticulate formulations of radiopharmaceuticals: Strategy to improve targeting and biodistribution properties.* 2020.

[66] Dovgan, I., et al., *Antibody–oligonucleotide conjugates as therapeutic, imaging, and detection agents.* 2019. **30**(10): p. 2483-2501.

[67] Baldo, B.A. and N.H. Pham, *Biologics: Monoclonal Antibodies for Non-cancer Therapy, Cytokines, Fusion Proteins, Enzymes, and Hormones*, in *Drug Allergy*. Springer. p. 533-593.

Chapter 6

Antibody Therapy Targeting Cancer-Specific Cell Surface Antigen AGR2

Alvin Y. Liu, Tatjana Crnogorac-Jurcevic, James J. Lai and Hung-Ming Lam

Abstract

For anterior gradient 2 (AGR2), normal cells express the intracellular form iAGR2 localized to the endoplasmic reticulum while cancer cells express the extracellular form eAGR2 localized on the cell surface and secreted. Antibodies targeting eAGR2$^+$ cancer cells for eradication will spare normal cells. Two AGR2 monoclonal antibodies, P1G4 and P3A5, were shown to recognize specifically eAGR2$^+$ pancreatic tumors implanted in mice. In addition, P1G4 showed enhancement in drug inhibition of tumor growth. Human:mouse chimeric antibodies of IgG1, IgG2, IgG4 were generated for both antibodies. These human IgG were shown to lyse eAGR2$^+$ prostate cancer cells in vitro with human serum. AGR2 has an important function in distal spread of cancer cells, and is highly expressed in prostate, pancreatic, bladder metastases. Therefore, immunotherapy based on AGR2 antibody-mediated ADCC and CDC is highly promising. Cancer specificity of eAGR2 predicts possibly minimal collateral damage to healthy tissues and organs. Moreover, AGR2 therapy, once fully developed and approved, can be used to treat other solid tumors since AGR2 is an adenocarcinoma antigen found in many common malignancies.

Keywords: anterior gradient 2, adenocarcinoma antigen, solid tumors, metastasis, chimeric AGR2 antibodies, antibody enhancement of drug inhibition

1. Introduction

The adenocarcinoma antigen anterior gradient 2 (AGR2) is expressed by prostate, pancreatic and bladder cancer as well as many other solid tumor types. In 2018, close to 1.3 million new cases of prostate cancer worldwide were diagnosed and 360,000 deaths were recorded, mostly in the developed countries [1]. In the same year, nearly 460,000 new cases of pancreatic cancer were diagnosed [2]. Patients with pancreatic cancer seldom exhibit symptoms until at advanced stages making 5-year survival dismal. Bladder cancer represents only 3% of global cancer diagnoses, and 5-year survival decreases from >75% to 5% when the cancer has metastasized [3].

Since the FDA approval of IFNα2 in 1986, a number of immunotherapeutic agents have been developed for cancer treatment. In prostate cancer, antigens such as PSA, PAP, PSCA, MUC1, PAGE/GAGE were used to impart T cell-mediated immunity [4]. Lack of consistent success could be partly attributed to non-prostate specific expression of these proteins. PSCA (prostate stem cell antigen), for example, is misidentified as a stem cell marker, and is expressed by the bladder, colon, kidney and stomach as well [5]. Vaccines against PSA (prostate-specific antigen) in PROSTVAC-VF and PAP (prostatic acid phosphatase) in Provenge were used to prime immune cells. However, inconsistent trial results with modest survival benefits were reported [6]. Strategies to target immune checkpoints (CTLA-4, PD-1, PD-L1) with the intention to amplify T cell responses in eradicating tumors have not been particularly successful in prostate cancer, with one of the main side effects being immune-related adverse events with tissue damage caused by overly activated T cells [6]. These potential therapies are beset by response monitoring although a subset of patients with advanced disease did show some benefits. There are even fewer similar types of immunotherapeutic approaches developed for pancreatic and bladder cancer, which is largely due to fewer suitable targets identified. Immunotherapy based on antibodies, on the other hand, would not require tinkering the immune system to achieve an outcome. Tumor-associated antigens (TAA) [7] constitute a pool of candidates for targeted cancer therapies. Antibodies raised against TAA mediate cancer cell killing through antibody-dependent cellular cytotoxicity (ADCC) by recruiting cytotoxic T cells [8] and complement-dependent cytotoxicity (CDC) by assembling complement components into a membrane attack complex [9]. The antibody-bound cancer cells are lysed by T-cell secreted enzymes and water uptake through a perforated cell membrane, respectively. A major complication is the cancer non-specificity of most TAA identified to date, because other normal cell types also express these TAA leading to unintended collateral damage of healthy tissue. Therefore, the quest for a truly cancer-specific targetable molecule is an ongoing endeavor.

Our work in Urologic Cancer Biomarker Development identified AGR2 as a TAA for prostate cancer. AGR2 is present in prostate cancer cells but absent in the normal luminal cells [10, 11]. Similarly, AGR2 expression is detected in various cancers including pancreatic [12], breast [13], lung [14], colorectal [15], oral [16], subsets of ovarian [17], and bladder [18]. What makes AGR2 attractive for cancer therapy besides its ubiquity in solid tumors is its differential subcellular localization between cancer and normal cells [19] as we demonstrated previously for bladder cancer [18]. Intracellular iAGR2 is localized to the endoplasmic reticulum (ER) of normal cells where, as a protein disulfide isomerase, it functions in protein folding [19]. Extracellular eAGR2 is localized to the cell surface of and secreted by cancer cells. Thus, eAGR2 is a unique TAA that it is not found on normal cells.

Antibodies targeting eAGR2 on cancer cells would thus spare normal cells as the iAGR2 antigen is cell interior. We have generated mouse monoclonal antibodies, P1G4 (mIgG1) and P3A5 (mIgG2a), recognizing two epitopes of AGR2 [20]. The use of mouse monoclonal antibodies for therapeutics is problematic. Mouse antibodies, besides being immunogenic in human, do not interact efficiently with human immune system components. To overcome these drawbacks, we have replaced the constant domains of AGR2 antibodies by the analogous human constant domains via recombinant DNA technology [21], generating human:mouse chimeric hIgG1, hIgG2, hIgG4 for both P1G4 and P3A5 for potential therapeutic development [22].

With these chimeric human:mouse antibodies, direct antigenic stimulation of T cells via CAR-T cell therapy can potentially also be achieved [23]. We could link via the engineered restriction enzyme sites the antigen-binding V_H and V_L domains of the AGR2 antibodies to T cell activator molecules for triggering response upon binding of the T cells via eAGR2 on the cancer cell surface. In the future, one might be able to use patient-derived induced pluripotent stem (iPS) cells to differentiate into dendritic cells in vitro (by bone marrow factors and interaction with bone marrow stromal cells) rather than leukapheresis to isolate dendritic cells from patients. The derived dendritic cells can then be stimulated with AGR2 antigens. The use of AGR2 to transduce dendritic cells via expression vectors to generate cytotoxic T lymphocytes capable of lysing AGR2$^+$ (colorectal) cancer cells has been reported [24].

In this review, we will discuss the role of AGR2 in various cancers, the development and therapeutic evidence of chimeric AGR2 antibodies, and the future use of AGR2 in biomarker and therapeutic applications.

2. AGR2 as a cancer biomarker

We used comparative transcriptomic analysis between sorted CD26$^+$ prostate cancer cells from a Gleason pattern 3 (well-differentiated glandular adenocarcinoma) tumor focus and CD26$^+$ luminal cells of benign glands to identify differentially expressed genes that encode secreted proteins for use as urine biomarkers [10]. AGR2 was the top candidate with elevated expression in cancer cells, which was verified by immunohistochemistry (**Figure 1**). A similar analysis was carried out between CD9$^+$ urothelial cancer cells and CD9$^+$ normal urothelial cells [25]. In this case, AGR2 was down-regulated in cancer. AGR2 is expressed by urothelial cells (iAGR2 for normal cells) and was found absent in 75% of bladder cancer cases [18]. Although the AGR2 gene contains a leader signal peptide characteristic of secreted proteins, in normal cells iAGR2 is retained in the ER (via a *C*-terminus ER-retention motif). Over-expression of AGR2 in cancer cells provides a possible explanation for its secretion due to saturation of ER anchorage [26]. For example, urothelial cells were immunostained for AGR2 at moderate intensity *vs*. prostate cancer cells. The immunostaining corroborated a 35-fold difference in expression levels measured

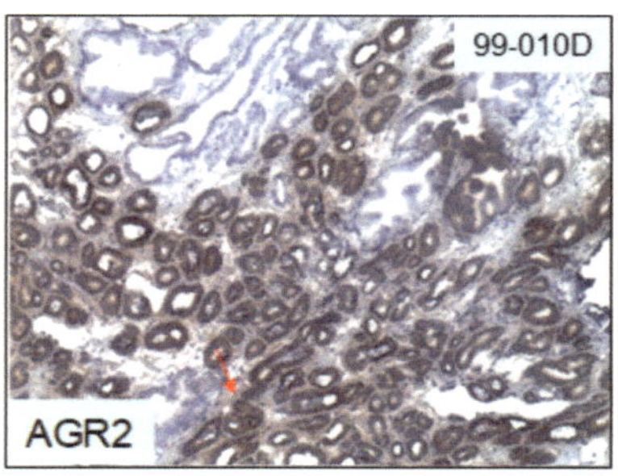

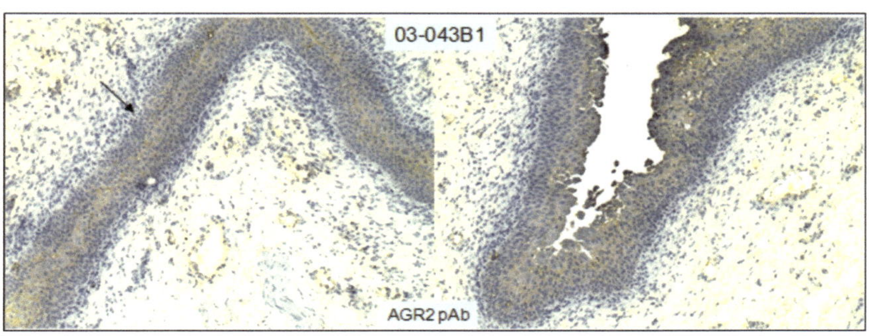

Figure 1.
AGR2 in prostate cancer and bladder. The prostate tumor glands (specimen 99-010D, top) are stained positive for AGR2 while benign glands are negative. Faint staining in the cancer-associated stroma (red arrow) suggests AGR2 secretion from the adjacent cancer cells. The urothelium (specimen 03-043B1, bottom) is stained at moderate intensity. Two different parts of the specimen indicate uniform expression throughout the entire urothelium. Black arrow indicates the lamina propria below the urothelium.

by DNA microarray analysis of CD9$^+$ urothelial cells (signal value = 105.54) [25] and CD26$^+$ prostate cancer cells (signal value = 4168.03) [10]. A previous study estimated that adenocarcinoma cells had 80% iAGR2 and 20% eAGR2 while in all non-tumor cells AGR2 was located intracellularly [19]. Faint AGR2 staining of the stroma surrounding prostate tumor glands could be evidence of AGR2 secretion [27] (**Figure 1**, top panel). No such staining was detectable in the lamina propria next to the iAGR2$^+$ urothelium [18] (**Figure 1**, bottom panel) or benign glands of the prostate. In prostate cancer cells, AGR2 could be activated by ER stress with down-regulation of unfolded protein response genes leading to an accumulation of misfolded proteins like that in pancreatic cancers cells [28].

In summary, three AGR2 expression patterns have been described in solid tumors: (1) iAGR2 positive for normal urothelial cells, eAGR2 positive for 25% primary tumors [18]; (2) no AGR2 for prostate epithelial cells, eAGR2 positive for >95% primary tumors [10], similar to pancreas [12] and breast [13]; (3) iAGR2 positive for normal bronchial epithelial cells, eAGR2 positive for>95% non-small cell lung tumors [14].

3. Differential subcellular localization of AGR2

The contrasting localization of eAGR2 and iAGR2 is well illustrated by the bladder. The entire urothelium is positive for AGR2 expression as shown by immunostaining [18] (**Figure 1**). If AGR2 is secreted, then a substantial amount of this protein would be found in voided urine. In fact, little AGR2 is released by normal iAGR2$^+$ urothelial cells as detected by ELISA [18]. This result was supported by urine proteome database queries that AGR2 was not listed in the *UrinePA-PeptideAtlas* of 2,500 proteins profiled by large-scale proteomics [29], and in the core urinary proteome of 587 proteins obtained from healthy people [30]. In contrast, we found that AGR2$^+$ bladder cancer cells secreted AGR2. Urine from a bladder cancer patient was scored 7.5-fold higher than buffer control for AGR2. Five of 20 bladder cancer patient urine in one cohort were tested positive (AUC = 0.75), which matched the 25% bladder cancer being positive for AGR2 expression [18]. Our urine assay also detected AGR2 secreted by prostate cancer producing a similar AUC [31]. For serum, level of AGR2 is near background in healthy people [32]. Query of the *PeptideAtlas* database yielded very low AGR2 signature peptide counts. However, when sera of five prostate cancer patients were analyzed for AGR2, there was a strong correlation, $R^2 = 0.93$, found between levels of AGR2 (in pg/ml) and those of PSA (in ng/ml) [32]. This result would not be possible if there was a basal level of blood AGR2 arising from possible secretion by AGR2$^+$ cells of normal tissue such as the urothelium and lung epithelium into the circulatory system [32].

4. Differential expression of AGR2 in prostate cancer – primary vs. metastasis

AGR2 in prostate cancer shows two seemingly conflicting features in tumor biology. High expression in primary tumors is linked to better patient survival. Together with cell surface CD10 (membrane metallo-endopeptidase), four cancer phenotypes can be distinguished: AGR2$^+$CD10$^-$, AGR2$^-$CD10$^+$, AGR2$^-$CD10$^-$, and AGR2$^+$CD10$^+$; normal luminal cells are AGR2$^-$CD10$^+$. For high-grade disease, the AGR2$^+$CD10$^-$ phenotype is associated with a near 10-fold survival advantage than that of AGR2$^-$CD10$^+$; those of AGR2$^-$CD10$^-$ and AGR2$^+$CD10$^+$ in between [27]. Not unexpectedly, a majority of these tumors were typed AGR2$^-$CD10$^+$ (**Figure 2**). It appears that CD10 plays an important role in the extraprostatic

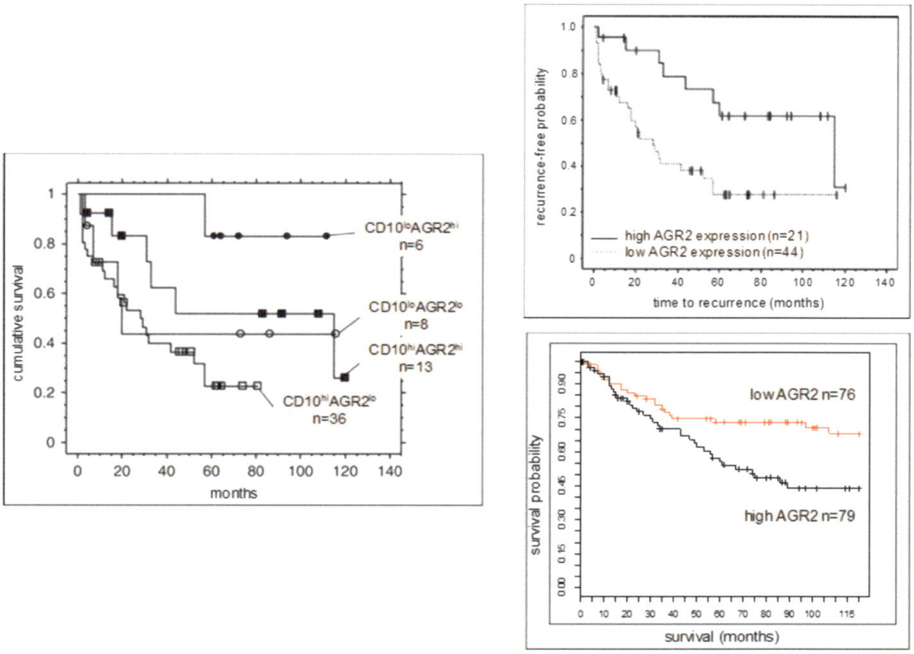

Figure 2.
AGR2 expression and patient survival. Left: the plot shows the outcome of high-stage patients grouped by AGR2 and CD10. At 5 years, 85% of AGR2^{hi}CD10^{lo} were recurrence-free compared with just 25% of AGR2^{lo}CD10^{hi}. Right: survival analyses for prostate cancer (top) and lung cancer (bottom) patients (<65y) show a contrasting trend.

spread of cancer cells to local lymph nodes because cancer cells in involved regional lymph nodes are invariably CD10^{+}(AGR2$^{-/lo}$) [33]. Node metastasis-derived cancer cell line LNCaP and patient-derived xenograft (PDX) LuCaP 35 are CD10^{+}AGR2^{-} and CD10^{+}AGR2^{lo}, respectively. A notable feature is the localization of CD10 to cell interior in cancer cells of higher grades where it appears to interact with cytosolic heat shock proteins [34]. As in the case for AGR2, CD10 has extracellular eCD10 and intracellular iCD10, but in this case, iCD10 is specific to cancer cells. This suggests that protein trafficking is abnormal in cancer cells. AGR2 expression is also associated with prostate cancer differentiation, with Gleason grade 3 (well-differentiated) cancer cells showing a 10-fold higher level than Gleason grade 4 (less differentiated) cancer cells [10]. Its association with lower tumor grade predicts better survival for patients harboring AGR2^{+} tumors [11] (**Figure 2**). Similarly, in breast cancer AGR2 is associated with better survival [35]. In contrast to AGR2, CD10 is more prominent in higher grade prostate tumors, and is associated with poorer survival for patients [33, 36].

However, most of the distal bone and soft tissue metastases contain cancer cells with the AGR2^{+}CD10^{-} phenotype, the exception being tumors of small cell carcinoma (AGR2^{-}CD10^{-}) [27], (**Figure 3**). PDX LuCaP lines established from samplings of these metastases are also AGR2^{+} [27]. These results underscore the important role of AGR2 in cancer spread as we reported for pancreatic cancer [37]. Possible mechanisms on how AGR2 promotes metastasis include disruption of epithelial cell adhesion, imparting invasive behavior to tumor cells [19], inducing apoptosis in susceptible normal cells by secreted AGR2 to undergo apoptosis [38], and through activating matrix metalloproteases, cathepsins B and D [37], which could facilitate tumor cells access to the circulatory system. Importantly, inhibition of AGR2 expression in lung cancer cells leads to their loss of metastatic capability [19].

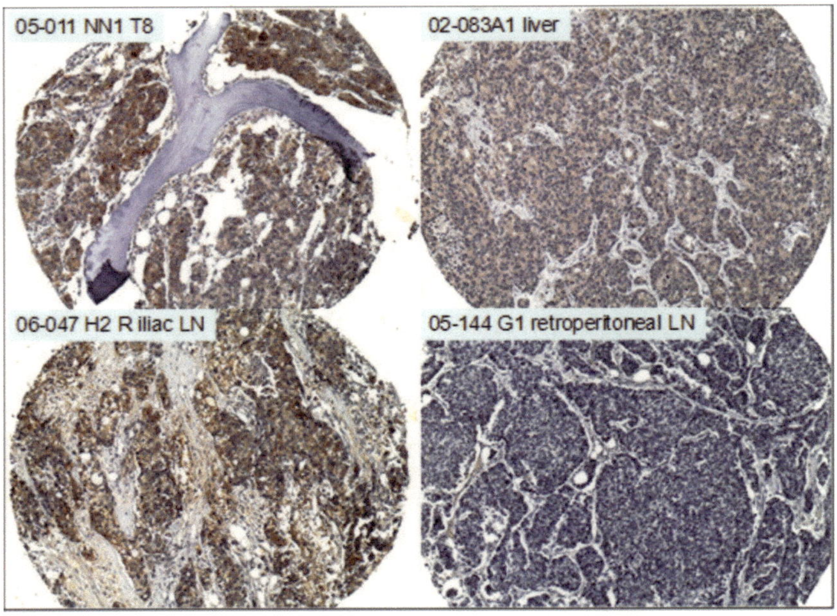

Figure 3.
AGR2 in prostate cancer metastases. Tumor cells in distal metastases – bone (top left), liver (top right), lymph node (bottom left) – are strongly stained for AGR2. A metastasis containing small cell carcinoma (bottom right) is not stained.

5. AGR2 in bladder cancer and lung cancer

Although 25% primary bladder tumors of a study cohort were found positive for AGR2, this percentage increased to 45% in the synchronous lymph node metastases [18]. The discordance between primary cancer and lymph node metastasis could involve a phenotypic change [39], which could occur in bladder cancer cells going from $AGR2^-$ to $AGR2^+$. AGR2 in bladder cancer, unlike prostate cancer, showed no link to patient survival in one cohort analyzed [18]. A role for CD10 in lymph node spread of bladder cancer was also not apparent [18]. Recently, UW Urology initiated the bladder cancer rapid autopsy program modeled on the Department's success in obtaining>40 prostate cancer LuCaP lines with various characteristics [40], and has established lines, dubbed CoCaB, from primary and metastatic urothelial cancer. To date, seven lines are available: CoCaB 1, CoCaB 8 urothelial carcinoma, CoCaB 11, CoCaB 19 squamous carcinoma, CoCaB 12 urothelial with sarcomatoid component; three lines from metastases of deceased patients: CoCaB 10 (liver metastasis) urothelial carcinoma, CoCaB 14.1 (omentum metastasis) and CoCaB 14.2 (liver metastasis) urothelial carcinoma with squamous features. These lines were profiled by RNAseq and exome sequencing. Notably, the lines derived from metastases showed high AGR2 expression (**Figure 4**). This is in line with our result on prostate cancer metastases where, except for small cell carcinoma, all tumors as well as the LuCaP lines derived from metastases showed high AGR2 expression [27]. Likewise, pancreatic cancer metastases invariably showed high AGR2 expression [37].

In non-small cell lung cancer, higher AGR2 expression in primary tumors is associated with a poorer outcome for patients under 65 [14, 19], though over 90% of the tumors are $AGR2^+$ (**Figure 2**). This is in contrast to the finding for prostate cancer. Thus, depending on the microenvironment, the metastatic function of AGR2 is not predominant in differentiated prostate tumors. When cancer cells have escaped the prostatic capsule (via CD10), AGR2 appears to be essential for distal

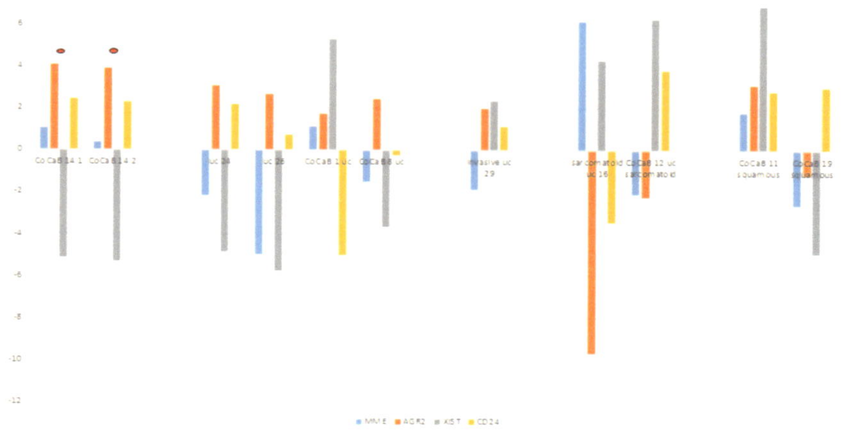

Figure 4.
Bladder cancer cell types. Cancer cell lines are identified on the x-axis (CoCaB and uc). Histogram represents fold in expression difference as scored by RNAseq signal values on the y-axis for MME/CD10, AGR2, XIST (X-inactive specific transcript) and CD24. The two CoCaB lines established from metastases are indicated by small red oval.

colonization of other organs for prostate cancer cells. In the disease course, AGR2 expression could be down- or up-regulated in cancer cells through mechanisms yet to be elucidated.

A meta-analysis of the published data on the clinical utility of AGR2 expression in various solid tumors summarizes the link to survival findings [41]. AGR2 expression in primary cancer can be associated with better survival for prostate cancer, no survival advantage in bladder cancer, poorer survival for lung cancer. While AGR2 in pancreatic cancer could have a significant impact in treating both early and advanced diseases, anti-AGR2 therapy in prostate cancer could prove promising in treating advanced disease as 96.4% metastatic lesions of adenocarcinoma being $AGR2^+$ against 0.7% of $AGR2^-$ small cell carcinoma and 2.9% of mixed carcinoma type [42].

6. Chimeric human:mouse AGR2 antibodies

Mouse monoclonal antibodies to AGR2 were generated by inoculating bacterially produced recombinant AGR2 in RBF/DnJ mice [20]. Two of eleven clones collected, P1G4 (mIgG1) and P3A5 (mIgG2a), were tested positive for binding to native AGR2. These antibodies perform well in immunostaining of frozen tissue sections but not formalin-fixed tissue. ELISA based on these two antibodies was able to detect 17 pg of cancer-secreted AGR2 in 100 μg of total urinary protein isolated from a patient diagnosed with a tumor of 5.5 cc in size [20].

Based on our published design [43], the mouse antibodies were converted to chimeric human:mouse. The mouse variable V_H and V_κ of P3A5 and P1G4 sequences were determined via reverse transcriptase-polymerase chain reaction (RT-PCR) with designed primers from mIg mRNA isolated from the respective hybridoma cell lines. The V sequences were-matched to known murine Ighv and Igkv genes. The human constant C_γ and C_κ domain cDNA were cloned by using designed primers from white blood cells of healthy donors. The hIg cDNA were verified by DNA sequencing and restriction enzyme digestion. The C_γ (digested by *Apa* I and *Bam* HI) and C_κ (*Hind* III and *Avr* II) modules were joined to the V_H (*Eco* RV and *Apa* I) and V_κ (*Bam* HI and *Hind* III) modules, respectively, in plasmid vector pVITRO1*neo*. Each cDNA contained a Kozak box. Plasmids of chimeric P1G4 hIgG1, hIgG2, hIgG4; P3A5 hIgG1, hIgG2, hIgG4 were generated [22]. The different Cγ plasmids could be distinguished by *Sac* II and *Eco* RI digestion. Cγ3 sequences were not detected in the cDNA prepared from 1 ml of blood.

Human embryonic kidney fibroblasts, HEK293F, were transfected by the hIgG plasmids, selected for G418 (neomycin) resistance and cloned. RT-PCR analysis of the transfected cells showed equivalent mRNA levels for the 560 bp neo, 720 bp IgL and 1420 bp IgH [22]. The culture media supernatant was assayed for AGR2 binding. P1G4 was used to capture AGR2 (secreted by eAGR2$^+$ prostate cancer LuCaP 147 in tissue collagenase digestion media to obtain single cells from minced tumor pieces) followed by P3A5 (positive control) and culture supernatant containing the chimeric antibodies. HRP-conjugated anti-mIgG2a or anti-hIgG were used for detection. The chimeric antibodies were found similar to P3A5 in AGR2 binding [22]. Untransfected 293F cells or transfected with a defective L-chain construct produced no binding. Media from serial culture passages showed that hIgG synthesis continued indicating stable integration of the transgenes into the host genome. The hIgG-producing clones were weaned from fetal bovine serum supplement, and cultured in the absence of drug for G418 is toxic. The serum-free growth media contained few other proteins (293F cells are non-secretory fibroblasts compared to hybridoma cells), and a spin-filtration step using a 30 K molecular weight cut-off could readily concentrate the 150 kDa IgG proteins [22]. If necessary, each antibody can be purified further on protein G-sepharose. The chimeric hIgG1, hIgG2, hIgG4 and mIgG2a P3A5 detected similar amounts of AGR2 secreted by different LuCaP lines: 147, 35CR, 86.2, 105 (**Figure 5**). Thus, these chimeric antibodies retain specific antigen binding and can be produced more economically via large-scale cell culture (instead that of hybridoma cells, which also produce a defective non-specific mouse light chain, and potentially infectious murine bioactive agents).

To increase the production of hIgG by transfected 293F cells, we transferred the different hIgG gene cassettes into plasmid vector pVITRO1*bsr* (encoding blasticidin resistance). Selected hIgG-producing neo^R clones were transfected by the *bsr* constructs and selected for blasticidin resistance. The resultant neo^{R}bsr^R clones showed increased amounts of secreted hIgG in the culture media due to the increased gene dosage [22].

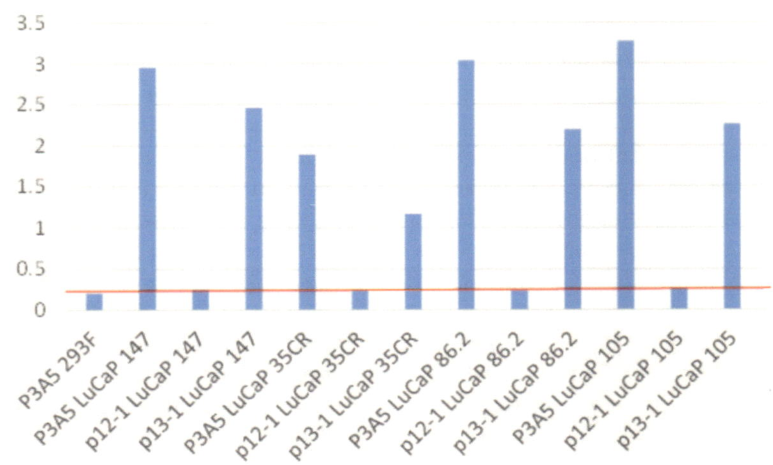

Figure 5.
Chimeric IgG binding to AGR2. Both chimeric (transfected HEK clone p13–1) and P3A5 detect varying amounts of AGR2 secreted by different LuCaP PDX lines. Clone p12–1 is a defective construct that produced untranslated L chain mRNA. Similar binding was also shown by the other IgG types. The absorbance units of ELISA are on the y-axis.

7. Cancer cell surface expression of eAGR2 and tumor localization

To demonstrate cancer cell surface expression, we used flow cytometry with our obtained monoclonal antibodies. The mouse Agr2$^+$ pancreatic cell line DT6606 [44], derived from an engineered C57BL/6 mouse strain to develop pancreatic cancer [45], was incubated with P3A5 followed by dye-conjugated anti-mIgG2a. Antibody binding to the cell surface was indicated by fluorescence shift (*vs*. isotype-matched control) [22]. Most available anti-human AGR2 antibodies, like P3A5, recognize both human AGR2 and murine Agr2 as the two proteins share a high degree of sequence homology. Human pancreatic cells were previously shown to have cell surface expression of eAGR2 using a different antibody [37].

To demonstrate tumor localization, ^{111}In-radiolabeled P3A5 was injected into mice carrying DT6606 tumors. At 48 h post-injection, the implanted tumors showed intense labeling (**Figure 6**). There was minimal labeling of the iAgr2$^+$ bladder or lung, or elsewhere [22]. The imaging confirmed cancer cell surface localization as well as cancer cell specificity of eAgr2. The cross-reactivity between human AGR2 and mouse Agr2 allowed one to speculate that a similar result would be obtained in human patients, i.e., specific localization to eAGR2$^+$ pancreatic (or other solid) tumors and not to iAGR2$^+$ organs. With cancer-specific localization, there is a strong likelihood that ant-AGR2 would be highly effective against cancer with minimal reactivity towards non-cancer tissue.

8. Enhancement of chemodrug inhibition of tumor by antibody

Our P1G4 antibody was found to possess a clinically useful property. Using eAGR2$^+$ pancreatic PDX in mice, the combination of pancreatic cancer drug Gemcitabine (Gem) and P1G4 (P1) reduced tumor growth compared to Gem alone. This difference was statistically significant ($P < 0.05$) [22]. Immunostaining for Ki67 indicated less (AGR2$^+$) tumor cell proliferation in P1 + Gem, which was manifested by the size of the corresponding resected tumors (**Figure 7**). ELISA indicated that serum AGR2 levels could be correlated with tumor burden. Once Gem was discontinued, the tumors in the Gem-only group relapsed immediately, and grew at a faster rate than those in the P1 + Gem group despite an effectively reduced antibody concentration as antibody treatment was terminated after 28 days. The combination of P3A5 (P3) and Gem showed no such enhancement. Parenthetically, our data also confirmed that Agr2 was not secreted from normal mouse organs into blood. The

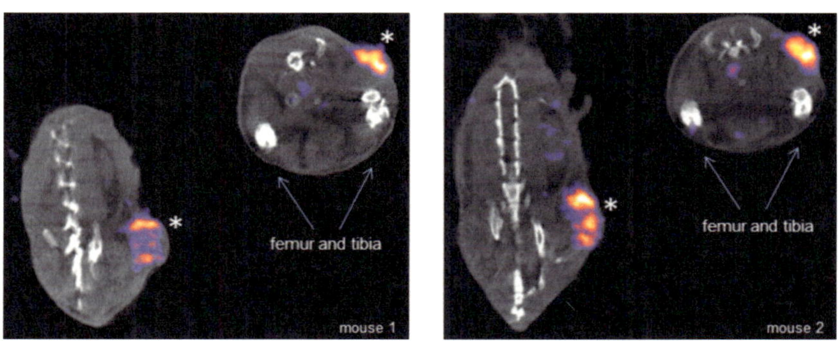

Figure 6.
Tumor localization of P3A5. The SPECT/CT scans show specific uptake of radiolabeled P3A5 by Agr2$^+$ DT606 tumors (*) in two C57BL/6 mice.

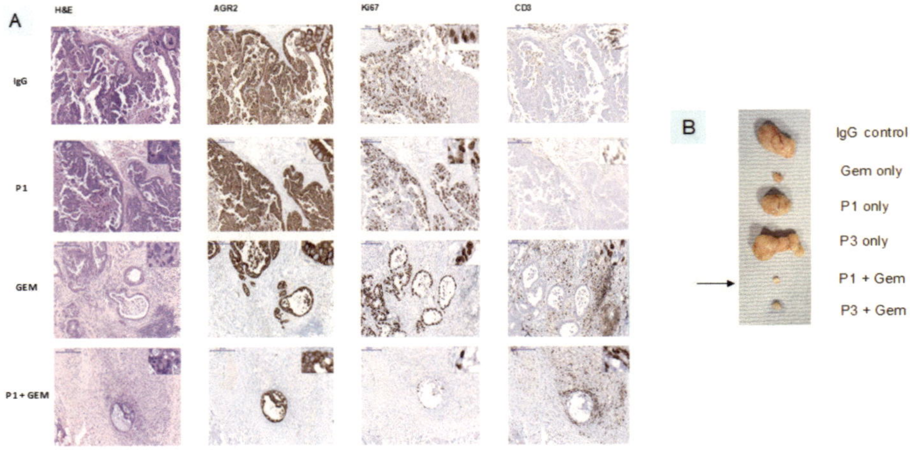

Figure 7.
Drug inhibition of tumor growth enhancement by P1G4. (A) Representative immunohistochemistry images show the effect (from top to bottom) of IgG control, P1G4 (P1) alone, Gemcitabine (GEM) alone, P1 + GEM. Ki67 staining indicates that tumors treated with drug still had high proliferation rate, which was limited in P1 + GEM tumors. CD3 shows T cell infiltration in the GEM and P1 + GEM groups. (B) Tumors resected at week 6 from the different treatment groups are compared. The smallest size is found in the P1 + GEM group (arrowed).

internal organs of liver, spleen, stomach, intestine, colon, and pancreas were histologically examined, and no visible pathologic changes were identified. The sparing of organs in anti-AGR2 tumor targeting was also reported by another group [46]. The mechanism behind this epitope-dependent phenomenon is unknown but could be related to a reported observation of increased tumor inhibition by an antibody to AGR3 in combination with the chemodrug cisplatin [47]. AGR3 is a close family member of AGR2. Both AGR2 and AGR3 tend to be elevated in cancer, though to different levels as found in prostate cancer [10]. The combination of monoclonal antibody plus biological inhibitors are being pursued to treat more successfully non-small cell lung cancer [48].

9. Tumor cell lysis in vitro

In our earlier work, ^{51}Cr radiolabeled target cancer cells were exposed to TAA antibodies and human serum (as a source of complement factors) or peripheral blood leukocytes [43, 49]. By CDC, the chimeric antibody generated higher cytotoxicity at all complement dilutions. By ADCC, at a ratio of 100:1 blood leukocytes to target cells, the chimeric lysed a greater fraction of the cancer cells and gave 50% cytolysis at 100-fold lower concentration than the mouse antibody. ADCC was observed at a 3:1 ratio of effector to target cells when the chimeric (at 2.5 μg/ml) was used. Cell killing was specific because ADCC was not observed with cell lines lacking the target antigen.

To test the anti-tumor effect of chimeric antibodies, we incubated PC3 prostate cancer cell line in the presence of donated human serum. Like pancreatic cancer cells, cell surface expression of eAGR2 was found on PC3 cells. Spin-concentrated chimeric IgG was used with human serum for CDC. PC3 cells were incubated with freshly donated human serum and added AGR2 antibodies. There was no observable effect on cell viability in the culture well with human serum only, as was the well with mouse P3A5 + serum. In the well with a cocktail of chimeric IgG1, IgG2, and IgG4, cell growth was inhibited with well surface showing areas devoid of cells, and clusters of pyknotic cells in suspension [22]. We postulate that a combination of IgG subtypes would be more effective than IgG1 alone since our normal immune response produces these IgG types, each exhibiting a unique profile with respect to immune complex formation, complement activation, recruitment of effector cells, and half-life [50]. For example, strong antitumor activities were observed for an IgG3 antibody targeting a melanoma-associated ganglioside [51]. We did not obtain chimeric IgG3 for our monoclonal antibodies. We will attempt to clone $C_{\gamma}3$ from a larger volume of blood or a pool of several donations using γ3-specific primer oligonucleotides. Our cloned human C_{γ} and C_{κ} can accept any new V_H and V_L of antibodies developed against novel TAA.

10. Antibody-drug conjugation

In addition to antibodies that rely on immune system components, a cytotoxic drug can be linked directly to the AGR2 antibodies to produce an antibody-drug conjugate (ADC). ADC delivers the drug payload to the target organs or tissues [52]. For anti-AGR2 ADC, drug compounds were constructed by covalently linking poly(N-isopropylacrylamide) to both P1G4 and P3A5 via carbodiimide chemistry. The linking polymer was synthesized by reversible addition fragmentation chain transfer (RAFT) with a carboxylate chain end [53]. To conjugate antibodies, the carboxylate was converted to an active ester for formation of an amide bond to lysine residues [53–56]. We have also developed a block copolymer with tetrafluorophenyl (TFP) ester monomers to drive the antibody conjugation [57]. The resulting anti-AGR2 ADC were confirmed by gel electrophoresis, which showed the larger molecular weight products compared to the unconjugated antibodies (**Figure 8**). After the size-exclusion chromatography, the purified ADC were shown by ELISA to bind AGR2 (**Figure 8**). Sample solutions containing a constant AGR2 concentration were mixed with ADC from 125 to 1,000 ng/ml. ELISA measured the unbound AGR2 with higher ADC concentrations resulting in less free AGR2 in the solution. Thus, our conjugation chemistry did not affect appreciably the antigen binding affinity of the antibodies. Polymer chains with improved loading capacity by incorporating functional groups [58] could be developed for conjugation to docetaxel, doxorubicin, and other drugs. To improve delivery efficiency, the polymer can be engineered to increase circulation time, and the polymer composition can be modulated.

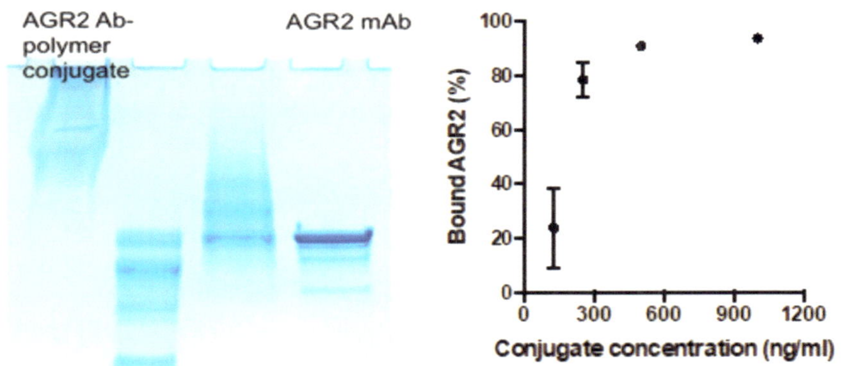

Figure 8.
Antibody drug conjugate. The left panel shows the conjugated products (lane 1) vs. unconjugated antibody (lane 4). The right plot shows more AGR2 bound (percentage, y-axis) with higher ADC concentrations of the conjugate (in ng/ml, x-axis).

11. Adaptation of PDX LuCaP lines to in vitro culture

For therapeutic testing, the LuCaP series of >40 different models established from patient tumor samples donated at autopsies and surgeries provide an invaluable resource than long-used cultured cell lines. They have been molecularly and pharmacologically characterized, and encompass a large spectrum of the disease course and representative of human prostate cancer [39]. Transcriptomics and genomics data have shown that the gene expression of these cancer cells was concordant with that of the human tumors from which they originated. Indeed, these models were used in the preclinical study to determine efficacy of anti-prostate-specific membrane antigen (PSMA) ADC as they show a range of PSMA expression [59]. For AGR2, concordant expression has been determined by DNA microarrays [40], immunostaining [27], and ELISA measurement of secreted AGR2 [20, 38]. Similar to prostate cancer patient specimens, the adenocarcinoma lines are positive for AGR2 while the small cell carcinoma including some non-adenocarcinoma are negative or low for AGR2.

Their utility could be increased if they can be grown outside the mouse for in vitro testing of ADCC and CDC. We showed that LuCaP cells prepared from freshly excised tumors could be successfully cultured long-term in the presence of irradiated mouse embryonic fibroblasts (MEF) as feeder [60]. Furthermore, LuCaP cells could be viably frozen using a protocol for stem cells [60], which makes constant harvests from animals unnecessary. Both adenocarcinoma and small cell carcinoma LuCaP lines could be thus grown in culture (unpublished data). The in vitro-adapted cell lines with differential AGR2 expression could be used to determine the molecular mechanism controlling AGR2 expression in cancer cells. The same methodology can be used to adapt CoCaB cells for in vitro growth and testing.

12. Future work and developments

12.1 Preclinical testing of chimeric antibodies

With the availability of chimeric antibodies and ADC, we can carry out animal studies to assess safety and efficacy of anti-AGR2 therapy, especially in PDX models available in prostate and bladder cancers. The LuCaP lines recapitulate the molecular heterogeneity of metastatic castration-resistant prostate cancer. Overall, a majority of molecular events characterized in human prostate tumors are found in LuCaP such as *AR* amplification, *PTEN* loss, *RB1* deletion, DNA damage response deficiencies [40, 61]. These LuCaP lines can be selected for study: AGR2$^+$ LuCaP 23.1, 35, 136, 147 and AGR2$^-$ LuCaP 145.1 to test P1G4-ADC, P3A5-ADC, P1G4 + docetaxel, P3A5 + docetaxel. With regard to AGR2 expression, LuCaP 23.1 and LuCaP 147 have relatively high levels, while small cell carcinoma LuCaP 145.1 as control has no expression [27]. Complete effect from anti-AGR2 would be expected for the former examples and no effect for the latter. For IgG control, we can transfect 293F cells with a construct containing H chain of P3A5 and L chain of P1G4 or H chain of P1G4 and L chain of P3A5, which would be expected to produce an AGR2 non-binding V domain. Green fluorescence protein (GFP)-labeled chimeric antibodies could be used for tumor localization (to show no labeling of iAgr2$^+$ normal organs) in place of radioisotopes, if necessary, to add to our pancreatic cancer PDX result. The study will also test if P1G4 has an enhancement effect in tumor growth inhibition by docetaxel as shown by this antibody in the Gemcitabine study. Response by LuCaP lines to docetaxel treatment varied substantially [40]. A high dose (20 mg/kg) generally produced growth suppression and survival benefits.

Only LuCaP 86.2 showed response at a low dose. Others like LuCaP 35 showed reduced survival as monitored by body weight loss despite tumor growth inhibition. We will test whether the response to docetaxel will be less variable and more pronounced with the addition of P1G4 (but not P3A5). The P1G4-docetaxel ADC may act in an equivalent way as P1G4 + docetaxel. Docetaxel was the first chemotherapeutic drug shown to prolong patient survival, and is in widespread use [62].

The different anti-AGR2-ADC are tested through intraperitoneal injection twice a week for four weeks. In our pancreatic cancer study, a 5 mg/kg antibody concentration was shown to be effective in the P1G4 + Gemcitabine arm. LuCaP tumor volume and body weight are monitored, and treatment will last four weeks. Tumors are collected at study end for histology, and the internal organs are examined for anti-Agr2 effect, if any. Serum is collected for AGR2 measurements by ELISA. Serum PSA may also be measured to see if there is concordance between these two biomarkers. Other parameters to try include higher antibody concentration, longer treatment time. The in vitro adapted LuCaP cells will allow us to determine the effective dose of serum and effector cell donations from multiple individuals (and if available, blood from cancer patients whose immune response may be compromised by their disease) in CDC and ADCC, respectively, mediated by the chimeric IgG. The optimal antibody concentration (μg/ml) for 10^6 cancer cells is determined. It is possible that a higher dose is required since AGR2 is secreted by the tumor cells where a portion of the antibodies might be bound to the free antigen. This in vitro assay is in effect an immune system model for the human body. PDX lines can also be grown as spheroids/organoids in vitro [63]. Organoids could be used to represent a solid tumor mass *vs*. monolayer culture to test the efficacy of chimeric antibodies.

In the past years, an ADC to PSMA was shown to produce clinically relevant decline in serum PSA and circulating tumor cell counts in metastatic castration resistant, taxane-experienced and chemo-naived prostate cancer patients [64]. At a working dose of 2.3 mg/kg, side effects reported in some patients include neutropenia, fatigue, electrolyte imbalance, anemia and neuropathy. A small number died from disease progression. PSMA is a membrane metalloenzyme (FOLH1) found in the kidney, small intestine, central and peripheral nervous systems [65]. Non-exclusivity of this TAA to prostate cancer likely accounts for the range of side effects observed. The co-targeting of normal cells has led to recall of, for example, gemtuzumab because of severe complications since the TAA, CD30, is present on both leukemic blast and normal cells [66]. Importantly, not all prostate cancer cells express PSMA. Anti-PSMA-MMAE (monomethyl auristatin E) was shown less or not effective against tumors with low or null PSMA expression [59]. In this efficacy study using LuCaP cells, complete tumor regression for LuCaP 96CR with the highest PSMA expression was found, and no response for LuCaP 58 with the lowest PSMA expression [59]. However, intermediate effect was found for LuCaP 77 and LuCaP 105, two lines with similar PSMA expression levels as LuCaP 96CR. Why the difference was not explained. Thus, the inherent pitfall in prescribing anti-PSMA therapy by itself is selection of PSMA-negative tumors. Nonetheless, this PSMA ADC is currently under large clinical trials [64, 67].

The rationale of our developing a second prostate cancer immunoreagent is that anti-eAGR2 could complement anti-PSMA when used in combination, which could be effective against $PSMA^-AGR2^+$, $PSMA^+AGR2^-$, and $PSMA^+AGR2^+$ cancer cells. Note LuCaP 35 is negative for PSMA. This particular model is used to show whether anti-AGR2 will inhibit its growth where anti-PSMA could not. Two other attributes additionally bolster our rationale. eAGR2, unlike PSMA, is tumor-specific as normal cells do not express eAGR2, and metastatic prostate cancer cells express high levels of eAGR2. The two AGR2 epitopes (P1G4 and P3A5) targeted could also ensure that allelic changes in one of the epitopes will not affect susceptibility of the cancer to anti-AGR2. For bladder cancer, we will carry out a similar study employing the AGR2⁺ CoCaB lines to test the ADC and P1G4 + cisplatin. Cisplatin is more commonly used to treat this cancer, sometimes in combination with Gemcitabine [68]. In vitro-adapted CoCaB lines are similarly used for CDC and ADCC testing.

Cancer treatment by antibody is well established and proven to be effective. One good example is trastuzumab to target HER2/EGFR (CD340) for a subset of breast cancer and non-small cell lung cancer [69, 70]. The major obstacle to more success in antibody therapy is the time-consuming need to discover TAA for each type of cancer that at a minimum is expressed by only a few normal cell types. eAGR2 is not only expressed in prostate cancer cells but also multiple tumor types so that anti-AGR2 would have a much wider application than just treating one or two cancers. Our experiments will demonstrate the validity of this claim.

12.2 Lineage relationship between $AGR2^+$ and $AGR2^-$ prostate cancer

The use of anti-AGR2 might lead to the selection of $AGR2^{lo/-}$ non-adenocarcinoma cancer including small cell carcinoma. The introduction of newer anti-androgen therapies of late has led to an almost 20% patients presenting small cell carcinoma at treatment failure [71]. Of critical importance is finding a means to prevent the emergence of $AGR2^-$ tumors.

Figure 9 shows our model of prostate cancer differentiation relating luminal-like $AGR2^+$ adenocarcinoma to $AGR2^-$ more stem-like small cell carcinoma [72]. Stem-like cancer cells could arise from de-differentiation of luminal-like cancer cells. This process is akin to reprogramming of somatic cells via forced expression of a set of stem cell transcription factors (scTF) to induced pluripotent stem (iPS) cells [73]. We demonstrated that prostate adenocarcinoma cells could be so reprogrammed to stem-like, small cell carcinoma-like derivatives with scTF LIN28A, NANOG, POU5F1, SOX2 [60]. A relevant clinical finding is that tumors with Gleason score ≥ 8, i.e., less differentiated, tended to show a shorter interval to the emergence of small cell carcinoma [74], as the non-glandular tumor cells are closer to stem-like in lineage. On the other hand, stem-like cancer cells could be induced to differentiate into luminal-like cancer cells by prostate stromal mesenchyme cell factors [75]. From early tissue recombinant studies, stromal cells were found to determine the specificity of urologic organ development [76, 77]. Thus, prostate stromal cells would induce stem/progenitor cells, regardless of tissue origin, to differentiate into prostate; bladder stromal cells into bladder. This induction involves secreted factors and heterotypic cell contact. We identified proenkephalin (PENK, 267 aa) and stanniocalcin 1 (STC1, 247 aa) as prostate stromal-specific genes encoding

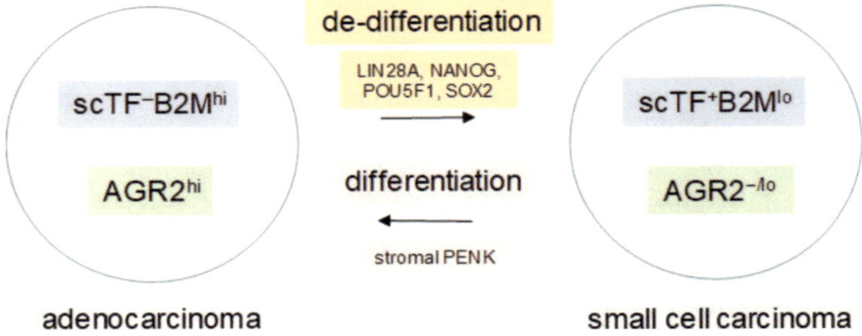

Figure 9.
Lineage of prostate cancer cell types. Luminal-like, non-stem-like adenocarcinoma $AGR2^{hi}$, $scTF^-B2M^{hi}$ and stem-like $AGR2^{-/lo}$, $scTF^+B2M^{lo}$ small cell carcinoma are related by de-differentiation with activation of scTF. The reverse of the process can be triggered by stromal cell factors such as PENK.

secreted hormones [78]. When cultured stem-like cells were incubated with prostate stromal cell conditioned media (containing stromal secreted molecules) PENK and STC1 were specifically induced in the differentiating stem cells. The resultant cells showed a change in colony morphology as well as one in transcriptome [79]. PENK was not induced by $PENK^-$ bladder stromal cell or $PENK^-$ prostate cancer-associated stromal cell conditioned media [79, 80]. The absence of PENK in the stroma of tumor foci suggests that it could be an underlying contributing cause of cancer development.

PENK cDNA (803 bp) was cloned from microdissected benign prostate tissue [10], and was transfected into small cell carcinoma LuCaP 145.1 cells. LuCaP 145.1 is stem-like because of its expression of scTF, which are, as a quartet, absent in non-stem-like LuCaP adenocarcinoma lines [60, 81]. In addition, LuCaP 145.1 was found to share expression of other genes with stem cells, including the down-regulation of β2-microglobulin (B2M) [60, 81, 82]. Forced expression of PENK in LuCaP 145.1 down-regulated the scTF, and up-regulated in tandem B2M [75]. Thus, a phenotypic change of stem-likeness ($scTF^+B2M^{lo}$) exhibited by LuCaP 145.1 to a phenotype ($scTF^{lo/-}B2M^{hi}$) more characteristic of differentiated cancer cells was produced by PENK. In other words, PENK can counteract the activity of scTF. Therefore, PENK and other stromal factors could be envisioned as effective agents in differentiation therapy to maintain adenocarcinoma in the differentiated state with high AGR2 expression.

The effect of PENK on AGR2 expression could be seen when $scTF^-B2M^{hi}$ adenocarcinoma LuCaP 70CR (CR = castration resistant, a variant obtained from passages in castrated mice) was transfected by PENK. An increase in the expression of AGR2 was observed [75]. Increased production by LuCaP 70CR/PENK was validated by measurement of secreted AGR2 in the cell-free culture media [75]. The change in AGR2 expression indicated cancer cell differentiation induced from $AGR2^{lo}$ to $AGR2^{hi}$ by PENK in LuCaP 70CR. In contrast, AGR2 expression was down-regulated in reprogrammed LuCaP 70CR by scTF transfection to small cell carcinoma-like [60]. These results show that preventing or even reversing prostate cancer de-differentiation from luminal-like $scTF^-B2M^{hi}AGR2^{hi}$ to stem-like $scTF^+B2M^{lo}AGR2^-$ through stromal factor influence could keep anti-AGR2 therapy a viable treatment option in the disease course.

12.3 Cancer vaccine based on cancer-specificity of eAGR2

The cancer specificity of eAGR2 could allow us to develop a cancer vaccine in the future. Treated patients can be immunized by AGR2. Any emergent cells with eAGR2 expression are, by reasoning, cancerous and will be eliminated by a primed immune system. The result shown in **Figure 6** indicates no iAgr2-positive mouse organs were targeted outside non-specific background, which was non-overlapping in the study mice. Besides the bladder and lung, the intestinal tract containing $Agr2^+$ mucus-producing cells [83] also did not show labeling. Secreted AGR2 is known to function in early development where it signals cell differentiation such as that described in limb regeneration of lower vertebrates [84]. Introduction of AGR2 was reported to accelerate wound healing through recruitment of fibroblasts and migration of keratinocytes [85]. So a possibility exists that AGR2-immunized patients would experience difficulty in tissue repair after damage. For these patients, one could treat injuries with local administration of AGR2 protein.

To show the potential of an AGR2 cancer vaccine, we could immunize C57BL/6 mice with recombinant (r)AGR2 as was done in the generation of P1G4 and P3A5 (although a different mouse strain was used) [20]. After rAGR2 injection, mice are boosted at intervals and bled for ELISA testing of serum anti-AGR2 activity.

IgM-to-IgG switch is monitored. Once an adequate antibody titer is measured, syngeneic mouse bladder cancer cells MB49 [86] are implanted *vs*. into control animals without AGR2 immunization. MB49 was derived from DMBA-transformed (presumably iAgr2$^+$) bladder epithelial cells of C57BL. Whether these cancer cells express eAgr2 will be determined. If eAgr2 is not detected, we can transfect these cells with our AGR2 plasmid construct (550-bp full length cDNA cloned from prostate cancer tissue). AGR2$^-$ LNCaP cells when transfected by this plasmid produced secreted and cell surface AGR2 [81]. Note we do not need to transfect the murine Agr2 gene because the antibodies produced would recognize both human AGR2 and mouse Agr2 as shown for P3A5. We expect that the immunized mice would show no tumor growth. AGR2 vaccination will, in principle, prevent recurrence and metastasis.

12.4 AGR2 antibody in early detection

Since AGR2 expression is an early event in cancer, AGR2 antibodies could be used in early detection through imaging for example. Small foci of eAGR2$^+$ lung or pancreatic tumor can be visualized through binding of labeled chimeric P1G4. The antibody might even eradicate the detected tumors through ADCC and CDC. The iAGR2$^+$ non-involved lung epithelium would not be detected, and as would AGR2$^-$ pancreatic cells. Proposed studies will determine the minimum number of cells in a tumor mass to produce a detectable signal. Given the pg/ml detection levels of our antibodies and the high levels of AGR2 in cancer cells, this potential clinical application is promising. In addition, one could envision a reliable blood test on cancer-secreted AGR2 as a means towards cancer detection and disease monitoring.

Acknowledgements

We thank our colleagues for their contribution to the research that resulted in this writing. We thank Dr. Eva Corey and the UW Genitourinary Laboratory for help in the establishment of bladder cancer PDX lines and for donating the LuCaP tumors for study. Our research was supported in part by UW CoMotion Fund, NCI grant U01CA111244, DoD W81XWH-16-1-0614.

Author details

Alvin Y. Liu[1]*, Tatjana Crnogorac-Jurcevic[3], James J. Lai[4] and Hung-Ming Lam[2]

1 Department of Urology and Institute for Stem Cell and Regenerative Medicine, University of Washington, USA

2 Department of Urology, University of Washington, USA

3 Centre for Cancer Biomarkers and Biotherapeutics, Barts Cancer Institute, Queen Mary University of London, UK

4 Department of Bioengineering, University of Washington, USA

*Address all correspondence to: aliu@uw.edu

References

[1] Rawla P. Epidemiology of prostate cancer. *World J Oncol* 2019, **10**:63-89. doi 10.14740/wjon119.1

[2] Rawla P, Sunkara T, Gaduputi V. Epidemiology of pancreatic cancer: global trends, etiology and risk factors. *World J Oncol* 2019, **10**:10-27. doi: 10.14740/wjon1166

[3] Saginala K, Barsouk A, Aluru JS, Rawla P, Padala SA, Barsouk A. Epidemiology of bladder cancer. *Med Sci* 2020, **8**:15. doi: 10.3390/medsci8010015

[4] Baxevanis CN, Papamichail M, Perez SA. Prostate cancer vaccines: the long road to clinical application. *Cancer Immunol Immunother*, 2015, **64**:401-408. doi: 10.1007/s00262-015-1667-7

[5] Santos PB, Patel HR. Prostate stem cell antigen – novel biomarker and therapeutic target? *Expert Rev Anticancer Ther* 2014, **14**:5-7. doi: 10.1586/14737140.2014.870481

[6] Goswami S, Aparicio A, Subudhi SK. Immune checkpoint therapies in prostate cancer. *Cancer J* 2016, **22**:117-120. doi: 10.1097/PPO.0000000000000176

[7] Zhang J, Looi KS, Tan EM. Identification of tumor-associated antigens (TAAs) as diagnostic and predictive biomarkers in cancer. *Methods Mol Biol* 2009, **520**:1-10. doi: 10.1007/978-1-60327-811-9_1

[8] Bournazos S, Chow SK, Abboud N, Casadevall A, Ravetch JV. Human IgG F_c domain engineering enhances antitoxin neutralizing antibody activity. *J Clin Invest* 2014 **124**:725-729. doi: 10.1172/JCI72676

[9] Derer S, Beurskens FJ, Rosner T, Peipp M, Valerius T. Complement in antibody-based tumor therapy. *Crit Rev Immunol* 2014, **34**:199-214. doi: 10.1615/critrevimmunol.2014009761

[10] Pascal LE, Vêncio RZN, Page LS, Liebeskind ES, Shadle CP, Troisch P, Marzolf B, True LD, Hood LE, Liu AY. Gene expression relationship between prostate cancer cells of Gleason 3, 4 and normal epithelial cells as revealed by cell type-specific transcriptomes. *BMC Cancer* 2009, **9**:452. doi: 10.1186/1471-2407-9-452

[11] Maresh EL, Mah V, Alavi M, Horvath S, Bagryanova L, Liebeskind ES, Knutzen LA, Zhou Y, Chia D, Liu AY, Goodglick L. Differential expression of anterior gradient gene AGR2 in prostate cancer. *BMC Cancer* 2010, **10**:680. doi: 10.1186/1471-2407-10-680

[12] Ramachandran V, Arumugam T, Wang H, Logsdon CD. Anterior gradient 2 is expressed and secreted during the development of pancreatic cancer and promotes cancer cell survival. *Cancer Res* 2008, **68**:7811-7818. doi: 10.1158/0008-5472.CAN-08-1320

[13] Ann P, Seagle BL, Shilpi A, Kandpal M, Shahabi S. Association of increased primary breast tumor *AGR2* with decreased disease-specific survival. *Oncotarget* 2018, **9**:23114-23125. doi: 10.18632/oncotarget.25225

[14] Alavi M, Mah V, Maresh EL, Bagryanova L, Horvath S, Chia D, Goodglick L, Liu AY. High expression of AGR2 in lung cancer is predictive of poor survival. *BMC Cancer* 2015, **15**:655. doi: 10.1186/s12885-015-1658-2

[15] Tian S, Hu J, Tao K, Wang J, Chu Y, Li J, Liu Z, Ding X, Xu L, Li Q, Cai M, Gao J, Shuai X, Wang G, Wang L, Wang Z. Secreted AGR2 promotes invasion of colorectal cancer cells via Wnt11-mediated non-canonical Wnt signaling. *Exp Cell Res* 2018, **364**:198-207. doi: 10.1016/j.yexcr.2018.02.004

[16] Ma S, Wang W, Huang C, Zhang W, Sun Z. Anterior gradient protein 2 expression in high grade head and neck squamous cell carcinoma correlated with cancer stem cell and epithelial mesenchymal transition. *Oncotarget* 2015, 6:8807-8821. doi: 10.18632/oncotarget.3556

[17] Armes JE, Davies CM, Wallace S, Taheri T, Perrin LC, Autelitano DJ. AGR2 expression in ovarian tumours: a potential biomarker for endometrioid and mucinous differentiation. *Pathology* 2013, **45**:49-54. doi: 10.1097/PAT.0b013e32835bd561

[18] Ho ME, True LD, Seiler R, Fleischmann A, Bagryanova L, Kim SR, Chia D, Goodglick L, Shimizu Y, Rosser CJ, Gao Y, Liu AY. Bladder cancer cells secrete while normal bladder cells express but do not secrete AGR2. *Oncotarget* 2016, 7:15747. doi: 10.18632/oncotarget.7400

[19] Fessart D, Domblides C, Avril T, Eriksson LA, Begueret H, Pineau R, Malrieux C, Dugot-Senant N, Lucchesi C, Chevet E, Delom F. Secretion of protein disulphide isomerase AGR2 confers tumorigenic properties. *eLIFE* 2016, **5**:e13887. doi: 10.7554/eLife.13887

[20] Wayner EA, Quek S, Ahmad R, Ho ME, Loprieno MA, Zhou Y, Ellis WJ, True LD, Liu AY. Development of an ELISA to detect the secreted prostate cancer biomarker AGR2 in voided urine. *Prostate* 2012, **72**:1023-1034. doi: 10.1002/pros.21508

[21] Clark DP, Pazdernik NJ. Immune technology. In: *Biotechnology* 2016, pp. 181-217. Elsevier. doi: 10.1016/B978-0-12-385015-7.00006-5

[22] Liu AY, Kanan AD, Radon TP, Shah S, Weeks ME, Foster JM, Sosabowski JK, Dumartin L, Crnogorac-Jurcevic T. AGR2, a unique tumor-associated antigen, is a promising candidate for antibody targeting. *Oncotarget* 2019, **10**:4276-4289. doi: 10.18632/*Oncotarget*.26945

[23] Magee MS, Snook AE. Challenges to chimeric antigen receptor (CAR)-T cell therapy for cancer. *Discov Med* 2014 **18**:265-271.

[24] Lee HJ, Hong CY, Kim MH, Lee YK, Nguyen-Pham TN, Park BC, Yang DH, Chung IJ, Kim HJ, Lee JJ. In vitro induction of anterior gradient-2-specific cytotoxic T lymphocytes by dendritic cells transduced with recombinant adenoviruses as a potential therapy for colorectal cancer. *Exp Mol Med* 2012, **44**:60-67. doi: 10.3858/emm.2012.44.1.006

[25] Liu AY, Vêncio RZN, Page LS, Ho ME, Loprieno MA, True LD. Bladder expression of CD cell surface antigens and cell-type-specific transcriptomes. *Cell Tissue Res* 2012, **348**:589-600. doi: 10.1007/s00441-012-1383-y

[26] Gupta A, Dong A, Lowe AW. AGR2 gene function requires a unique endoplasmic reticulum localization motif. *J Biol Chem* 2012, **287**:4773-4782. doi: 10.1074/jbc.M111.3051531

[27] Ho ME, Quek S, True LD, Morrissey C, Corey E, Vessella RL, Dumpit R, Nelson PS, Maresh EL, Mah V, Alavi M, Kim SR, Bagryanova L, Horvath S, Chia D, Goodglick L, Liu AY. Prostate cancer cell phenotypes based on AGR2 and CD10 expression. *Mod Pathol* 2013, **26**:849-859. doi: 10.1038/modpathol.2012.238

[28] Dumartin L, Alrawashdeh W, Trabulo SM, Radon TP, Steiger K, Feakins RM, di Magliano MP, Heeschen C, Esposito I, Lemoine NR, Crnogorac-Jurcevic T. ER stress protein AGR2 precedes and is involved in the regulation of pancreatic cancer initiation. *Oncogene* 2017, **36**:3094-3103. doi: 10.1038/onc.2016.459

[29] Farrah T, Deutsch EW, Omenn GS, Sun Z, Watts JD, Yamamoto T, Shteynberg D, Harris MM, Moritz RL. State of the human proteome in 2013 as viewed through PeptideAtlas: comparing the kidney, urine, and plasma proteomes for the biology- and disease-driven Human Proteome Project. *J Proteome Res* 2014, **13**:60-75. doi: 10.1021/pr4010037

[30] Nagaraj N, Mann M. Quantitative analysis of the intra- and inter-individual variability of the normal urinary proteome. *J Proteome Res* 2011, **10**:637-645. doi: 10.1021/pr100835s

[31] Shi T, Quek S, Gao Y, Nicora CD, Nie S, Fillmore TL, Liu T, Rodland KD, Smith RD, Leach RJ, Thompson IM, Vitello EA, Ellis WJ, Liu AY, Qian W. Multiplexed targeted mass spectrometry assays for prostate cancer-associated urinary proteins. *Oncotarget* 2017, **8**:101887-101898. doi: 10.18632/oncotarget.21710

[32] Shi T, Gao Y, Quek S, Fillmore TL, Nicora CD, Su D, Zhao R, Rodland KD, Liu T, Smith RD, Chan DW, Camp DG, Liu AY, Qian WJ. A highly sensitive targeted mass spectrometric assay for quantification of low-abundance AGR2 in human urine and serum. *J Proteome Res* 2014, **13**:875-882. doi: 10.1021/pr400912c

[33] Dall'Era MA, True LD, Siegel AF, Porter MP, Sherertz TM, Liu AY. Differential expression of CD10 in prostate cancer and its clinical implication. *BMC Urol* 2007, **7**:3. doi: 10.1186/1471-2490-7-3

[34] Dall'Era MA, Oudes A, Martin DB, Liu AY. Identification of HSP27 and HSP70 as CD10 binding proteins in prostate cancer cells. *Prostate* 2007, **67**:714-721. doi: 10.1002/pros.20558

[35] Fritzsche FR, Dahl E, Pahl S, Burkhardt M, Luo J, Mayordomo E, Gansukh T, Dankof A, Knuechel R, Denkert C, Winzer K, Dietel M, Kristiansen G. Prognostic relevance of AGR2 expression in breast cancer. *Clin Cancer Res* 2006, 12:1728-1734. doi: 10.1158/1078-0432.CCR-05-2057

[36] Fleischmann A, Schlomm T, Huland H, Köllermann J, Simon P, Mirlacher M, Salomon G, Chun FHK, Steiber T, Simon R, Sauter G, Graefen M, Erbersdobler A. Distinct subcellular expression patterns of neutral endopeptidase (CD10) in prostate cancer predict diverging clinical courses in surgically treated patients. *Clin Cancer Res* 2008, **14**:7838-7842. doi: 10.1158/1078-0432.CCR-08-1432

[37] Dumartin L, Whiteman HJ, Weeks ME, Hariharan D, Dmitrovic B, Iacobuzio-Donahue CA, Brentnall TA, Bronner MP, Feakins RM, Timms JF, Brennan C, Lemoine NR, Crnogorac-Jurcevic T. AGR2 is a novel surface antigen that promotes the dissemination of pancreatic cancer cells through regulation of cathepsins B and D. *Cancer Res* 2011, **71**:7091-7102. doi: 10.1158/0008-5472.CAN-11-1367

[38] Vitello EA, Quek S, Kincaid H, Fuchs T, Crichton DJ, Troisch P, Liu AY. Cancer-secreted AGR2 induces programmed cell death of normal cells. *Oncotarget* 2016, **7**:49425-49434. doi: 10.18632/oncotarget.9921

[39] Sjödahl G, Eriksson P, Lövgren K, Marzouka N, Bernardo C, Nordentoft I, Dyrskjøt L, Liedberg F, Höglund M. Discordant molecular subtype classification in the basal-squamous subtype of bladder tumors and matched lymph-node metastases. *Mod Pathol* 2018, **31**:1869-1881. doi: 10.1038/s41379-018-0096-5

[40] Nguyen HM, Vessella RL, Morrissey C, Brown LG, Coleman IM, Higano CS, Mostaghel EA, Zhang X, True LD, Lam HM, Roudier M, Lange PH, Nelson PS, Corey E. LuCaP prostate cancer patient-derived xenografts reflect the molecular

heterogeneity of advanced disease and serve as models for evaluating cancer therapeutics. *Prostate* 2017, 77:654-671. doi: 10.1002/pros.23313

[41] Tian S, Tao K, Hu J, Liu Z, Ding X, Chu Y, Cui J, Shuai X, Gao J, Cai K, Wang J, Wang G, Wang L, Wang Z. The prognostic value of AGR2 expression in solid tumours: a systematic review and meta-analysis. *Sci Rep* 2017, 7:15500. doi 10.1038/s41598-017-15757-z

[42] Robinson D, Van Allen EM, Wu YM, Schultz N, Lonigro RJ, Mosquera JM, Montgomery B, Taplin ME, Pritchard CC, Attard G, Beltran H, Abida W, Bradley RK, Vinson J, Cao X, Vats P, Kunju LP, Hussain M, Feng FY, Tomlins SA, Cooney KA, Smith DC, Brennan C, Siddiqui J, Mehra R, Chen Y, Rathkopf DE, Morris MJ, Solomon SB, Durack JC, Reuter VE, Gopalan A, Gao J, Loda M, Lis RT, Bowden M, Balk SP, Gaviola G, Sougnez C, Gupta M, Yu EY, Mostaghel EA, Cheng HH, Mulcahy H, True LD, Plymate SR, Dvinge H, Ferraldeschi R, Flohr P, Miranda S, Zafeiriou Z, Tunariu N, Mateo J, Perez-Lopez R, Demichelis F, Robinson BD, Schiffman M, Nanus DM, Tagawa ST, Sigaras A, Eng KW, Elemento O, Sboner A, Heath EI, Scher HI, Pienta KJ, Kantoff P, de Bono JS, Rubin MA, Nelson PS, Garraway LA, Sawyers CL, Chinnaiyan AM. Integrative clinical genomics of advanced prostate cancer. *Cell* 2015, **161**:1215-1228. doi: 10.1016/j.cell.2015.05.001

[43] Liu AY, Robinson RR, Hellström KE, Murray ED, Chang CP, Hellström I. Chimeric mouse-human IgG1 antibody that can mediate lysis of cancer cells. *Proc Natl Acad Sci USA* 1987, **84**:3439-3443. doi: 10.1073/pnas.84.10.3439

[44] Celesti G, Di Caro G, Bianchi P, Grizzi F, Marchesi F, 36. Basso G, Rahal D, Delconte G, Catalano M, Cappello P, Roncalli M, Zerbi A, Montorsi M, Novelli F, Mantovani A. Allavena P, Malesci A, Laghi L. Early expression of the fractalkine receptor CX3CR1 in pancreatic carcinogenesis. *Br J Cancer* 2013, **109**:2424-2433. doi: 10.1038/bjc.2013.565

[45] Hingorani SR, Wang L, Multani AS, Combs C, Deramaudt TB, Hruban RH, Rustgi AK, Chang S, Tuveson DA. *Trp53*^{R172H} and *Kras*^{G12D} cooperate to promote chromosomal instability and widely metastatic pancreatic ductal adenocarcinoma in mice. *Cancer Cell* 2005, 7:469-483. doi: 10.1016/j.ccr.2005.04.023

[46] Negi H, Merugu SB, Mangukiya HB, Li Z, Zhou B, Sehat Q, Kamle S, Yunus F, Mashausi DS, Wu Z, Li D. Anterior gradient-2 monoclonal antibody inhibits lung cancer growth and metastasis by upregulating p53 pathway and without exerting any toxicological effects: a preclinical study. *Cancer Lett* 2019, **449**:125-134. doi: 10.1016/j.canlet.2019.01.025

[47] Gray TA, MacLaine NJ, Michie CO, Bouchalova P, Murray E, Howie J, Hrstka R, Maslon MM, Nenutil R, Vojtesek B, Langdon S, Hayward L, Gourley C, Hupp TR. Anterior gradient-3: a novel biomarker for ovarian cancer that mediates cisplatin resistance in xenograft models. *J Immunol Methods* 2012, **378**:20-32. doi: 10.1016/j.jim.2012.01.013

[48] Silva APS, Coelho PV, Anazetti M, Simioni PU. Targeted therapies for the treatment of non-small-cell lung cancer: monoclonal antibodies and biological inhibitors. *Hum Vaccin Immunother* 2017, **13**:843-853. doi: 10.1080/21645515.2016.1249551

[49] Liu AY, Robinson RR, Murray ED, Ledbetter JA, Hellström I, Hellström KE. Production of a mouse-human chimeric monoclonal antibody to CD20 with potent F_c-dependent biologic activity. *J Immunol* 1987, **139**:3521-3526.

[50] Vidarsson G, Dekkers G, Rispens T. IgG subclasses and allotypes: from structure to effector functions. *Front*

Immunol 2014, **5**:520. doi: 10.3389/fimmu.2014.00520

[51] Hellström I, Brankovan V, Hellström KE. Strong antitumor activities of IgG3 antibodies to a human melanoma-associated ganglioside. *Proc Natl Acad Sci USA* 1985, **82**:1499-1502. doi: 10.1073/pnas.82.5.1499

[52] Ringsdorf H. Structure and properties of pharmacologically active polymers. *J Polym Sci Pol Sym* 1975, **51**:135-153.

[53] Hoffman JM, Stayton PS, Hoffman AS, Lai JJ. Stimuli-responsive reagent system for enabling microfluidic immunoassays with biomarker purification and enrichment. *Bioconjug Chem* 2015, **26**:29-38. doi: 10.1021/bc500522k

[54] Nehilla BJ, Hill JJ, Srinivasan S, Chen YC, Schulte TH, Stayton PS, Lai JJ. A stimuli-responsive, binary reagent system for rapid isolation of protein biomarkers. *Anal Chem* 2016, 88:10404-10410. doi: 10.1021/acs.analchem.6b01961

[55] Phan JC, Nehilla BJ, Srinivasan S, Coombs RW, Woodrow KA, Lai JJ. Human immunodeficiency virus (HIV) separation and enrichment via the combination of antiviral lectin recognition and a thermoresponsive reagent system. *Pharm Res-Dordr* 2016, 33:2411-2420. doi: 10.1007/s11095-016-1980-7

[56] Jauregui R, Srinivasan S, Vojtech LN, Gammill HS, Chiu DT, Hladik F, Stayton PS, Lai JJ. Temperature-responsive magnetic nanoparticles for enabling affinity separation of extracellular vesicles. *ACS Appl Mater Interfaces* 2018, 10:33847-33856. doi: 10.1021/acsami.8b09751

[57] Roy D, Nehilla BJ, Lai JJ, Stayton PS. Stimuli-responsive polymer-antibody conjugates via RAFT and tetrafluorophenyl active ester chemistry. *Acs Macro Lett* 2013, 2:132-136. doi: 10.1021/mz300620v

[58] Frankel M, Liwschitz Y, Zilkha A. Acyl chlorides of amino acids and peptides as monomers for the preparation of polymeric polypeptides. *J Amer Chem Soc* 1954, 76:2814-2816. doi: 10.1021/ja01639a062

[59] DiPippo VA, Olson WC, Nguyen HM, Brown LG, Vessella RL, Corey E. Efficacy studies of an antibody-drug conjugate PSMA-ADC in patient-derived prostate cancer xenografts. *Prostate* 2015, **75**:303-313. doi: 10.1002/pros.22916

[60] Borges GT, Vêncio EF, Quek S, Chen A, Salvanha DM, Vêncio RZN, Nguyen HM, Vessella RL, Cavanaugh C, Ware CB, Troisch P, Liu AY. Conversion of prostate adenocarcinoma to small cell carcinoma-like by reprogramming. *J Cell Physiol* 2016, **231**:2040-2047. doi: 10.1002/jcp.25313

[61] Kumar A, Coleman I, Morrissey C, Zhang X, True LD, Gulati R, Etzioni R, Bolouri H, Montgomery B, White T, Lucas JM, Brown LG, Dumpit RF, DeSarkar N, Higano C, Yu EY, Coleman R, Schultz N, Fang M, Lange PH, Shendure J, Vessella R, Nelson PS. Substantial interindividual and limited intraindividual genomic diversity among tumors from men with metastatic prostate cancer. *Nat Med* 2016, **22**:369-378. doi: 10.1038/nm.4053

[62] Petrylak DP, Tangen CM, Hussain MH, Lara PN, Jones JA, Taplin ME, Burch PA, Berry D, Moinpour C, Kohli M, Benson MC, Small EJ, Raghavan D, Crawford ED. Docetaxel and estramustine compared with mitoxantrone and prednisone for advanced refractory prostate cancer. *N Eng J Med* 2004, **351**:1513-1520. doi: 10.1056/NEJMoa041318

[63] Young SR, Saar M, Santos J, Nguyen HM, Vessella RL, Peehl DM.

Establishment and serial passage of cell cultures derived from LuCaP xenografts. *Prostate* 2013, **73**:1251-1262. doi: 10.1002/pros.22610

[64] Petrylak DP, Kantoff P, Vogelzang NJ, Mega A, Fleming MT, Stephenson JJ, Frank R, Shore ND, Dreicer R, McClay EF, Berry WR, Agarwal M, DiPippo VA, Rotshteyn Y, Stambler N, Olson WC, Morris SA, Israel RJ. Phase 1 study of PSMA ADC, an antibody-drug conjugate targeting prostate-specific membrane antigen, in chemotherapy-refractory prostate cancer. *Prostate* 2019, **79**:604-613. doi: 10.1002/pros.23765

[65] Barinka C, Šácha P, Sklenář J, Man P, Bezouška K, Slusher BS, Konvalinka J. Identification of the *N*-glycolysis sites in glutamate carboxypeptidase II necessary for proteolytic activity. *Protein Sci* 2004, **13**:1627-1635. doi: 10.1110/ps.04622104

[66] Bennett CL, Nebeker JR, Lyons A, Samone MH, Feldman MD, McKoy JM, Carson KR, Belknap SM, Trifilio SM, Shumock GT, Yamold PR, Davidson CJ, Evens AM, Kuzel TM, Parada JP, Cournoyer D, West DP, Sartor O, Tallman MS, Raisch DW. The Research on Adverse Drug Events and Reports (RADAR) project. *JAMA* 2005, **293**:2131-2140. doi: 10.1001/jama.293.17.2131

[67] Cho S, Zammarchi F, Williams DG, Havenith CEG, Monks NR, Tyrer P, D'Hooge F, Fleming R, Vashisht K, Dimasi N, Bertelli F, Corbett S, Adams L, Reinert HW, Dissanayake S, Britten CE, King W, Dacosta K, Tammali R, Schifferli K, Strout P, Korade M, Masson Hinrichs MJ, Chivers S, Corey E, Liu H, Kim S, Bander NH, Howard PW, Hartley JA, Coats S, Tice DA, Herbst R, van Berkel PH. Antitumor activity of MEDI3726 (ADCT-401), a pyrrolobenzodiazepine antibody-drug conjugate targeting PSMA, in preclinical models of prostate cancer. *Mol Cancer Ther* 2018, **17**:2176-2186. doi: 10.1158/1535-7163.MCT-17-0982

[68] Kamat AM, Hahn NM, Efstathiou JA, Lerner SP, Malmström P, Choi W, Guo CC, Lotan Y, Kassouf W. Bladder cancer. *Lancet* 2016, **388**:2796-2810. doi: 10.1016/S0140-6736(16)30512-8

[69] Tai W, Mahato R, Cheng K. The role of HER2 in cancer therapy and targeted drug delivery. *J Control Release* 2010, **146**:264-275. doi: 10.1016/j.jconrel.2010.04.009

[70] Pirker R, Filipits M. Monoclonal antibodies against EGFR in non-small cell lung cancer. *Crit Rev Oncol Hematol* 2011, **80**:1-9. doi: 10.1016/j.critrevonc.2010.10.008

[71] Aggarwal R, Huang J, Alumkal JJ, Zhang L, Feng FY, Thomas GV, Weinstein AS, Friedl V, Zhang C, Witte ON, Lloyd P, Gleave M, Evans CP, Youngren J, Beer TM, Retting M, Wong CK, True L, Foye A, Playdle D, ryan CJ, Lara P, Chi KN, Uzunangelov V, Sokolov A, Newton Y, Beltran H, Demichelis F, Rubin MA, Stuart JM, Small EJ. Clinical and genomic characterization of treatment-emergent small-cell neuroendocrine prostate cancer: a multi-institutional prospective study. *J Clin Oncol* 2018, **36**:2492-2503. doi: 10.1200/JCO.2017.77.6880

[72] Pascal LE, Vêncio RZN, Vessella RL, Ware CB, Vêncio EF, Denyer G, Liu AY. Lineage relationship of prostate cancer cell types based on gene expression. *BMC Medical Genomics* 2011, **4**:46. doi: 10.1186/1755-8794-4-46

[73] Takahashi K, Tanabe K, Ohnuki M, Narita M, Ishisaka T, Tomoda K, Yamanaka S. Induction of pluripotent stem cells from adult human fibroblasts by defined factors. *Cell* 2007, **131**:861-872. doi: 10.1016/j.cell.2007.11.019

[74] Wang HT, Yao YH, Li BG, Tang Y, Chang JW, Zhang J. Neuroendocrine prostate cancer (NEPC) progressing from conventional prostatic adenocarcinoma: factors associated

with time to development of NEPC and survival from NEPC diagnosis – a systematic review and pooled analysis. *J Clin Oncol* 2014, **32**:3383-3390. doi: 10.1200/JCO.2013.54.3553

[75] Liu AY, Borges GT, Kanan AD, Pascal LE, Vêncio EF, Vêncio RZN. Prostate cancer de-differentiation and reprogramming of cancer cells to pluripotent stem cells. In *Cell Sources for iPSCs*, vol. 7. Ed. A. Birbrair. Elsevier, 2021, in press.

[76] Aboseif S, El-Sakka A, Young P, Cunha GR. Mesenchymal reprogramming of adult human epithelial differentiation. *Differentiation* 1999, **65**:113-118. doi: 10.1046/j.1432-0436.1999.6520113.x

[77] Oottamasathien S, Wang Y, Williams K, Franco OE, Wills ML, Thomas JC, Saba K, Sharif-Afshar AR, Makari JH, Bhowmick NA, DeMarco RT, Hipkens S, Magnuson M, Brock JW, Hayward SW, Pope JC, Matusik RJ. Directed differentiation of embryonic stem cells into bladder tissue. *Dev Biol* 2007, **304**:556-566. doi: 10.1016/j.ydbio.2007.01.010

[78] Goo YA, Goodlett DR, Pascal LE, Worthington KD, Vessella RL, True LD, Liu AY. Stromal mesenchyme cell genes of the human prostate and bladder. *BMC Urol* 2005, **5**:17. doi: 10.1186/1471-2490-5-17

[79] Pascal LE, Vêncio RZN, Goo YA, Page LS, Shadle CP, Liu AY. Temporal expression profiling of the effects of secreted factors from prostate stromal cells on embryonal carcinoma stem cells. *Prostate* 2009, **69**:1353-1365. doi: 10.1002/pros.20982

[80] Pascal LE, Ai J, Vêncio RZN, Vêncio EF, Zhou Y, Page LS, True LD, Wang Z, Liu AY. Differential inductive signaling of $CD90^{+}$ prostate cancer-associated fibroblasts compared to normal tissue stromal mesenchyme cells. *Cancer Microenvironment* 2011, **4**:51-59. doi: 10.1007/s12307-010-0061-4

[81] Kanan AD, Corey E, Vêncio RZN, Ishwar A, Liu AY. Lineage relationship between prostate adenocarcinoma and small cell carcinoma. *BMC Cancer* 2019, 19:518. doi: 10.1186/s12885-019-5680-7

[82] Vêncio EF, Nelson AM, Cavanaugh C, Ware CB, Miller DG, Garcia JCO, Vêncio RZN, Loprieno MA, Liu AY. Reprogramming of prostate cancer-associated stromal cells to embryonic stem-like. *Prostate* 2012, **72**:1453-1463. doi: 10.1002/pros.22497

[83] Park SW, Zhen G, Verhaeghe C, Nakagami Y, Nguyenvu LT, Barczak AJ, Killeen N, Erle DJ. The protein disulfide isomerase AGR2 is essential for production of intestinal mucus. *Proc Nat Acad Sci USA* 2009, **106**:6950-6955. doi 10:1073/pnas.0808722106

[84] Tereshina MB, Ivanova A, Eroshkin FM, Korotkova DD, Nesterenko AM, Bayramov AV, Solovieva EA, Parshina EA, Orlov EE, Martynova NY, Zaraisky AG. Agr2-interacting Prod1-like protein Tfp4 from *Xenopus laevis* is necessary for early forebrain and eye development as well as for the tadpole appendage regeneration. *Genesis* 2019 **57**:323293. doi: 10.1002/dvg.23293

[85] Zhu Q, Mangukiya HB, Mashausi DS, Guo H, Negi H, Merugu SB, Wu Z, Li D. Anterior gradient 2 is induced in cutaneous wound and promotes wound healing through its adhesion domain. *FEBS J* 2017, **284**:2856-2869. doi 10.1111/febs.14155

[86] Summerhayes IC, Frank IM. Effects of donor age on neoplastic transformation of adult mouse bladder epithelium in vitro. *J Nat Cancer Inst* 1979, **62**:1017-1023.

Chapter 7

Advances in Adoptive Cellular Therapy (ACT)

Rajesh Kumar Yadav, Bandana Kumari, Pritanjali Singh, Asgar Ali, Sadhana Sharma and Krishnan Hajela

Abstract

Adoptive T cell therapy (ACT) is getting acknowledged as the Advanced Therapy Medicinal Products (ATMPs) in many countries and it has evolved as one of the newest regimens to treat cancer. Developed gradually by the basic understanding of cells, involved in innate and adaptive immunity, ACT has emerged as one of the successful immunotherapies in recent times. It broadly includes various cell types such as stem cells, T cells, dendritic cells and Natural Killer cells. By the applications of genetic engineering and advanced cell culture techniques, these cells from patients' blood, can be manipulated to train them for better efficacy against specific tumor cells. However, only some cells' subsets have shown promising regression for certain cancer cells types. To understand the reason behind this, technical knowledge about the tumor antigens presentation, tumor microenvironment (TME), hosts' immune responses and possible issues in the manufacturing of adoptive cellular material for infusion in patients are being explored further. This chapter brings together development of immune cells from basic research to clinical use, newer approaches which have been taken to address the resistance of ACT and future promises of this therapy.

Keywords: immunotherapy, advanced therapy medicinal products, adoptive T cell therapy, tumor microenvironment, TCR T cell Therapy, CAR T cell therapy

1. Introduction

Human body has a natural tendency to fight against diseases including cancer, aided by its immune system. So far, the journey of understanding mechanisms of tumor suppression by immune system and immune suppression by tumor cells, has been overwhelming. The ability of immune cells to differentiate between self and non-self is the key for immune response against cancer cells [1]. However, as cancer cell is actually a transformed self-cell, its ability to escape immune recognition is quite probable and a reason of cancer progression.

The treatment of cancer in the new era has shifted its focus from conventional treatment to physiological treatment, which involves the modification of immune system. This has also led to a concept of personalized treatment where an individual immune system of patient is manipulated rather immune responses obtained based on general population. The efficacy of the immune cells is modified so that its tumor suppression function is improved. This strategy has shown better outcomes and therefore has drawn attention of researchers and clinicians and is now a preferred choice for cancer treatment. The efforts to design universal immune cell-based immunotherapy are also being explored besides personalized immunotherapy [2]. Numbers of approaches have been developed to treat cancer cells using immune-based technology broadly known as cancer immunotherapy (**Figure 1** and **Table 1**).

Among all these immunotherapies, cell-based cancer immunotherapy is getting popular day by day [18–20]. The ability of immune system to inhibit tumor growth and cure it, has been exploited in the development of anti-neoplastic immunotherapy. The immune cells play a key role in adoptive cell therapy (ACT). This is achieved by either expanding the autologous cancer-cognate lymphocytes or empowering them by genetic modifications. These alterations are done *ex-vivo* and then these cells are infused back to patient to fight against the cancer (**Figure 2**).

Cancer treatments by general immunotherapy have their own limitations due to personal variation in the immune response. In such cases, precision medicine through adoptively modified cellular transfers is being preferred lately. The cells to be transferred may be autologous (self-derived) or allogeneic (donor derived) depending upon the availability. These cells undergo various genetic modifications to suit the cancer types. Allogeneic cells are chosen on the basis of haplo-identical donors, or immune-suppressive conditioning to the patient.

This chapter outlines the emergence and evolvement of ACT, advancements particularly with genetic engineering of autologous cells, treatment approaches, evidences for its effectiveness in refractory patients, and future directions of ACT.

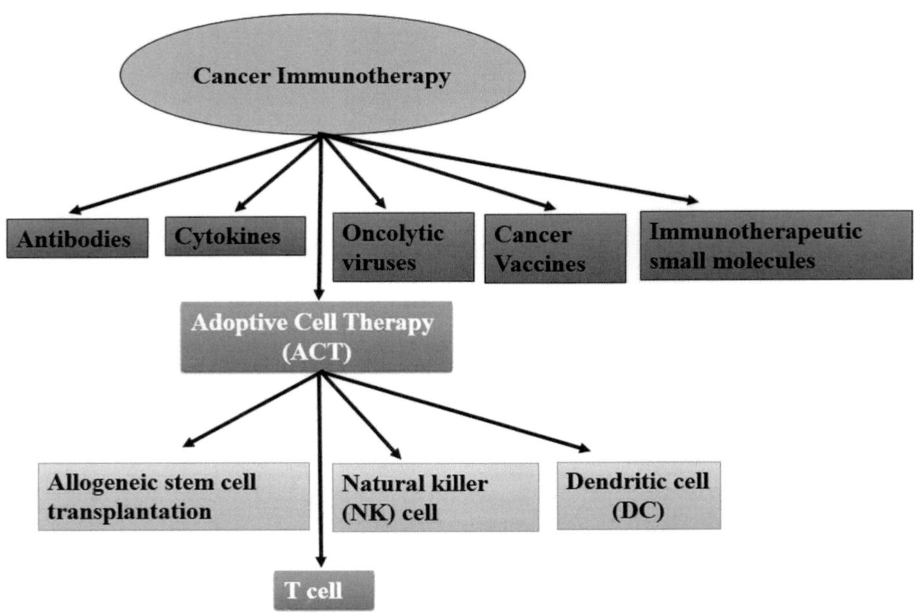

Figure 1.
Different approaches to cancer immunotherapy. Arrow indicates different modes through which immunotherapy can be performed. Application of T cells is the foremost choice of the cellular advancement for ACT.

Types	Salient features	Ref.
Antibody	• Therapeutic use of monoclonal antibodies (mAbs) • Tumor killing by cytotoxicity; Fc mediated immune effector engagements, non-restricted activation of T-cells and blockade of inhibitory signaling.	[3–5]
Cytokines	• Molecular messengers with anti-tumor property, majorly secreted by immune cells • Pro-inflammatory cytokines limit tumor cell growth by stimulating the cytotoxic activity of immune cells against tumor cells. • Recombinant interferon-alpha (IFN-α) and interleukin-2 (IL2)	[6]
Oncolytic Viruses	• Genetically engineered viruses carrying tumor suppressor genes • Work like the gene therapy • When administered, self-replicate in the tumor and induce apoptosis. • Modulate tumor microenvironment and provide anti-cancer immunity	[7]
Vaccine	• Meant to treat cancer as a personalized cancer vaccine • Helps the patient's immune system for cancer killing and relapses. • May consist of dendritic cells, tumor cell lysate, nucleic acids (DNA and mRNA), or neoantigens. • Approaches: dendritic cells engineered to express high levels of tumor-associated target antigens, and delivered to relevant lymph nodes to activate T-cells • The DNA and mRNA-based vaccines: taken up by APCs and present to T-cells to induce their activation • Tumor neoantigen: tumor specific antigens for the development of cancer vaccines without 'off-target' adverse effects.	[8–15]
Small molecules	• Chemotherapeutics as regulator of immune cells • Indoleamine 2,3-dioxygenase-1 inhibitors boost cellular immunity	[16, 17]

The salient features with examples of various approaches toward the cancer immunotherapy have been discussed. The bullets points highlight their primary modes and mechanisms.

Table 1.
Cancer immunotherapy.

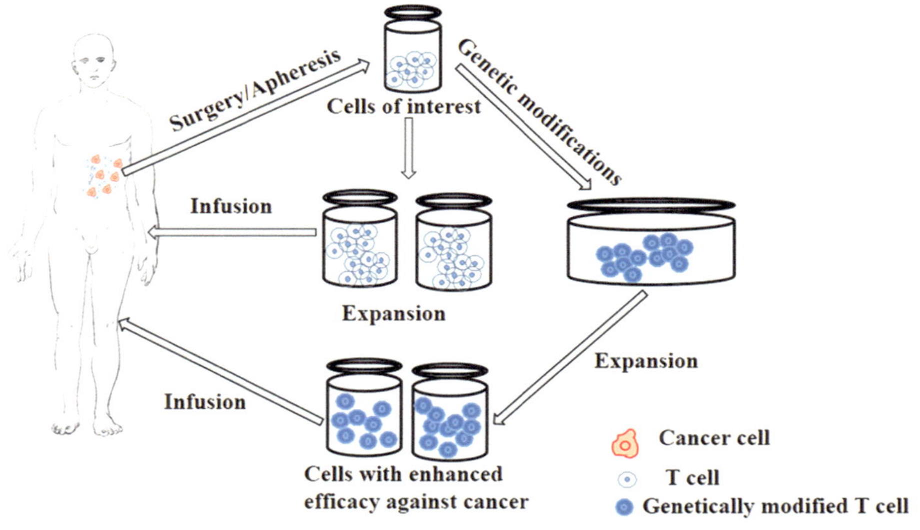

Figure 2.
Approach toward adoptive cellular therapy. Cells of interest to perform ACT may be collected through surgery or apheresis. Next, either these cells can be re-infused to patient after its proper expansion or genetic manipulations depending upon cancer types.

2. Emergence of ACT

The concept of ACT was first developed more than fifty-five years back when immune lymphocytes were successfully used to inhibit growth of sarcoma in an animal model [21].

Further, efforts were made to augment the potential of ACT by inducing activation and proliferation of immune cells in use, which was achieved by the use of recombinant IL2. The IL-2 has been known to potentiate immunological functions and later, its use as T cell growth factor were also recommended [22].

In cell based or cellular therapy, autologous or allogenic stem cells, progenitor or primary cells were the choice of possible cell types, which were modified *ex-vivo* and transfused into the patient for disease regression [2, 18, 19]. Cellular therapy's outcomes were better studied in the case of cancer as it was easy to readout its regression and thus, cancer was chosen first for treatment by cellular therapy. However, lately, this strategy has also been tested for treating cardiovascular, neurological and bone diseases [23]. The choice of cells to develop immunotherapy was from innate and adaptive immune systems as these cells play a key role in controlling cancer progression [24].

Further, initial failures of cell- based therapy were reported due to the role of T cells as the mediators of allograft rejection and also due to the host immune inhibitory factors [2, 25]. Therefore, measures were taken prior to ACT such as use of syngeneic lymphocytes for transfer to minimize the failures of the same [25]. Thus, ACT was developed as a biomedical procedure where the immune cells of the cancer patient, which have high anticancer activity, are expanded, modified and returned to the patients [2, 18, 19].

During eighties, the antitumor activities were reported in cells like natural killer (NK) and lymphokine-activated killer cells [26–30]. These cells directly recognize antigens present on tumor cells and kill them, whereas T cells recognize tumor antigens when presented with major histocompatibility complex (MHC) [31]. However, each cell has different anti-tumor potential. With advancements in immuno-technologies, such as fluorescence activated cell sorter, molecular markers were assigned on various immune cells to define them properly [32, 33]. This led to the classification of lineages and subtypes of immune cells. Thus, selection of cells was made and this followed their manipulation *ex-vivo* for ACT.

So far various cell types such as stem cells, T cells, dendritic cells and NK cells from patients are successfully used and have shown promising results in cancer regression (**Figure 1**). Dendritic cells (DCs) regulate innate immune response and due to its nature of antigen presentation, it may induce adaptive response. Tumor antigen exposed DCs may play a critical role in enhancing cytotoxic activities of immune cells. Therefore, DCs are used as an anti-tumor therapeutic vaccines or to enhance the stimulation of cytotoxic T cells by appropriate antigen presentation [34].

Different subset of T cells (gamma/delta T cells, regulatory T cells, helper and cytotoxic T lymphocytes) respond differently for various tumor subtypes [35]. Interestingly, some T cell subtypes confer advantage over other in reducing tumor volume [36].

3. Evolving modes and mechanisms of ACT

ACT developed in different ways has different mechanisms to target cancer cells. These are the foremost cellular technology adopted for cancer treatment after their validations and regulations through various clinical trials.

3.1 Tumor infiltrating lymphocytes (TILs)

Under the immune surveillance, lymphocytes differentiate between self and non-self-cells and antigens. Any self-cell when gets transformed and starts proliferating as cancer, lymphocytes infiltrate into that site, recognize abnormally growing cells and activate themselves to remove these *not so self*, cancerous cells. These lymphocytes are named as Tumor Infiltrating Lymphocytes (TILs). It so happens sometimes that these TILs fail to perform their function efficiently which may lead to cancer progression. In such cases, it was found that the TILs are not enough in number to show effective cytotoxicity, though have ability to specifically recognize tumor cells, stop their growth and eventually kill them. Thus, to develop any cellular therapy, the first and the foremost approach was to expand TILs, which have infiltrated into the tumor site with anti-tumor potential. These cells can be isolated from cancer origin tissue by resection and expanded *ex-vivo* to a sufficient number to improve their anti-tumor activity. These are then infused back into the patient as ACT therapy (**Figure 3a**). The TILs used in the therapy are autologous lymphocytes as these are derived from the tumor site.

Hence, for the development of ACT, antitumor lymphocytes are grown *in-vitro* up to a number of 10^{11}–10^{12}, followed by a process of selection of specific tumor recognizing cells with effector functions. These cells when infused in the patient, behave like live drug, which proliferate when encounter tumor antigen in the host and help in tumor regression. Though the process of cellular expansion *in-vitro* does not absolutely match with *in-vivo* environment around the tumor, which has certain immune inhibitory responses. Thus, in ACT, a favorable tumor microenvironment is necessary prior to the therapy which should support the anti-tumor immune function of the infused TILs [37].

3.2 Genetic manipulations of T cells

Sometimes in certain cases, tumor infiltrated T cells do not recognize tumor cells and hence they neither get activated nor proliferated *in-vivo*. In such cases, T cells' usefulness becomes redundant. To improve the functional properties of these cells including recognition of antigen on cancer cells, an alternative approach is adopted

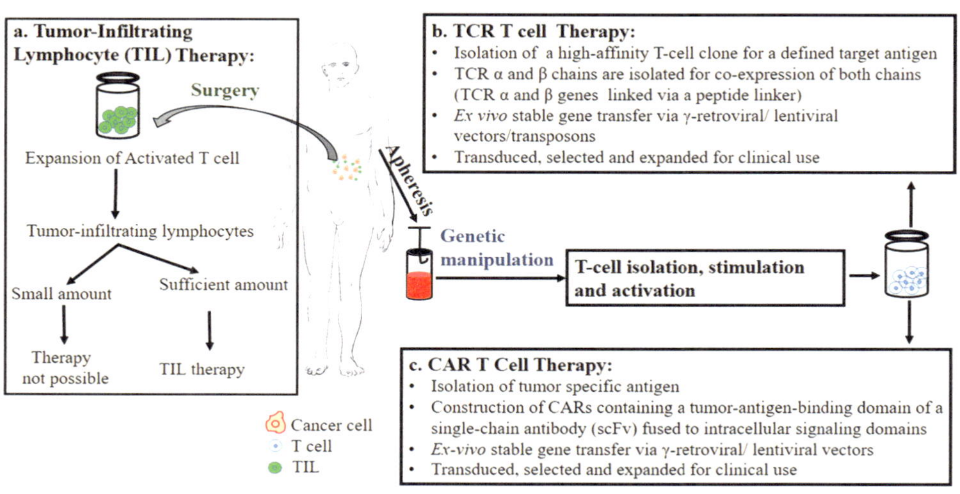

Figure 3.
Leading adoptive cellular therapy. Patients' T cells utilized in TILs, TCR T cells and CAR T cell therapy. Major steps of these therapies discussed in the boxes.

where patient's T cells are genetically manipulated using gene editing technology. This also overcomes the problem of isolating pre-existing tumor-reacting T cells from patients with tumors of other types. Here the cells are made to express tumor antigen-specific TCRs, thus are effective in anti-tumor cytotoxic function [38].

There are two strategies to genetically modify the specificity of T cells. The patient's cells can be genetically modified by integrating genes encoding either conventional alpha-beta TCRs, or Chimeric Antigen Receptors (CARs), specific for tumor antigen(s). To develop ACT by these mechanisms, TCR T cells or CAR T cells are manufactured by autologous T cells which are amended *ex-vivo,* expanded and re-injected in patient to fight against cancer cells (**Figure 3b** and **c**). The only difference remains in the mode of recognition of tumor antigen by these T cells (**Figure 4**).

3.2.1 TCR T cell therapy

The TCR is a specific receptor as well as characteristic marker on T cell surface. TCR complex is a di-sulphide linked membrane anchored heterodimer protein, consisting of two different peptide chains, TCR α and TCR ß encircled by four CD3 chains [39]. These TCR α and ß chains recognize the polypeptide fragment presented by MHC molecule on cancer cells. The principal objective behind TCR T cell technology is to modify TCR binding to tumor antigen which as such shows poor affinity for antigens making them incompetent to recognize and kill tumor cells effectively [40]. Thus, making of high affinity TCR T cell requires identification of specific targets on cancer cells. This way the genetically engineered TCR shows augmented recognition specificity and affinity for tumor cells.

In a study done by Rapoport AP et al., an autologous T cell was engineered to express a high affinity TCR specific to identify naturally processed peptide shared by cancer-testis antigen New York Esophageal Squamous Cell Carcinoma-1 (NY-ESO-1) and L antigen family member 1 (LAGE-1) to be used for multiple myeloma patients showing encouraging clinical response in 16 of 20 (80%) patients with advanced disease [41].

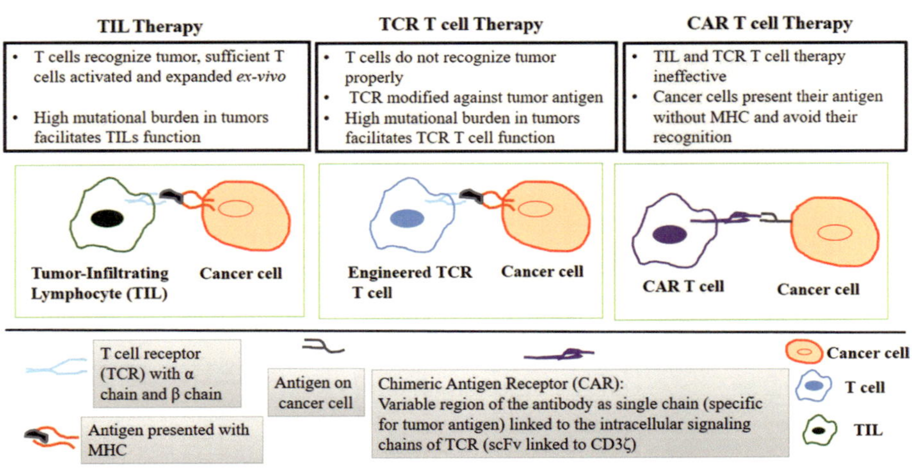

Figure 4.
Molecular insights of cellular therapy. The boxes illustrate the salient features to determine the choice of ACT. In TILs and TCR T cells, the TCR α and ß chains recognize the antigen presented with MHC molecule on cancer cells whereas CAR T cells recognize the tumor antigen independent of MHC. In TCR T cell, genetically engineered high affinity TCR recognizes tumor cells. In CAR T cell, a CAR, a scFv derived from variable regions of heavy and light chains of a monoclonal antibody against tumor antigen recognize tumor cells. CAR also consists of a trans-membrane domain; a hinge; one or more than one intracellular co-stimulatory molecules and a CD3z signaling domain. TCR T cell and CAR T cell therapy highly depend upon identification of unique antigen on cancer cells.

In above mentioned TIL and TCR T cell-based therapies, there may be yet another problem which may be encountered when these expanded/modified cells still do not so efficiently recognize cancer cells. This happens when cancer cells smartly down regulate expression of specific MHC molecules and tumor antigen is presented without MHC complex and thus these T cells fail to recognize the target cancer cells. Fortunately, emergence of recombinant DNA technology and novel cell isolation techniques from blood have paved newer ways to cancer immunotherapy. Hence, to overcome this evading mechanism by cancer cells, T cells are genetically modified in such a way that they recognize cancer cells by a mechanism independent of MHC [2, 42, 43].

3.2.2 CAR T cell therapy

This newer modality of modifying T cells is yet another type of ACT, where T cell are armed with a CAR, which can now make the T cells recognize cancer antigen without MHC molecules. Use of such modified T cells bearing CAR is called as CAR T cell for therapy. The concept of CAR T cell is based on the ability of genetically engineered patient's own T cells to express a CAR, which is specific for a tumor antigen and therefore better in fighting cancer cells. A CAR consists of a scFv derived from variable region of heavy and light chains of a monoclonal antibody against tumor antigen to recognize tumor cells. Apart from this, a trans-membrane domain; a hinge; one or more than one intracellular co-stimulatory molecules and a CD3 zeta signaling domain are the part of CAR construct to make fully activated and functional T cell [2, 44].

Four generations of CARs have been developed, with subsequent generations being better than the previous ones with respect to cytotoxicity and shelf-life. First generation CARs had only single chain variable fragment (scFv) linked to CD3ζ or Fc receptor gamma signaling domain. With the subsequent additions of co-stimulatory domains like CD28, CD 137, or OX40, second and third generation CARs have been created. Fourth generation CARs also called TRUCK (T cell redirected for universal cytokine killing) are armed with immune stimulatory cytokines that ameliorate the performance of CAR T cell with respect to its expansion, persistence, and resistance even in immunosuppressive tumor microenvironment [45, 46]. This therapy harnesses the power of immune system to fight the cancer but in contrast to the regular T cell receptor (TCRs), that recognize Ag, only when presented with MHC, CARs have the aptitude to redirect the effector function of T cell toward any tumor associated antigen (TAA) expressed on the tumor surface even without MHC. Once CAR of the T cell binds to its specific TAA, T cell gets activated through phosphorylation of immune receptor tyrosine-based activation motifs leading to cytokine secretion, T cell proliferation and cytotoxicity [47]. The word chimeric here signifies both, antigen binding, independent of MHC and T cell activation function into a single receptor (**Figure 4**).

Advantage of TCR T cell therapy over CAR T cell therapy is that these can recognize even deep-seated antigens fragment presented on MHC molecule in contrast to CAR T cell that recognize only cell surface proteins. So, TCR T cell therapy offer wider range of application but it is also MHC restricted and recognizes only those antigens presented on MHC molecule, a major drawback of TCR T cell therapy.

4. Opportunities and challenges

Like any other therapy, ACT also has success and failures. The therapy deals with T cells in two different ways, firstly, the natural T cell with antitumor activity and secondly, the genetically manipulated T cells, either the TCRs engineered or the receptor is chimeric. Thus, T cells' immune responsiveness for tumor targeting functions discretely. Also, during the therapy, responsiveness and un-responsiveness of host is guided by many factors. Similarly, many criteria in preparation of the cells for therapy are the deciding factor for the effectiveness of the therapy, which in turn is decided by extent of tumor regression.

4.1 Tumor regression

Dramatic regression of variety of cancers, like melanoma, cervical cancer, lymphoma, leukemia, bile duct cancer, and neuroblastoma has been reported by the use ACT based approaches [2]. A number of cancer patients showed success using TILs, however, TIL therapy requires surgery and to obtain enough TILs is always a huge challenge technically. TILs expansion approach has been best used for the treatment of metastatic melanoma by Rosenberg et al. [48].

Applications of genetic manipulations in ACT have greatly contributed in improving the remission rate of treatment of various type of cancers [49]. For relapsed and refractory B-cell precursor Acute Lymphoblastic Leukemia in children and young adults, CAR T cell therapy was successful in 52 of 63 patients and three of every four patients did not show relapse in six months [50]. In another trial to treat refractory large B-cell lymphoma, CAR T cell therapy has shown promising results as it completely cured 54% patients, slowed tumor growth in 82% patients and there was no relapse in 40% patient even after 15.4 months [51]. CAR T cell therapy using B cell maturation antigen was tried on multiple myeloma patients and showed remission in 74% of patients [52].

4.2 Challenges

The failures of the therapy in any form have been associated with many factors. The extent to which the tumor cells can evade immune recognition and successfully employ immune suppression mechanisms leads to failure of ACT.

4.2.1 Cell selection

One of the factors which guards the successful use of ACT in humans is the identification of cells that can target antigens selectively expressed on the cancer and not on essential normal tissues. This criterion is the basis of the success of ACT. Also, sometimes immune cells lose their natural tendency to recognize and kill the tumor cells, leads to failure of therapy. Therefore, even though the cell selection is appropriate, sometimes success is not achieved.

4.2.2 Tumor microenvironment

Activities of tumor cells also play a key role in suppressing the effector function of immune cells used in ACT. The tumor cells along with their neighborhood constitute a unique environment which is called as tumor microenvironment (TME). This has an ability to suppress host's immune system by various mechanisms such as a) T cell exhaustion due to continuously changing antigen signatures on them; b) affects the cytotoxic function of T cells at the site of tumor and c) also the T cell trafficking [53]. To counter these immune suppressive mechanisms of TME, there are possible technologies available that locally deliver T cells to the TME and increase their proliferation, thus, could provide a means to treat inoperable solid tumors [54].

4.2.3 Technical glitches

ACT involves different stages to generate clinical grade therapeutic cells and trained personnel to execute the technology. Therefore, it needs great care and precautions to avoid technological pitfalls.

4.2.3.1 Manufacturing

The technical issues are related to the manufacturing process of adoptive cellular material and the delivery platforms which also account for the success or failure of the ACT. During the *ex-vivo* expansion and genetic modification process, factors such as cell culture time, use of cytokines and use of vectors for gene transfer are the major concerns deciding the efficacy and survival of T cells being used in the therapy. Besides sometimes cancer specific T cells may not grow that well and not sufficient for infusion. At the same time efficacy of T cell may also change in *ex-vivo* growth conditions [55].

Major hurdle with regard to TCR T cell technology is related to its expansion which includes identifying of a good target, along with specific TCRs, screening for desirable TCR affinity. Also, TCR T cell therapy is MHC dependent and there is grave peril of hybridization between exogenous and endogenous chain causing recognition of auto-antigens thereby leading to graft-versus host disease [43].

Failures of the therapy with adverse outcomes have been reported due to some chromosomal DNA translocations and rearrangements during the preparation of the cells [56, 57].

4.2.3.2 Delivery system

A major limitation of adoptive T cell therapies is the delivery technology used in the patient. It is noted that the viability and function of the transplanted cells rapidly decline after administration [58]. Hence, different delivery technologies (nanoparticles or scaffolds) have been explored to improve success of ACT. Adjuvant-loaded nanoparticles, chemically conjugated to the surface of T cells to stimulate transplanted cells and minimize the systemic side effects have been designed [59]. Advantages of having a delivery system of T cells which has some immune stimulating mechanisms linked, may help the T cells to enter the tumor site and perform better results of the therapy. Apart from systemic administration route, biomaterials-based strategies have also been explored to locally deliver adoptive T cells to solid tumors [60, 61] as successful targeting of T cells to most solid cancers remain challenging [62]. To overcome the barrier of secluded location of solid tumors, local injection of T cell in brain tumors in mouse model has been tried and has shown better outcome than systemic administration [54].

Overall, biomaterial-mediated local T cell delivery approaches could improve the efficiency of adoptive T cell therapies for treating inoperable solid tumors by overcoming local immunosuppressive barriers. The usefulness of these therapies depends on how quickly T cells can be generated in tumors *in-vivo* using this approach relative to the time it takes to expand T cells *ex-vivo*.

4.2.4 Regulatory guidelines and cost

Regulatory guidelines are other part of the story that limit the use of any therapy where biological samples are used for therapeutic. There are certain considerations to be followed for minimal manipulation and homologous use of human cells, tissues, and cellular and tissue-based products. Cellular & Gene Therapies are complex products which are regulated by the Food and Drug Administration (FDA) in the United States. The European Union (EU), governs the regulation of all medicinal products for human use, including advanced therapy medicinal products (ATMPs), i.e., medicinal products comprised of cells, genes, or tissues to ensure the quality, safety, and efficacy of medicines placed on the market in the EU. The aims of EU are to ensure the quality, efficacy and most importantly safety of public health.

A very high treatment cost of ACT based immunotherapies has been another concern for its limited use [20, 63]. Cost of CAR-T cell has been curtailed by developing Universal CAR-T cell and CAR NK cell so that this therapy can be a hope for majority of cancer patients [64].

4.3 Advantages

There are many advantages with ACT that outweigh the conventional therapy.

One major advantage of TCR-T cell therapy is that it can target many TAA, even when these lie intracellular and are deep seated. Site directed injection of T cells into tumor giving superior result than systemic administration, is yet another favorable approach in cell-based therapies. A successful example of such application is reported in brain tumors where T cells are injected into CSF directly [43, 54]. Similarly, next generation of CARs have enhanced the ability of T cells to destroy tumor by infiltrating into diseased tissue site and have potential to moderate tumor microenvironment by secreting pro-inflammatory cytokines and expand their own life span *in-vivo* [64].

CARs have another unique ability to recognize not only peptide but also carbohydrate and glycolipid antigens, thus increasing their target antigen number and are also not MHC restricted.

5. Enhancing efficacy of ACT

The journey of development of ACT for cancer treatment has faced success and failures of the therapy in different cancer types. This has led to newer researches and explorations in various domains of the treatment by ACT. Work on improving effectiveness of therapy has contributed enormously and made difference in its outcomes. Following are some areas, which have been mentioned in this section about the efforts made toward enhancing efficacy of ACT.

5.1 Measuring effectiveness

Measuring effectiveness of any therapy is an essential part of it. It is critical to measure of cellular therapy's effectiveness as variations may occur in various steps, starting from isolation of cells to its re-infusion and homing of effective cells to target the cancer cells (**Figure 5**). For this purpose, a therapeutic index (TI) has been developed [65].

TI of a drug is a quantitative assessment of the ratio of a drug dose that produces toxicity to the dose that yields a clinically effective response. ACT has complex biodistribution and also content dependent potency, so for this TI estimation depends on other factors as well. These include functional fitness of the product, vague pharmacokinetics due to trapping, sequestration and extravasations in nearby tissue and inconstant rate of expansion *in-vivo*. Addition factors also influence pharmacokinetics in case of solid tumors like difference in trafficking to benign and cancer tissue, immune suppression and cellular dysfunction due to unfavorable hostile metabolic state.

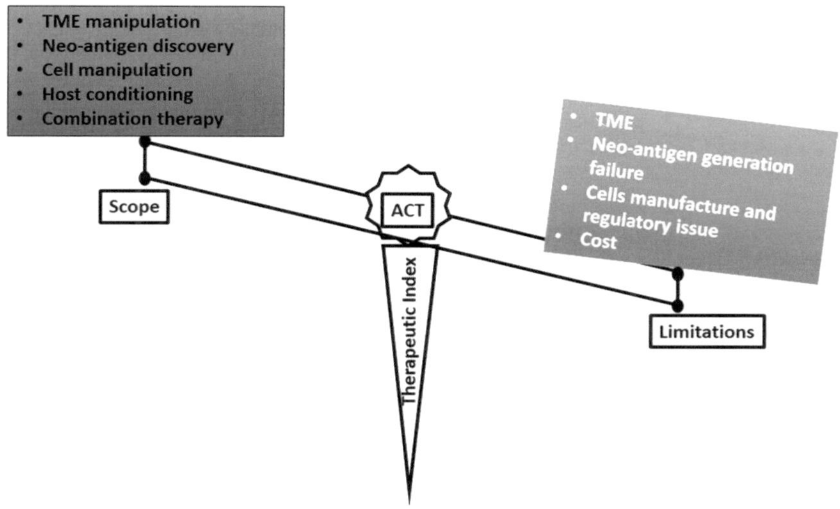

Figure 5.
Scope to enhance therapeutic efficacy of ACT. The scope and limitations are two ends ACT. It may be viewed as the seesaw game. Increasing the scope will determine its future.

Thus, TI of the ACT largely depends on generic factors (T cell potency and fitness, Dispersion, Dysfunction, combinatorial therapies, comorbidities and microbiome) and TME-specific factors (Antigen availability, tumor, immune response related) [65].

5.2 Host conditioning

It is important to understand that anti-tumor efficacy of ACT greatly depends on the persistence of adoptively transferred T cells in the host. This is achieved by an optimal pre-conditioning of the host, an important part of pre-treatment protocol where lymphodepletion by chemotherapy and/or radiation therapy is done prior to therapy. The process of lymphodepletion is important to deplete T regulatory cells and lymphocytes, as these cells compete with the transferred cells for homeostatic cytokines, interleukin 7 and IL15 and this needs to be minimized [66]. This may also be important to avoid excessive cytokine release by lymphocytes which causes adverse effect during the therapy. Host conditioning by either nonmyeloablative chemotherapy or irradiation may induce high levels of IL-1β which increase the number and functionality of adoptively transferred T cells within the tumor and thus improves efficacy of ACT [67]. An FDA-approved reagent, fludarabine has predictable lymphodepleting kinetics and duration of action. Its use in a conditioning regimen, promotes homeostatic upregulation of cytokines and growth signals for T cell persistence [6]. The use of cytokine IL2 has also been recommended for better proliferation of the cells being used in this cellular therapy [2, 6].

5.3 Affinity of T cells

5.3.1 Selection of CARs with moderate affinity

Affinity of the immune cells in ACT is a highly critical criterion while using them for therapy. Optimum affinity is ensured during making of the cells. In TILs based therapy, it may not be that critical as there are no manipulations involved as such except increasing their numbers. However, while doing genetic manipulations, it needs care especially when a gene fragment is being incorporated into the cell to express a chimeric receptor as in the case of CAR T cell therapy. High affinity CAR bearing cells are *not* the choice of cells as these might recognize the TAA present on the normal cells too and may cause *on target/off tumor* effect, an effect occurs when CAR T cells attack non-tumor cells expressing the target antigen. Thus, CAR selection is very important and ensured to be of low affinity so that it recognizes the antigen when it is present in high number as in case of tumor cells. This helps in recognizing *only* tumor cells and sparing normal cells [68].

5.3.2 Countering loss of antigen on cancer cells

Sometimes problem of therapy arises when the cancer cells start losing CAR-targeted antigen on them and escape their detection by CAR T cells, thus avoid their killing. Such situation is countered by targeting multiple antigens with multiple CARs [69]. For this, anti-tag CARs (AT-CARs) have been developed by adding affinity-enhanced monomeric streptavidin2 (mSA2) biotin-binding domain in the CAR construct. Such novel mSA2CARs have an advantage that the T cells expressing such CARs can bind cancer cells coated with biotinylated antibodies [69]. Binding of such antibodies to cancer cells probably avoids the loss of antigen being targeted on them. Thus, recognition of cancer cells occurs followed by their killing by such CAR T cells without fail.

5.3.3 Formation of synapse

To further improve efficacy of CARs, small sized antibodies (variable heavy homodimers) or nanobodies are recommended to be used with CAR T cell preparation for infusion. These antibodies cause tight synapse formation between the target and effector cell, which is important for the initiation of immune signaling, thus effective T cell mediated killing [70].

5.3.4 CARs expressing Heparanase

It has been discovered that heparanase enzyme expression needs to be upregulated in CAR T cells to penetrated tumor stroma which consists of heparin sulfate proteoglycane. In vitro expanded T cells show reduced heparanase expression as compared to activated immune cell, suggesting their compromised migration [71]. This drawback has been overcome by designing better CAR T cells which were engineered to express heparanase enzyme and therefore show greater capacity to infiltrate tumor stroma with enhanced anti-tumor activity in neuroblastoma xenograft model [72].

5.4 Dose

Next important part of therapy is the dose, i.e., number of the cells in the prepared fraction/dose. The dose frequency and the number of cells per dose to be used for infusion, both play a crucial role in outcome of the therapy. Proportion of immune cells responsible for tumor regression controls the success of ACT. Such as CD8+ enriched "young" tumor infiltrating lymphocytes show better response in the regression of metastatic melanoma compared to the crude fraction containing both CD8+ and CD4+ both proportions [73].

It has also been reported that the number of transfused CAR T cell needed for single transfusion is much less than that needed for TCR T cell therapy to produce equivocal response [43].

5.5 Minimizing toxicities

ACT involves manipulation of immune system to improve its efficacy for specific killing of cancer cells. Such alterations may lead to exaggerated immune response and cause toxicities which are different from other cancer therapies. Thus, depending upon the type of mechanisms involved in these toxicities, discrete approaches are needed to minimize them. The possible toxicities observed and their management are as follow:

a. On target/off tumor recognition develops a toxicity due to shared expression of target antigens by normal tissue leading to varying severity of adverse event from B cell aplasia to death. Hypogammaglobulinemia in B cell aplasia can be treated with intravenous immunoglobulin replacement therapy.

b. Anaphylaxis is seen in patients receiving genetically modified T cell as their antigen recognition domain in derived from murine mAb. Efforts are being made to humanize the expressed protein [74].

c. Graft versus host disease is commonly observed phenomena in immunotherapies. Infusion of isolated autologous TILs is the way to curtail it.

d. Cytokine Release Syndrome (CRS) is associated with overt activation of T cell, which leads to immune activation process with markedly elevated cytokines. It is seen in CAR T cell therapy and called as CAR T cell toxicity. CRS can be minimized by controlling the activity of CAR T cells. For this a bispecific adaptor has been designed which is a cancer specific ligand conjugated with fluorescein. This specifically binds with cancer cells and tag them with fluorescein. CAR is so devised that it recognizes fluorescein and not tumor antigen. Thus, the bispecific adaptor bridges CAR T cell and its tumor target. Thus, availability of bispecific adaptor regulates the killing of tumor cells and can control the CRS. Also, to subdue any CRS, rupture of bridge between CAR T cell to cancer cell can be lifesaving [74]. Other successful approaches to control CRS are immuno-suppression by systemic corticosteroids, IL-6 receptor blockade with mAb or lymphodepleting chemotherapy.

e. Immune effector cell associated neurotoxicity syndrome has also been reported, plausible explanation being elevated cytokine level.

f. Toxicity of T cell activation is also managed by inclusion of an “on switch” in CAR design which can make a hold on functional intensity and T cell activation. This requires selection of two target antigens that are co-expressed on malignant tissue making dual antigen binding a must for complete T cell activation. So normal tissue expressing one target antigen cannot provide complete activation and so limits this toxicity. Conversely, if dual antigens presentation is exclusive to normal tissue, inhibitory signaling in CAR design allow for selective targeting of malignant tissue expressing one antigen while normal tissue is spared.

g. Severe neurological side effects leading to coma and death are reported in patients treated with ACT using autologous T cell when T cells were modified with Melanoma-associated antigen 3 (MAGE-A3) antigen specific TCRs (MAGE-A3 is cancer testis antigen never expressed in normal tissue). These TCRs recognize the different but similar epitopes of especially MAGE-A12 and possibly MAGE-A1, A8, A9 expressed in human brain. So unfortunately, strategies to enhance TCR affinity to neoantigens on tumor may lead to unanticipated toxicities thus warrants need of improved preclinical testing methods to better enable prediction of TCRs specificity.

6. Conclusions

Cancer is a multifactorial disease with varieties of treatment options available, depending upon the location, drug delivery and stage of cancer. Optimization of immune response to curb the growth, proliferation and containment of cancer has been chosen in TIL, TCR T cell and CAR T cell therapy. Growing technologies in cell biology are improving the future promises for further breakthroughs in the T cell ACT field. Various future domains, which are being explored for further improvements are being discussed below [75]:

a. The TME and other immune escape mechanisms are the challenges to ACT for solid tumors. For this, individualized approaches and strategies combining treatments targeting different immunotherapeutic aspects will be needed in order to expand the applicability and improve the response rates in future.

b. Cross reactivity is seen in antigen specific TCRs, which leads to fatal outcomes, needs newer platforms for preclinical screening, such as X-scan.

c. Newer approaches to manage abnormalities of blood vessels and endothelial cells that hinder T cell infiltration into tumors may be tried with inhibitory molecules.

d. Scope to make ACT more effective in solid tumors can be tested by reducing high interstitial pressure and dense extracellular matrix of solid tumor tissue by angiotensin inhibition.

e. Another strategy to enhance the antitumor immunity of infused T cell may be explored through depletion of tumor-associated macrophages.

f. Also, combination of these therapies is providing newer opportunities to personalized immunotherapy due to individual variation in immune response.

In short, advantages versus toxicities of the anti-cancer therapy have to be considered before deciding the treatment modalities. Ultimately, successful implementation of ACT as the clinical program and cost minimization will determine its success across the globe.

Acknowledgements

Dr. Rajesh Kumar Yadav is a Ramalingaswami Re-entry Fellow and his fellowship had been awarded by Department of Biotechnology, Government of India.

Conflict of interest

The authors declare no conflict of interest.

DOI: http://dx.doi.org/10.5772/intechopen.95854

Author details

Rajesh Kumar Yadav[1*], Bandana Kumari[1], Pritanjali Singh[2], Asgar Ali[1], Sadhana Sharma[1*] and Krishnan Hajela[3]

1 Department of Biochemistry, All India Institute of Medical Sciences, Patna, India

2 Department of Radiotherapy, All India Institute of Medical Sciences, Patna, India

3 School of Life Sciences, Devi Ahilya Vishwavidyalaya, Indore, MP, India

*Address all correspondence to: biochemrajesh.yadav@gmail.com and drsadhanas@aiimspatna.org

References

[1] Pillai M, Davies MM, Thistlethwaite FC. Delivery of adoptive cell therapy in the context of the health-care system in the UK: challenges for clinical sites. Ther Adv Vaccines Immunother. 2020; 8:2515135520944355.

[2] Lee DW, Kochenderfer JN, Stetler-Stevenson M, Cui YK, Delbrook C, Feldman SA, et al. T cells expressing CD19 chimeric antigen receptors for acute lymphoblastic leukaemia in children and young adults: a phase 1 dose-escalation trial. Lancet. 2015; 385(9967):517-28.

[3] Hodi FS, O'Day SJ, McDermott DF, Weber RW, Sosman JA, Haanen JB, et al. Improved survival with ipilimumab in patients with metastatic melanoma. N Engl J Med. 2010; 363(8):711-23.

[4] Wolchok JD, Kluger H, Callahan MK, Postow MA, Rizvi NA, Lesokhin AM, et al. Nivolumab plus ipilimumab in advanced melanoma. N Engl J Med. 2013; 369(2):122-33.

[5] Weiner LM, Murray JC, Shuptrine CW. Antibody-based immunotherapy of cancer. Cell. 2012;148(6):1081-4.

[6] Berraondo P, Sanmamed MF, Ochoa MC, Etxeberria I, Aznar MA, Perez-Gracia JL, et al. Cytokines in clinical cancer immunotherapy. Br J Cancer. 2019;120(1):6-15.

[7] Ylosmaki E, Cerullo V. Design and application of oncolytic viruses for cancer immunotherapy. Curr Opin Biotechnol. 2020; 65:25-36.

[8] Chiang CL, Coukos G, Kandalaft LE. Whole Tumor Antigen Vaccines: Where Are We? Vaccines (Basel). 2015; 3(2):344-72.

[9] Guo C, Manjili MH, Subjeck JR, Sarkar D, Fisher PB, Wang XY. Therapeutic cancer vaccines: past, present, and future. Adv Cancer Res. 2013; 119:421-75.

[10] Srivatsan S, Patel JM, Bozeman EN, Imasuen IE, He S, Daniels D, et al. Allogeneic tumor cell vaccines: the promise and limitations in clinical trials. Hum Vaccin Immunother. 2014; 10(1):52-63.

[11] Garg AD, Coulie PG, Van den Eynde BJ, Agostinis P. Integrating Next-Generation Dendritic Cell Vaccines into the Current Cancer Immunotherapy Landscape. Trends Immunol. 2017; 38(8):577-93.

[12] Butterfield LH. Dendritic cells in cancer immunotherapy clinical trials: are we making progress? Front Immunol. 2013; 4:454.

[13] Li L, Goedegebuure SP, Gillanders WE. Preclinical and clinical development of neoantigen vaccines. Ann Oncol. 2017; 28(suppl_12):xii11-xii7.

[14] Pardi N, Hogan MJ, Porter FW, Weissman D. mRNA vaccines - a new era in vaccinology. Nat Rev Drug Discov. 2018; 17(4):261-79.

[15] Schreibelt G, Bol KF, Westdorp H, Wimmers F, Aarntzen EH, Duiveman-de Boer T, et al. Effective Clinical Responses in Metastatic Melanoma Patients after Vaccination with Primary Myeloid Dendritic Cells. Clin Cancer Res. 2016;22(9):2155-66.

[16] Liu X, Shin N, Koblish HK, Yang G, Wang Q, Wang K, et al. Selective inhibition of IDO1 effectively regulates mediators of antitumor immunity. Blood. 2010;115(17):3520-30.

[17] Adams JL, Smothers J, Srinivasan R, Hoos A. Big opportunities for small molecules in immuno-oncology. Nat Rev Drug Discov. 2015; 14(9):603-22.

[18] Choi D, Kim TG, Sung YC. The past, present, and future of adoptive T cell therapy. Immune Netw. 2012; 12(4):139-47.

[19] Cohen JE, Merims S, Frank S, Engelstein R, Peretz T, Lotem M. Adoptive cell therapy: past, present and future. Immunotherapy. 2017; 9(2):183-96.

[20] Yadav RK, Ali A, Kumar S, Sharma A, Baghchi B, Singh P, et al. CAR T cell therapy: newer approaches to counter resistance and cost. Heliyon. 2020;6(4):e03779.

[21] Delorme EJ, Alexander P. Treatment of Primary Fibrosarcoma in the Rat with Immune Lymphocytes. Lancet. 1964; 2(7351):117-20.

[22] Vormittag P, Gunn R, Ghorashian S, Veraitch FS. A guide to manufacturing CAR T cell therapies. Curr Opin Biotechnol. 2018; 53:164-81.

[23] Buzhor E, Leshansky L, Blumenthal J, Barash H, Warshawsky D, Mazor Y, et al. Cell-based therapy approaches: the hope for incurable diseases. Regen Med. 2014;9(5):649-72.

[24] Vesely MD, Kershaw MH, Schreiber RD, Smyth MJ. Natural innate and adaptive immunity to cancer. Annu Rev Immunol. 2011; 29:235-71.

[25] Thangavelu G, Blazar BR. Achievement of Tolerance Induction to Prevent Acute Graft-vs.-Host Disease. Front Immunol. 2019; 10:309.

[26] Grimm EA, Mazumder A, Zhang HZ, Rosenberg SA. Lymphokine-activated killer cell phenomenon. Lysis of natural killer-resistant fresh solid tumor cells by interleukin 2-activated autologous human peripheral blood lymphocytes. J Exp Med. 1982; 155(6):1823-41.

[27] Yron I, Wood TA, Jr., Spiess PJ, Rosenberg SA. In vitro growth of murine T cells. V. The isolation and growth of lymphoid cells infiltrating syngeneic solid tumors. J Immunol. 1980; 125(1):238-45.

[28] Herberman RB, Nunn ME, Lavrin DH. Natural cytotoxic reactivity of mouse lymphoid cells against syngeneic acid allogeneic tumors. I. Distribution of reactivity and specificity. Int J Cancer. 1975; 16(2):216-29.

[29] Kiessling R, Klein E, Pross H, Wigzell H. "Natural" killer cells in the mouse. II. Cytotoxic cells with specificity for mouse Moloney leukemia cells. Characteristics of the killer cell. Eur J Immunol. 1975; 5(2):117-21.

[30] Kiessling R, Klein E, Wigzell H. "Natural" killer cells in the mouse. I. Cytotoxic cells with specificity for mouse Moloney leukemia cells. Specificity and distribution according to genotype. Eur J Immunol. 1975; 5(2):112-7.

[31] Davis ZB, Felices M, Verneris MR, Miller JS. Natural Killer Cell Adoptive Transfer Therapy: Exploiting the First Line of Defense against Cancer. Cancer J. 2015;21(6):486-91.

[32] Maecker HT, McCoy JP, Nussenblatt R. Standardizing immunophenotyping for the Human Immunology Project. Nat Rev Immunol. 2012; 12(3):191-200.

[33] Pitoiset F, Cassard L, El Soufi K, Boselli L, Grivel J, Roux A, et al. Deep phenotyping of immune cell populations by optimized and standardized flow cytometry analyses. Cytometry A. 2018;93(8):793-802.

[34] Sabado RL, Balan S, Bhardwaj N. Dendritic cell-based immunotherapy. Cell Res. 2017; 27(1):74-95.

[35] Wesch D, Kabelitz D, Oberg HH. Tumor resistance mechanisms and their

consequences on gammadelta T cell activation. Immunol Rev. 2020.

[36] Klebanoff CA, Gattinoni L, Torabi-Parizi P, Kerstann K, Cardones AR, Finkelstein SE, et al. Central memory self/tumor-reactive CD8+ T cells confer superior antitumor immunity compared with effector memory T cells. Proc Natl Acad Sci U S A. 2005; 102(27):9571-6.

[37] Restifo NP, Dudley ME, Rosenberg SA. Adoptive immunotherapy for cancer: harnessing the T cell response. Nat Rev Immunol. 2012; 12(4):269-81.

[38] Ikeda H. T-cell adoptive immunotherapy using tumor-infiltrating T cells and genetically engineered TCR-T cells. Int Immunol. 2016; 28(7):349-53.

[39] Xu Y, Yang Z, Horan LH, Zhang P, Liu L, Zimdahl B, et al. A novel antibody-TCR (AbTCR) platform combines Fab-based antigen recognition with gamma/delta-TCR signaling to facilitate T-cell cytotoxicity with low cytokine release. Cell Discov. 2018; 4:62.

[40] Barrett DM, Grupp SA, June CH. Chimeric Antigen Receptor- and TCR-Modified T Cells Enter Main Street and Wall Street. J Immunol. 2015; 195(3):755-61.

[41] Rapoport AP, Stadtmauer EA, Binder-Scholl GK, Goloubeva O, Vogl DT, Lacey SF, et al. NY-ESO-1-specific TCR-engineered T cells mediate sustained antigen-specific antitumor effects in myeloma. Nat Med. 2015; 21(8):914-21.

[42] Kershaw MH, Westwood JA, Darcy PK. Gene-engineered T cells for cancer therapy. Nat Rev Cancer. 2013; 13(8):525-41.

[43] Zhao L, Cao YJ. Engineered T Cell Therapy for Cancer in the Clinic. Front Immunol. 2019; 10:2250.

[44] Kenderian SS, Porter DL, Gill S. Chimeric Antigen Receptor T Cells and Hematopoietic Cell Transplantation: How Not to Put the CART Before the Horse. Biol Blood Marrow Transplant. 2017; 23(2):235-46.

[45] Sadelain M, Brentjens R, Riviere I. The basic principles of chimeric antigen receptor design. Cancer Discov. 2013; 3(4):388-98.

[46] Zhang Q, Zhang Z, Peng M, Fu S, Xue Z, Zhang R. CAR-T cell therapy in gastrointestinal tumors and hepatic carcinoma: From bench to bedside. Oncoimmunology. 2016; 5(12):e1251539.

[47] Kershaw MH, Westwood JA, Slaney CY, Darcy PK. Clinical application of genetically modified T cells in cancer therapy. Clin Transl Immunology. 2014;3(5):e16.

[48] Rosenberg SA, Yang JC, Sherry RM, Kammula US, Hughes MS, Phan GQ, et al. Durable complete responses in heavily pretreated patients with metastatic melanoma using T-cell transfer immunotherapy. Clin Cancer Res. 2011; 17(13):4550-7.

[49] Heyman B, Yang Y. New developments in immunotherapy for lymphoma. Cancer Biol Med. 2018; 15(3):189-209.

[50] Ruella M, Kenderian SS. Next-Generation Chimeric Antigen Receptor T-Cell Therapy: Going off the Shelf. BioDrugs. 2017; 31(6):473-81.

[51] Neelapu SS, Locke FL, Bartlett NL, Lekakis LJ, Miklos DB, Jacobson CA, et al. Axicabtagene Ciloleucel CAR T-Cell Therapy in Refractory Large B-Cell Lymphoma. N Engl J Med. 2017; 377(26):2531-44.

[52] Cohen AD. CAR T Cells and Other Cellular Therapies for Multiple Myeloma: 2018 Update. Am Soc Clin Oncol Educ Book. 2018; 38:e6-e15.

[53] Lu C, Rong D, Zhang B, Zheng W, Wang X, Chen Z, et al. Current perspectives on the immunosuppressive tumor microenvironment in hepatocellular carcinoma: challenges and opportunities. Mol Cancer. 2019;18(1):130.

[54] Kavunja HW, Lang S, Sungsuwan S, Yin Z, Huang X. Delivery of foreign cytotoxic T lymphocyte epitopes to tumor tissues for effective antitumor immunotherapy against pre-established solid tumors in mice. Cancer Immunol Immunother. 2017; 66(4):451-60.

[55] Grigor EJM, Fergusson D, Kekre N, Montroy J, Atkins H, Seftel MD, et al. Risks and Benefits of Chimeric Antigen Receptor T-Cell (CAR-T) Therapy in Cancer: A Systematic Review and Meta-Analysis. Transfus Med Rev. 2019; 33(2):98-110.

[56] Basecke J, Griesinger F, Trumper L, Brittinger G. Leukemia- and lymphoma-associated genetic aberrations in healthy individuals. Ann Hematol. 2002; 81(2):64-75.

[57] McLean AR, Michie CA. *In-vivo* estimates of division and death rates of human T lymphocytes. Proc Natl Acad Sci U S A. 1995; 92(9):3707-11.

[58] Riley RS, June CH, Langer R, Mitchell MJ. Delivery technologies for cancer immunotherapy. Nat Rev Drug Discov. 2019; 18(3):175-96.

[59] Stephan MT, Moon JJ, Um SH, Bershteyn A, Irvine DJ. Therapeutic cell engineering with surface-conjugated synthetic nanoparticles. Nat Med. 2010;16(9):1035-41.

[60] Smith TT, Moffett HF, Stephan SB, Opel CF, Dumigan AG, Jiang X, et al. Biopolymers codelivering engineered T cells and STING agonists can eliminate heterogeneous tumors. J Clin Invest. 2017; 127(6):2176-91.

[61] Stephan SB, Taber AM, Jileaeva I, Pegues EP, Sentman CL, Stephan MT. Biopolymer implants enhance the efficacy of adoptive T-cell therapy. Nat Biotechnol. 2015; 33(1):97-101.

[62] Fesnak AD, June CH, Levine BL. Engineered T cells: the promise and challenges of cancer immunotherapy. Nat Rev Cancer. 2016; 16 (9):566-81.

[63] Lindenberg M, Retel V, Rohaan M, van den Berg J, Haanen J, van Harten W. Evaluating different adoption scenarios for TIL-therapy and the influence on its (early) cost-effectiveness. BMC Cancer. 2020; 20 (1):712.

[64] Huang R, Li X, He Y, Zhu W, Gao L, Liu Y, et al. Recent advances in CAR-T cell engineering. J Hematol Oncol. 2020; 13(1):86.

[65] Wang E, Cesano A, Butterfield LH, Marincola F. Improving the therapeutic index in adoptive cell therapy: key factors that impact efficacy. J Immunother Cancer. 2020; 8(2).

[66] Rosenberg SA, Restifo NP, Yang JC, Morgan RA, Dudley ME. Adoptive cell transfer: a clinical path to effective cancer immunotherapy. Nat Rev Cancer. 2008; 8(4):299-308.

[67] Lee PH, Yamamoto TN, Gurusamy D, Sukumar M, Yu Z, Hu-Li J, et al. Host conditioning with IL-1beta improves the antitumor function of adoptively transferred T cells. J Exp Med. 2019; 216(11):2619-34.

[68] Haso W, Lee DW, Shah NN, Stetler-Stevenson M, Yuan CM, Pastan IH, et al. Anti-CD22-chimeric antigen receptors targeting B-cell precursor acute lymphoblastic leukemia. Blood. 2013; 121(7):1165-74.

[69] Lohmueller JJ, Ham JD, Kvorjak M, Finn OJ. mSA2 affinity-enhanced biotin-binding CAR T cells for universal tumor targeting. Oncoimmunology. 2017;7(1):e1368604.

[70] Bever CS, Dong JX, Vasylieva N, Barnych B, Cui Y, Xu ZL, et al. VHH antibodies: emerging reagents for the analysis of environmental chemicals. Anal Bioanal Chem. 2016; 408(22):5985-6002.

[71] Tsunekawa N, Higashi N, Kogane Y, Waki M, Shida H, Nishimura Y, et al. Heparanase augments inflammatory chemokine production from colorectal carcinoma cell lines. Biochem Biophys Res Commun. 2016; 469(4):878-83.

[72] Caruana I, Savoldo B, Hoyos V, Weber G, Liu H, Kim ES, et al. Heparanase promotes tumor infiltration and antitumor activity of CAR-redirected T lymphocytes. Nat Med. 2015; 21(5):524-9.

[73] Dudley ME, Gross CA, Langhan MM, Garcia MR, Sherry RM, Yang JC, et al. CD8+ enriched "young" tumor infiltrating lymphocytes can mediate regression of metastatic melanoma. Clin Cancer Res. 2010; 16(24):6122-31.

[74] Bonifant CL, Jackson HJ, Brentjens RJ, Curran KJ. Toxicity and management in CAR T-cell therapy. Mol Ther Oncolytics. 2016; 3:16011.

[75] Magalhaes I, Carvalho-Queiroz C, Hartana CA, Kaiser A, Lukic A, Mints M, et al. Facing the future: challenges and opportunities in adoptive T cell therapy in cancer. Expert Opin Biol Ther. 2019; 19(8):811-27.

Chapter 8

Mathematical Modeling and Dynamics of Oncolytic Virotherapy

Abdullah Abu-Rqayiq

Abstract

Oncolytic virotherapy is a cancer treatment that uses competent replicating viruses to destroy cancer cells. This field progressed from earlier observations of accidental viral infections causing remission in many malignancies to virus drugs targeting and killing cancer cells. In this chapter, we study some basic models of the oncolytic virotherapy and their dynamics. We show how the dynamical system's theory can capture the behavior of the solutions of those models and provide different approaches to studying the models. We study the thresholds that enable us to classify asymptotic dynamics of the solutions. Fractional-derivative approach tells us about the memory of the derivative and related solutions of the models. We also study the affect of introducing control parameters on the cost of the therapy.

Keywords: Oncolytic Virotherapy, Stability, Bifurcation, Burst Size, Optimization, Immunotherapy

1. Introduction

Oncolytic viruses are a form of immunotherapy that uses viruses to infect and destroy cancer cells. These viruses can selectively replicate in cancer cells but leave healthy normal cells largely intact. In oncolytic virotherapy, the free viruses infect tumor cells and replicate themselves in tumor cells; upon analysis of infected tumor cells, new virion particles burst out and proceed to infect additional tumor cells. This idea was initially tested in the middle of the last century and merged with renewed ones over the last three decades due to the technological advances in virology and in the use of viruses as vectors for gene transfer. Over the last decade, great efforts have been made for understanding dynamics and molecular mechanics of viral cytotoxicity of oncolytic viruses. Those efforts provided an interesting possible alternative therapeutic approach to help cure cancer patients. However, the outcomes of virotherapy depends in a complex way on interactions between viruses and tumor cells [1]. One of the main advantages of applying the oncolytic virotherapy is that it can selectively damage cancerous tissues leaving normal cells unharmed. In addition, oncolytic viruses can mediate the killing of the normal cells by indirect mechanisms such as the destruction of tumor blood vessels, the amplification of specific anticancer immune responses or through the specific activities of transgene-encoded proteins expressed from engineered viruses.

During the last two decades, several mathematical models have been applied to understanding oncolytic virotherapy. For example, Wu et al. [2] and Wein et al. [3]

proposed and analyzed some partial differential equations models to study some aspects of cancer virotherapy. For ordinary differential equations models, Wodarz in [4, 5], Komarova and Wodarz [6], Novozhilov et al. [7], and Bajzer et al. [8], Tian in [9, 10], and others. Wodarz and Komarova [11] have modeled the dynamics of the oncolytic virus replication by ordinary differential equations that describe the development of the average population sizes of cells and viruses over time. For this purpose, they used a generalized approach and considered a class of models instead of a specific model and took into account two populations: uninfected tumor cells, denoted by x and infected tumor cells, denoted y. The general model is based on the law of mass action and is given by

$$\begin{aligned} \frac{dx}{dt} &= xF(x,y) - \beta yG(x,y) \\ \frac{dy}{dt} &= \beta yG(x,y) - ay, \end{aligned} \tag{1}$$

where the function F describes the growth properties of the uninfected tumor cells, and the function G describes the rate at which tumor cells become infected by the virus. The two functions can take several forms depending on the biological content and meaning that we may want to incorporate into the model. The parameter β represents the infectivity of the virus, and the death rate ay represents the virus-infected cells die.

Then, a three populations model was introduced by Wodarz [12] as

$$\begin{aligned} \frac{dx}{dt} &= rx\left(1 - \frac{x+y}{C}\right) - dx - \beta xv \\ \frac{dy}{dt} &= \beta xv - (d+a)y \\ \frac{dv}{dt} &= \alpha y - \gamma v, \end{aligned} \tag{2}$$

in which v stands for the free virus population and C is maximal tumor size. The term αy models the release of virions by infected tumor cells, and γv is the clearance rate of free virus particles by various causes including non-specific binding and generation of defective interfering particles. The death rate of tumor cells dx seems redundant, since it is included in the logistic model.

2. A basic model of oncolytic virotherapy

Tian [10] has proposed a modified model where the burst size was incorporated. The burst size of a virus is the number of new viruses released from a lysis of an infected cell. It us known that different types of viruses have different burst sizes. Viruses of the same type have almost the same burst size. The burst size is an important parameter of virus replicability.

$$\begin{aligned} \frac{dx}{dt} &= \lambda x\left(1 - \frac{x+y}{C}\right) - \beta xv \\ \frac{dy}{dt} &= \beta xv - \delta y \\ \frac{dv}{dt} &= b\delta y - \beta xv - \gamma v. \end{aligned} \tag{3}$$

Considering this last model as a starting point of our discussion of mathematical models of oncolytic virotherapy, we first show some analytical results. In this model, there are two threshold values for the burst size. When the burst size is smaller than the first threshold value, virotherapy always fails. When the burst size is in the between of the two threshold values, we have a partial success of virotherapy represented by the stable positive equilibrium solution. Since the tumor load is a decreasing function of the burst size, the minimum tumor load can be reached by genetically increasing the burst size of the virus up to the second threshold value. If the set in which the positive equilibrium solution is stable has more than one open intervals, we can increase the burst size up to the supreme value of this set, and still have stable partial therapeutic success with even lower tumor load. Once the burst size is greater than the second threshold value, there are one or three families of stable periodic solutions to the system of virotherapy dynamics.

For simplicity, the above system can be non-dimensionalized by setting $\tau = \delta t$, $x = K\hat{x}, y = K\hat{y}, v = K\hat{v}$, and rename parameters $r = \lambda, a = \beta K$, and $c = \gamma$.

Then dropping all hats over the variables and write τ as t, we have

$$\begin{aligned}\frac{dx}{dt} &= rx(1-x-y) - axv \\ \frac{dy}{dt} &= axv - y \\ \frac{dv}{dt} &= by - axv - cv\end{aligned} \tag{4}$$

It is assumed that all parameters are nonnegative.

Model (4) has three equilibrium points, $E_0 = (0,0,0)$, $E_1 = (1,0,0)$, and the positive equilibrium $E_+ = (x^*, y^*, v^*)$. The equilibrium E_0 is always unstable for all positive values of the burst size b. The equilibrium E_1 is globally asymptotically stable when $0 < b < \mu_1$, and it is unstable when $b \geq \mu_1$.

At $b = \mu_1$, the positive equilibrium E_+ moves into the domain $D = \{(x,y,v) : x \geq 0, y \geq 0, v \geq 0, 0 \leq x + y \leq 1\}$, a type of transcritical bifurcation occurs with E_1 and E_+. As the parameter b increases, while $\mu_1 < b < \mu_2$ and $b \in I_p$, E_+ is locally asymptotically stable. When $b > \mu_1$ and $b \in I_n$, E_+ is unstable. Hopf bifurcations occur for some $b \geq \mu_2$, and these bifurcations give rise to one or three families of periodic solutions. Here, μ_1 and μ_2 are thresholds, $I_p = \{b > \mu_1 : H(b) > 0\}$, $I_n = \{b > \mu_1 : H(b) < 0\}$, and $H(b)$ is defined next in formula (10).

- E_0 is unstable.
- E_1 is globally asymptotically stable when $b < 1 + \frac{c}{a}$; and unstable when $b \geq 1 + \frac{c}{a}$.
- When $\mu_1 < b < \mu_2$, the equilibrium solution E_+ is locally asymptotically stable

Two types of bifurcations occur in the system as the parameter b varies. A transcritical bifurcation at $b = \mu_1$ introduces the equilibrium point E_+ into the positive invariant domain D. The Hopf bifurcation at some value $b > \mu_1$ gives rise to the periodic solutions. The system (4) is a basic model of the oncplytic virotherapy. Three equilibrium points can be found: the trivial equilibrium

$E_0 = (0,0,0)$, $E_1(1,0,0)$, and the positive equilibrium $E_+(x^*, y^*, v^*)$, where $x^* = \frac{c}{a(b-1)}$, $y^* = \frac{rc(ab-a-c)}{a(b-1)(ab-a+rc)}$, and $v^* = \frac{r(ab-a-c)}{a(ab-a+rc)}$.

The Jacobian matrix is given by

$$J = \begin{pmatrix} r - 2rx - ry - av & -rx & -ax \\ av & -1 & ax \\ -av & b & -ax - c \end{pmatrix} \tag{5}$$

Proceeding in the linearization process and analyzing the eigenvalues, we find that the Jacobian matrix evaluated at E_0 is given as

$$J(E_0) = \begin{pmatrix} r & 0 & 0 \\ 0 & -1 & 0 \\ 0 & b & -c \end{pmatrix} \tag{6}$$

The obtained eigenvalues of this lower triangular matrix are $\lambda_1 = r$, $\lambda_2 = -1$, and $\lambda_3 = -c$. Note that λ_1 is positive due the r being positive. The other eigenvalues are negative. Therefore, E_0 is unstable. The local unstable invariant manifold lives in the $x-$axis. The stable invariant manifolds live in the $yv-$plane. This observation might be interpreted by saying that in the absence of viruses and the infected tumor cells, the tumor cells will grow away from E_0.

The Jacobian matrix evaluated at E_1 is given by

$$J(E_1) = \begin{pmatrix} -r & -r & a \\ 0 & -1 & a \\ 0 & b & -a - c \end{pmatrix} \tag{7}$$

The eigenvalues are $\lambda_1 = -r$, which is clearly negative, and $\lambda_{2,3} = \frac{1}{2}\left(-(1 + a + c) \pm \sqrt{(1 - a - c)^2 + 4ab}\right)$. λ_2, the eigenvalue with negative square root, is negative as well. However, for λ_3, it is not so clear when it is negative. Computations in [7], show that for $1 < b < 1 + \frac{c}{a}$, E_1 is a global asymptotically stable. This result can be obtained by applying appropriate Lyapunov functions such as $V_1(x, y, v) = y + v$ and $V_2(x, y, v) = \frac{1}{2}ab(a + c)y^2 + a^2byv + \frac{1}{2}a^2v^2$. When the value of b exceeds the threshold $\mu_1 = 1 + \frac{c}{a}$, E_1 becomes unstable. The system exhibits a transcritical bifurcation with bifurcation value μ_1 and changes stability as this parameter varies near the bifurcation value. When $b > \mu_1$, the positive equilibrium point E_+ appears. Proceeding with the linearization, the Jacobian materix at E_+ is given by

$$J(E_+) = \begin{pmatrix} r - 2rx - ry - av & -rx & -ax \\ av & -1 & ax \\ -av & b & -ax - c \end{pmatrix}. \tag{8}$$

To analyze the more complicated eigenvalue expressions, we apply the so called Routh-Hurwitz criterion on the associated characteristic polynomial $P(\lambda) = \lambda^3 + a_1\lambda^2 + a_2\lambda + a_3$, where $a_1 = \frac{rc+ab-a+abc}{a(b-1)}$, $a_2 = \frac{rc(bc+b-1)}{a(b-1)^2} + \frac{rc(ab-a-c)(r-a)}{a(b-1)(ab-a+rc)}$, and $a_3 = \frac{rc(ab-a-c)}{a(b-1)}$.

The R-H criterion requires

$$H_1 = a_1 > 0, \quad H_2 = \begin{vmatrix} a_1 & a_3 \\ 1 & a_2 \end{vmatrix} > 0, \quad \text{and} \quad H_3 = \begin{vmatrix} a_1 & a_3 & 0 \\ 1 & a_2 & 0 \\ 0 & a_1 & a_3 \end{vmatrix} > 0. \tag{9}$$

Computations based on the R-H stability criterion can lead to the following expression $\varphi(b) = \frac{a(b-1)(ab-a+rc)}{ab-a+rc+abc} - \frac{(bc+b-1)(ab-a+rc)}{(b-1)(ab-a-c)}$, [10]. the positive equilibrium E_+ is locally asymptotically stable if $\phi(b) < r - a$.

In addition to the transcritical bifurcation described above, the system develops a Hopf bifurcation for values of $b > \mu_1$ resulting in periodic solutions due to the pure imaginary eigenvalues $\pm i\sqrt{a_2}$.

In [10], bifurcation analysis was accomplished by the aid of defining a function

$$H(b) = \frac{rc\Phi(b-1)}{a^2(b-1)^3(ab-a+rc)}, \tag{10}$$

where

$$\begin{aligned}\Phi(x) &= -a(ax-c)(ax+rc)x^2 + ((a+ac)x + rc + ac)[((c+1)x+c)(ax+rc) \\ &\quad + x(ax-c)(r-a)] \\ &= -a^3x^4 + a^2(3c + c^2 + r - a - ac + 1)x^3 + ac(3rc + 3a + rc^2 + 3ac + r \\ &\quad + r^2 - a^2)x^2 + c^2(3ar + 2acr + r^2c + 2a^2)x + rc^3(r+a)\end{aligned}$$

Then, the another threshold, named μ_2 can be defined as the smallest number b of the set $I_0 = \{b > \mu_1 : H(b) = 0\}$.

The analysis presented in [10] also shows that if $\frac{c(1+r)}{ab-a+rc} < 1$, then E_+ represents a partial success of virotherapy at a modest value of b. The expression $\frac{c(1+r)}{ab-a+rc}$ is called the tumor load.

When the value of b satisfies $\mu_1 < b < \mu_2$, E_+ is locally asymptotically stable. For values of $b < \mu_1$ the positive equilibrium E_+ does not live in the positive invarient domain D, and as b increases to μ_1, the equilibrium point moves into the domain D and it coalecses with E_1. Finally, when $b > \mu_2$, periodic solutions will appear as a result of the Hope bifurcation (**Table 1**).

Parameter	Description	Value	Dimentions
λ	Tumor growth rate	2×10^{-2}	$1/h$
δ	Death rate of infected tumor cells	1/18	$1/h$
β	Infection rate of the virus	$7/10 \times 10^{-9}$	$mm^3h/$ virusl
k	Immune killing rate of virus	10^{-8}	$mm^3h/$ immune cell
b	Burst size of free virus	50	viruses/cell
γ	Clearance rate of virus	2.5×10^{-2}	$1/h$

Table 1.
Pameters' Description.

3. Model with innate immune response

Phan and Tian [13] developed the basic model by incorporating innate immune. The system is given by

$$\begin{aligned}\frac{dx}{dt} &= \lambda x\left(1-\frac{x+y}{C}\right)-\beta xv\\ \frac{dy}{dt} &= \beta xv-\mu yz-\delta y\\ \frac{dv}{dt} &= b\delta y-\beta xv-kvz-\gamma v\\ \frac{dz}{dt} &= syz-\rho z,\end{aligned}\tag{11}$$

where λ is tumor growth rate, C is the carrying capacity of tumor cell population, β is the infected rate of the virus, μ is immune killing rate of infected tumor cells, δ is death rate of infected tumor cells, b is the burst size of oncolytic viruses (i.e., the number of new viruses coming out from a lysis of an infected cell), k is immune killing rate of viruses, γ is clearance rate of viruses, s is the stimulation rate of the innate immune system, and ρ is immune clearance rate.

We non-dimensionalize the system by setting $\tau=\delta t, x=C\overline{x}, y=C\overline{y}, v=C\overline{v}, z=C\overline{z}$ and rename parameters $r=\lambda/\delta\; a=C\beta/\delta, c=\mu C/\delta, d=kC/\delta, e=\gamma/\delta, m=sC/\delta,$ and $n=\rho/\delta$. Then system (3.1) becomes

$$\begin{aligned}\frac{dx}{dt} &= rx(1-x-y)-axv\\ \frac{dy}{dt} &= axv-cyz-y\\ \frac{dv}{dt} &= by-axv-dvz-ev\\ \frac{dz}{dt} &= myz-nz.\end{aligned}\tag{12}$$

All parameters are assumed to be nonnegative. The effects of the innate immune system on the virotherapy in the model are encoded in the parameters $c, d,$ and m. To understand how the innate immune system affects the dynamics of oncolytic virotherapy, they use three combined parameters, the viral burst size b, the relative immune killing rate $K=c/d,$ and the relative immune response decay rate $N=n/m,$ to describe the solution behaviors of the model. Note that K represents the ratio of the rate of immune killing infected tumor cells over the rate of immune killing viruses, which can be considered as a relative immune killing rate of viral therapy since it describes the ability of the innate immune system destroying infection versus destroying viruses.

The system (12) have the following equilibrium points;

$E_0=(0,0,0,0)$,

$E_1=(1,0,0,0)$,

$E_2=\left(\frac{e}{a(b-1)}, \frac{re(ab-a-e)}{a(b-1)(ab-a+re)}, \frac{r(ab-a-e)}{a(ab-a+re)}, 0\right)$,

$E_3=\left(1-N-\frac{aA}{r}, N, A, \frac{(b-1)N-eA}{cN+dA}\right)$,

$E_4=\left(1-N-\frac{v_2}{q}, N, v_2, \frac{(b-1)N-ev_2}{cN+dv_2}\right)$, and

$E_5=\left(1-N-\frac{v_3}{q}, N, v_3, \frac{(b-1)N-ev_3}{cN+dv_3}\right)$.

Where $N = n/m$, $A = \left(-a_2 + \sqrt{a_2^2 - 3a_1}\right)/3$, $a_1 = \frac{rN}{a^2} \cdot \frac{c}{d}\left(-a + aN - e + \frac{d}{c}\right)$, and $a_2 = \frac{c}{d}N + \frac{r}{a}(N-1)$.

The analysis of model (12) is similar but more complicated than the basic model proposed by Tian. For details, see [13].

Now we describe some results of Phan and Tian work, [13]. It is clear that if no tumor cells existed, then there exists the equilibrium point E_0. If the effect of the immune system and the viruses is neglected, then the system has another equilibrium point E_1 with only tumor cells. This happens when the viruses are not powerful due to the burst size being smaller than some critical value. The equilibrium E_2 exists if the burst size is greater than the critical value (threshold), meaning that the viruses are powerful. With some conditions on the parameter K and with another burst size critical value, two newly formed equilibrium points will be born for values of b exceed the critical point.

Analysis and numerical simulation can show the existence of two types of bifurcations around the threshold values; the transcritical bifurcation which occurs with the equilibrium points E_1 and E_2, and a Hopf bifurcation that occurs for larger values of the burst size b.

Due to the complexity of expressions and knowing that it is impossible to find closed forms of bifurcation parameters, especially for the positive equilibrium points E_3, E_4, and E_5, numerical simulations become a need in order to capture the different behavior over the dynamical landscape.

Below the first threshold value of the burst size, the tumor always grows to its maximum size (carrying capacity), then as the bfurcation parameter b passes the first threshold value, the first locally stable positive equilibrium is born through the transcritical bifurcation. When the parameter value is at or exceeds the second threshold, families of periodic solutions arise from the Hopf bifurcation leading to undetectible level of tumor load.

4. Fractional derivative approach

Fractional derivative is a generalization of the usual derivative to include all orders of derivations. It can be traced back to the times of the invention of the calculus itself. The question about the 1/2 derivative was first asked by L'hopital as a reply to Leibniz letter which introduces the notation of the nth derivative. Most of biological systems have long-range temporal memory. Modeling such systems by fractional models provides the systems with a long-time memory and extra degrees of freedom. Despite of the fact that differential equations with integer-orders have long been used in modeling cancer, the fractional-order differential equations (FODEs) have been recently used to model many biological phenomena. One of the advantages of using FODEs to model such phenomena is that models become more consistent with the biological model. This is due to the fact that fractional order derivatives can capture the memory and hereditary properties of those models [14]. The classical mathematical models with integer-orders ignore the intermediate cellular interactions and memory effects. For example, the kinetic of the viral decline in patients responding to interferon is characterized by bi-phase shape following a delay about $8-9$ hours, likely to be the sum of interferono-pharmacokinetics and pharmaco-dynamics as well as the intracellular delay of the ciral life cycle [15]. Therefore, modeling of the biological systems by fractional order differential equations has more advantages than classical integer-order mathematical modeling, in which such effects are neglected. Abu-Rqayiq and Zannon [16] have formulated Tian's model using Caputo derivative definition. The system can be formulated as

$$\begin{aligned} D_t^{\alpha}x &= r^{\alpha}x(1-x-y) - a^{\alpha}xv \\ D_t^{\alpha}y &= a^{\alpha}xv - y \\ D_t^{\alpha} &= b^{\alpha}y - a^{\alpha}xv - c^{\alpha}v. \end{aligned} \tag{13}$$

where D_t^{α} is the Caputo fractional derivative and $0 < \alpha \le 1$. We assume that all parameters are nonnegative.

The fractional order integration and fractional order can be defined as: the definition of fractional order integration and fractional order. Let $L^1 = L^1[a,b]$ be the class of Lebesgue integrable functions on $[a,b]$, $a < b < \infty$. The fractional integral of order $\nu \in \mathbb{R}^+$ of the function $f(t), t > 0$ ($f : \mathbb{R} \to \mathbb{R}$) is defined by

$$I_a^{v} = \frac{1}{\Gamma(v)} \int_q^t (t-s)^{v-1} f(s) ds, \quad t > 0, \tag{14}$$

where $\Gamma(.)$ is the Gamma function.

The fractional derivative of order $\alpha \in (n-1, n)$ of the function $f(t)$ is defined by several ways, the most common ones are:

1. Riemann-Liouville fractional derivative: Take the fractional integral of order $(n-\alpha)$ and then apply the nth derivative

$$D_{a}^{a} f(t) = D_{\alpha}^{a} I_{n-\alpha}^{a},$$

where $D_n^* = \frac{d^n}{dt^n}, n = 1, 2, \ldots;$

2. Caputo's fractional derivative: Start with a nth derivative of the function, then take a fractional integral of order $(n-\alpha)$

$$D_{a}^{a} f(t) = I_{n-\alpha}^{a} D_{n}^{a} f(t), n = 1, 2, \ldots.$$

Since fractional-order models possess memory, FODE gives us a more realistic way to model oncolytic virotherapy and study their dynamics. The presence of a fractional derivative in a differential equation can lead to an increase in the complexity of the observed behavior. On the other hand, it can show how the solution is continuously dependent on all the previous states. The numerical results of applying the fractional approach will be show in **Figures 1–4**.

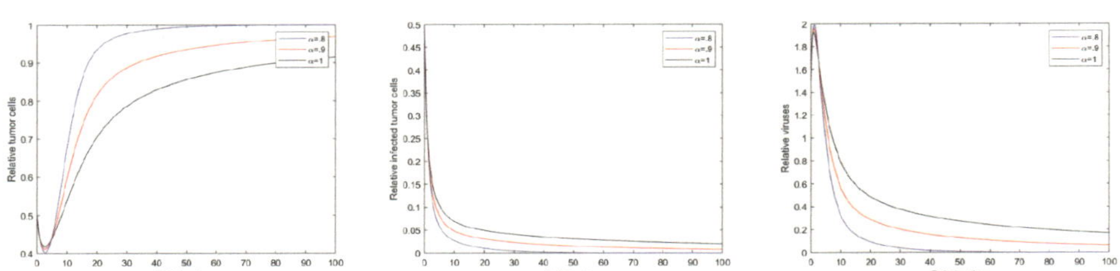

Figure 1.
Dynamics of virotherapy when $b = 4$ and initial values $x = 0.5$, $y = 0.5$, and $\nu = 1.5$, for $\alpha = 1$, $\alpha = .8$, and $\alpha = .9$.

DOI: http://dx.doi.org/10.5772/intechopen.96963

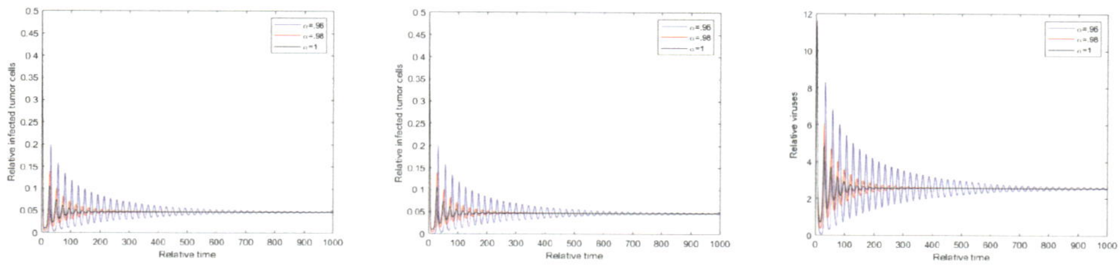

Figure 2.
Damped oscillators when $b = 27$ *and initial values* $x = 0.5$, $y = 0.5$, *and* $\nu = 1.5$, *for* $\alpha = .96$, $\alpha = .98$, *and* $\alpha = 1$.

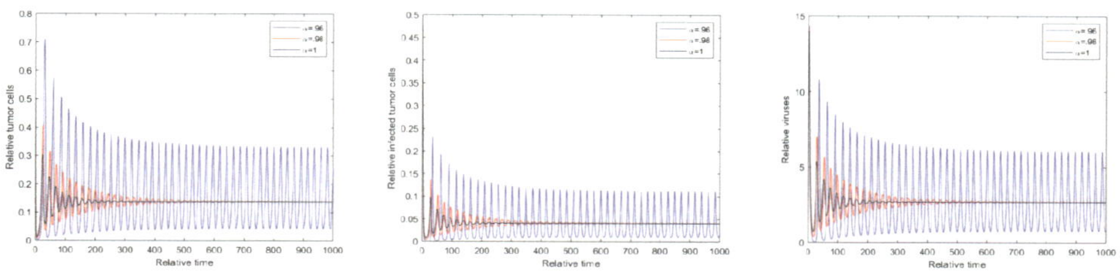

Figure 3.
Dynamics of model when $b = 28$ *and initial values* $x = 0.5$, $y = 0.5$, *and* $\nu = 1.5$, *for* $\alpha = .96$, $\alpha = .98$, *and* $\alpha = 1$.

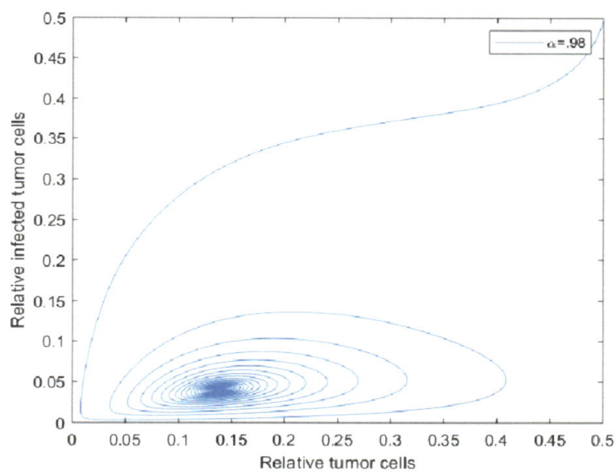

Figure 4.
Dynamics of Tumor cells vs infected tumor cells of the model when $\alpha = .98$.

5. Optimization by control theory

In this section, we develop a model for the controlled infected brain tumor cells. optimal control theory is applied to the cost functional and is supposed to achieve the ultimate goal of optimizing that functional and find a best strategy for minimizing the cost of the virotherapy. The goal here is to model, analyze, and explore optimal ways that can minimize a tumor and the cost of the virotherapy.

Optimal control theory is a branch of the applied mathematics that deals with finding the best possible control that can take a dynamical system from one state to another. The Hamiltonian of optimal control theory was developed by the Russian mathematician Lev Pontryagin as a part of his investigation into the maximum principle. Pontryagin proved that the necessary condition for solving certain optimal control problems is that the control should be chosen in such a way that minimizes the Hamiltonian, [17].

The general form of the control function $u(t)$ is given by

$$J(u(t)) = \Psi(x(T)) + \int_0^1 L(x(t), u(t), T(t))dt$$

where $x(t)$ is the system state which evolves according to the state equation

$$\dot{x} = \mathbf{f}(x(t), u(t), t) \quad x(0) = x_0 \quad t \in [0, T]$$

The Hamiltonian is defined as

$$H(x, \Psi, u, t) = \Psi^T(t)f(x, u, t) + L(x, u, t),$$

where $\Psi(t)$ is a vector of costate variables of the same dimension as the state variable $x(t)$ such that, [18]

$$\dot{\Psi}(t) = -\frac{\partial H}{\partial x}.$$

Applying the control theory approach, we reformulate the basic model by introducing a control function $u(t)$ which represents efforts on damaging the tumor cells AND $(1 - u(t))$ represents the growth rate of the infected cells. After incorporating the control u into the basic model, we obtain the following model with control

$$\begin{aligned} \frac{dx}{dt} &= (1 - u(t))\lambda x\left(1 - \frac{x + y}{K}\right) - \beta x v \\ \frac{dy}{dt} &= \beta x v - (1 - u(t))\delta y \\ \frac{dv}{dt} &= b\delta(1 - u(t))y - \beta x v - \gamma v. \end{aligned} \tag{15}$$

The control is usually assumed to be bounded by maximim value less than 1 and greater than 0. For our current model, we assume the maximum value is 0.9, a choice that make our proposed model more realistic from a medical view point.

The objective function will be the function that will host our optimal value u^* and it is given by

$$J(u(t)) = \int_0^T y(t) + \frac{1}{2}Bu^2\, dt.$$

Where B is a measure of the relative cost of interventions associated to the control $u(t)$. Our goal is to minimize the number of the infected tumor cells by choosing an appropriate strategy that can lower the number of free viruses as well. As a result of that, the cost of treatment will be lowered.

The admissible set of control functions is defined as

$$\Omega = \{u(\cdot) \in L^\infty(0, t_f) : 0 \leqslant u(t) \leqslant u_{\max}, \forall t \in [0, T]\}$$

Rescaling the system to ease mathematical treatment, we use same parameter rescaling that was used for the previous models and we get

$$\begin{aligned}\frac{\mathrm{d}x}{\mathrm{d}t} &= (1-u)rx(1-x-y) - axv \\ \frac{\mathrm{d}y}{\mathrm{d}t} &= axv - (1-u)y \\ \frac{\mathrm{d}v}{\mathrm{d}t} &= b(1-u)y - axv - cv.\end{aligned} \tag{16}$$

with fixed initial conditions $x(0), y(0), v(0)$ and a fixed final time T.

According to The Pontryagin's Maximum Principle, if $u(.) \in \Omega$ is optimal for the problem under consideration, the minimizer with the initial conditions and fixed final time T, then there exists a nontrivial absolutely continuous mapping $\Psi : [0, 1] \rightarrow \mathbb{R}^3$.

Now we come to the main result in this section, [19]

System (16) along with the initial conditions and the final time T has a unique optimal solution $(x^*(\cdot), y^*(\cdot), v^*(\cdot))$ associated to an optimal control (u^*) on $[0, T]$. Moreover, there exists adjoint functions Ψ_1^*, Ψ_1^*, and Ψ_3^*, such that with transversality conditions $\Psi_i^*(\mathrm{T}) = 0, i = 1, 2, 3$. Furthermore,

$$u^*(t) = \frac{rx(1-x-y)\Psi_1 - y(\Psi_2 + b\Psi_3)}{B}.$$

The proof is given in [19].

6. Numerical simulation and discussion

For the simulations and numerical results of the basic model and those of the fractional approach, we use the same parameter values used in [10] and summarized in **Table 1**. We also combing those results in the **Figures 1–4** below. Note that $\alpha = 1$ represents the simulation of the basic model (2.2), whereas the other values of α describe the memory of the derivatives of the basic model. The parameter values are $r = 0.36$, $a = 0.11$, and $c = 0.2$. By considering $b = 9$, the following equilibrium points can be obtained $E_0 = (0, 0, 0, 0)$, $E_1 = (1, 0, 0)$, $E_2 = (0.6, 0.0730, 2.5729)$. Here the bifurcation parameter values are $\mu_1 = 5$ and $\mu_2 = 27.766$. When $5 < b < 27.766$, E_+ is locally asymptotically stable while E_1 is unstable. The equilibrium point E_0 is always unstable. **Figure 1** shows the treatment will eventually reach the equilibrium point E_1 that is locally asymptotically stable. **Figures 2** and **3** show periodic solutions rising from Hopf bifurcation, and **Figure 4**

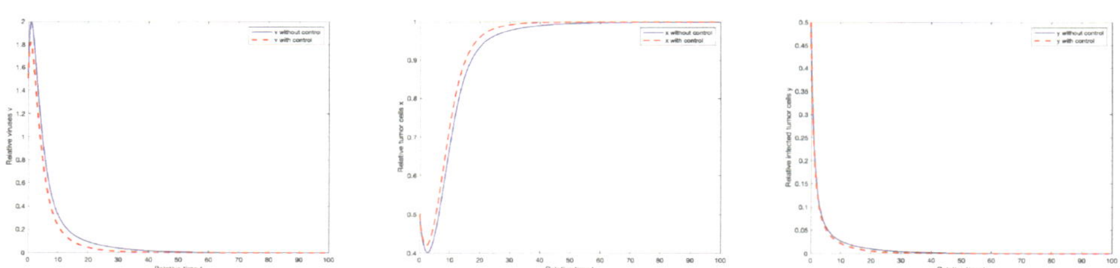

Figure 5.
Optimal state variables for the controlled and the uncontrolled systems subject to the initial values $x = 0.5, y = 0.5$, and $v = 1.5$, $b = 4$, and the admissible control set versus trajectories without control measures.

shows the dynamics of tumor cells vs infected tumor cells when $\alpha = 0.98$ which is almost the same as the result of the usual derivative $\alpha = 1$. E_+ is locally asymptotically stable when $5 < b < 27.766$.

The numerical results of the optimal control system (5.2) can be obtained by implementing forward fourth-order Runge-Kutta method for state system and the backward one for the adjoint system. The method depends on the choice of an initial guess for the value of the control u. The optimal control system is estimated to predict the evolution of the tumors cells relative to specific choices of virus bust size. Simulation shows the results in time scale of 100 days for burst size $b = 4$,

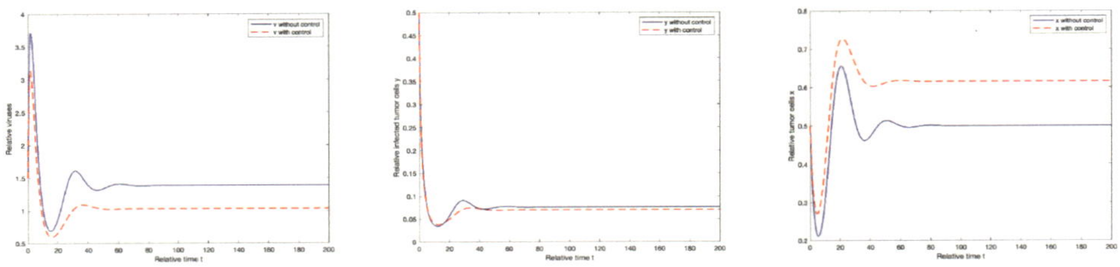

Figure 6.
Optimal state variables for the controlled and the uncontrolled systems subject to the initial values $x = 0.5, y = 0.5$, and $v = 1.5$, $b = 9$, and the admissible control set versus trajectories without control measures.

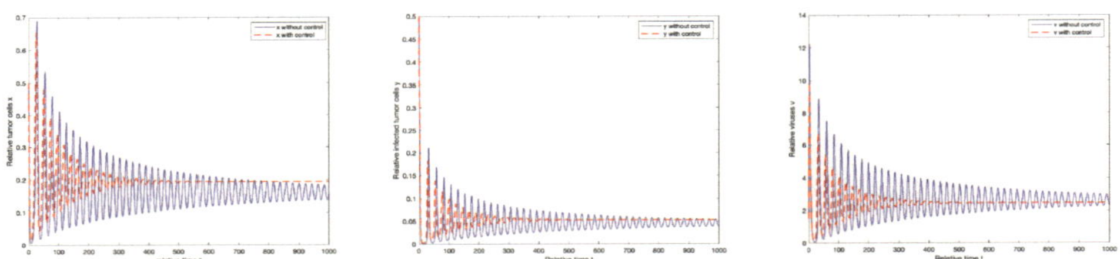

Figure 7.
Damped oscillators appear for the controlled and the uncontrolled systems subject to the initial values $x = 0.5, y = 0.5$, and $v = 1.5$, $b = 26$, and the admissible control set versus trajectories without control measures.

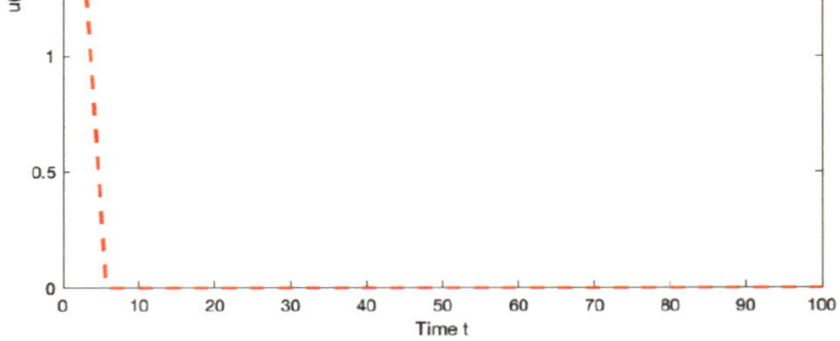

Figure 8.
The optimal control u^* for the Oncolytic virotherapy model subject to the initial values $x = 0.5, y = 0.5$, and $v = 1.5$, $b = 9$, and the admissible control.

200 days for burst size $b = 9$, and 1000 days for the oscillation to capture that behavior as shown in the **Figures 5–8**.

Numerical results show that the existence of the control can improve the growth of the normal cells until approximately 60 days of the therapy and will be stabilized after then. Whereas the number of the infected cells will be dropped significantly after the fifth day of the treatment until they are completely terminated in the day 50. The dynamics is hugely determined by the burst size in addition to the other control parameter values. The numerical results clearly show that the virotherapy can reduce the tumor load within days of the therapy and reduces number of the free viruses that are needed in the therapy. As a result, the cost of the therapy is minimized. See **Figures 5–8**.

Author details

Abdullah Abu-Rqayiq
Texas A&M University-Corpus Christi, United States

*Address all correspondence to: abdullah.aburqayiq@tamucc.edu

References

[1] E. A., Chiocca, *Oncolytic Viruses*, Nature Reviews Cancer, **2**, (2002), 938–950

[2] J. T. Wu, H. M. Byrne, D. H. Kirn, and L. M. Wein, *Modeling and analysis of a virus that replicates selectively in tumor cells*, Bulletin of Mathematical Biology, **63**, no. 4,(2001), 731–768

[3] L.M. Wein, J.T.Wu, and D.H.Kirn, *Validation and analysis of a mathematical model of a replication-competent oncolytic virus for cancer treatment: Implications for virus design and delivery*, Cancer Research, **63**, no. 6, (2003), 1317–1324

[4] D. Wodarz, *Computational approaches to study oncolytic virutherapy: insights and challenges*, Gene Ther Mol Biol, **8**(2004), 137–146.

[5] D. Wodarz, *Viruses as antitumor weapons: defining conditions for tumor remission*, Cancer Research, **61**, no 8, (2001), 3501–3507.

[6] L. Komarova and D. Wodarz, *ODE models for oncolytic virus dynamics*, Journal of Theoretical Biology, 263 (2010), 530–543

[7] A. S. Novozhilov, F., S. Berezovskaya, E. V. Koonin, and G.P. Karev, *Mathematical modeling of tumor therapy with oncolytic viruses: regimes with complete tumor elimination within the framework of deterministic models*, Biology Direct, 1, article 6,(2006), 1–18

[8] Z. Bajzer, T. Carr, K. Josic, S. J. Russell, and D. Dingli, *Modeling of cancer virotherapy with recombinant measles viruses*, Journal of Theoretical Biology, **252** (2008), 109–122

[9] A. Friedman, P. Tian, G. Fulci, A. Chiocca, and J. Wang, *Glioma Virotherapy: Effect of Innate Immune Suppression and Increased Viral Replication Capacity*, Cancer research, vol. 66, no. 4, (2006), 2314–2319

[10] P. Tian, *The Replicability of Oncolytic Virus: Defining Conditions in Tumor Virotherapy,* Mathematical Biosciences and Engineering, vol **8**, n0. 3, (2011), 841–860

[11] D. Wodarz and N. Komarova, *Towards predictive computational models of oncolytic virus therapy: Basis for experimental validation and model selection*, PloS ONE, **4** (2009), e4271.

[12] D. Wodarz, *Gene Therapy for Killing p53-Negative Cancer Cells: Use of Replicating Versus Nonreplicating Agents*, HUM. Gean Ther,, **14**, (2003), 143–159.

[13] T. Phan and P. Tian, *The Role of the Innate Immune System in Oncolytic Virotherapy*, Comp. & Math. Methods in Medicine, 6, (2017), 1–17.

[14] I. Podlubny, *Fractional Differential Equations*, Academic Press, San Diego, (1999)

[15] J. A. Machado, *Entropy analysis of integer and fractional dynamical systems*, Nonlinear Dynam., 62, (2010), 371–378.

[16] A. Abu-Rqayiq and M. Zannon, *On Dynamics of Fractional Order Oncolytic Virotherapy Models*, J. Math. Computer Sci., **20** (2020), 79–87.

[17] W. H. Fleming and R. W. Rishel, *Deterministic and Stochastic Optimal Control*, Springer Verlag, New York, (1975)

[18] R. Neilan, and S. Lenhart, *An Introduction to Optimal Control with an Application in Disease Modeling*, DIMACS Series in Discrete Mathematics and Theoretical Computer Science. Vol. 75, (2010)

[19] A. Abu-Rqayiq, H. Alayed, and M. Zannon, *Optimal Control of a Basic Oncolytic Virotherapy Model*, J. Math. Computer Sci., In Press

Section 2

Advances in Chemotherapy

Chapter 9

Molecular-Level Understanding of the Anticancer Action Mechanism of Anthracyclines

Manish Shandilya, Shrutika Sharma, Prabhu Prasad Das and Sonika Charak

Abstract

Anthracyclines drugs are used as a treatment regime to combat cancer owing to their great chemotherapeutic potential. They are characterized by the presence of a wide range of derivatives, the most famous are doxorubicin and daunorubicin. The proposed action mechanism of anthracyclines and their derivatives to exert cytotoxic effect involves the intercalation of the drug molecule into nucleic acid and inhibition of the activity of topoisomerases. These events consequences in halting DNA replication and transcription mechanisms of the cell. Understanding of the structural and conformational changes associated with nucleic acid after binding with drugs provides significant knowledge for the development of more effective drugs. A comprehensive elucidation of the molecular mechanism(s) of action of anthracyclines drugs plays a significant role in the rational drug designing to obtain an effective, selective, and safe anti-cancer drugs.

Keywords: anthracycline, anti-cancer activity, DNA, molecular mechanism

1. Introduction

Anthracyclines were primarily recognized as antibiotics due to their antibacterial properties in 1939 [1]. However, the chemical characterization of the anthracyclines which includes a rigid planar aromatic ring that remains bound to an amino-sugar by a glycosidic bond (**Figures 1** and **2**). Quinone and hydroquinone groups of these molecules on adjacent rings allow gain and loss of electrons in the conversion of quinone to the semiquinone radical [2, 3]. This semiquinone free radical converts back to quinine under aerobic conditions resulting in the formation of superoxide anion and hydrogen peroxide. The excessive formation of these free radical consequences in lipid peroxidation within cell membranes, DNA damage and finally cell death. This makes them the potent non-selective anti-cancer drugs i.e., they are used in the treatment of a wide range of cancer like small cell lung cancer, breast cancer, lymphoblastic and myeloblastic leukemia, etc. [1, 4–6]. There is a high probability that a cancer patient will be administered with anthracycline at some stage of their chemotherapy session. Daunomycin and doxorubicin were the earliest anthracyclines isolated from *Streptomyces peucetius* and were effective against a wide range of human cancers. Owing to significant antitumor potential, the World Health Organization (WHO) has included daunomycin and doxorubicin

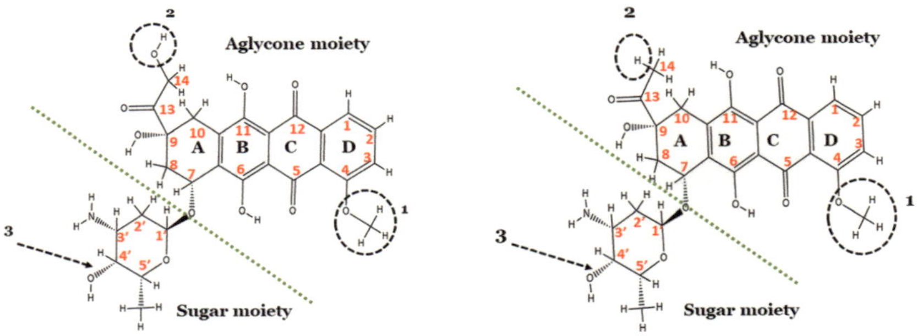

Figure 1.
Chemical structure of doxorubicin and daunorubicin. Dotted circle and dotted line arrow represents probable substitution position in anthracyclines. Doxorubicin and daunorubicin differ at C_{14} position encircled with 2. Green dotted line is used to depict aglycone and sugar moieties of anthracycline drugs. Chemical structures were rendered using ChemDeaw software.

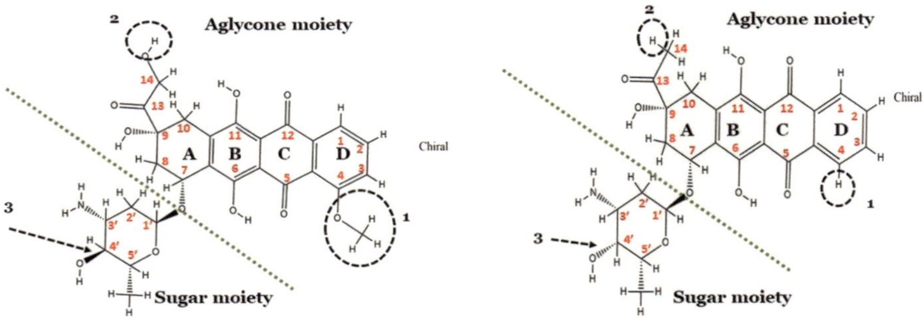

Figure 2.
*Chemical structure of epirubicin and idarubicin. Epirubicin and doxorubicin (**Figure 1**) differs at position no. 3 (C4′ of sugar moiety, stereoisomer). Idarubicin differs from daunorubicin (**Figure 1**) at position 1 by absence of methoxy group. Chemical structures were rendered using ChemDraw software.*

in the model list of medicines [7]. But it has been discovered that repeated administration of these drugs can impart chemotherapy-resistance to the tumors and cardiotoxicity [4]. To reduce or subside these side effects, major efforts are being done to find better alternatives. Therefore, the study of more than 2000 analogs has been done so far [8].

Regarding the chemical structure of daunomycin $C_{27}H_{29}NO_{10}$ and doxorubicin $C_{27}H_{29}NO_{11}$, they share the same carbon skeleton (**Figure 1**). The difference in their chemical structure comes at the side chain at C-14 position; daunomycin has a hydrogen atom whereas doxorubicin has an alcohol group (**Figure 1**) [5, 6].

2. Proposed action mechanisms

2.1 Anthracyclines as DNA intercalators

The exact mechanism of the anthracycline in the body is not known and still under investigation. However, DNA is recognized as the prime target of well-known anthracycline like doxorubicin. The primary mechanism involves the intercalation of planar tetracyclic chromophore between the DNA base pairs subsequently affecting the transcription and translation of DNA. The binding affinity of the drug to DNA is not only the factor contributing to the cytotoxic activity of anthracyclines but other factors like binding mode and binding site of anthracycline also play important role in exerting cytotoxic effects.

The specificity, binding affinity, and the binding mode of every anthracycline differ with the difference in the sequence of DNA bases (**Figures 3–5**). Structural, computational and solution studies on the daunomycin-DNA complex have provided the information that daunomycin has preferential binding where AT is present between two GC base pairs i.e. GCATGC [9, 10]. Equilibrium binding and DNase footprinting methods were utilized to study site and sequence specificity of daunorubicin to DNA. The results of these experiments demonstrate that daunomycin indeed recognizes specific DNA sequences and its binding affinity with DNA increases with an increase in GC content [11]. Moreover, the effect of daunorubicin in cleaving the linear pBR322 DNA by restriction endonuclease *Eco*RI and PvuI was investigated to assess the sequence-specific binding of daunorubicin [11]. The recognition sequence of *Eco*RI and PvuI are 5′-GAATTC-3′and 5′-CGATCG-3′ respectively. Chaires et al. observed that PvuI inhibits the rate of digestion of pBR322 DNA more than the *Eco*RI suggesting preferential sequence specificity of daunorubicin. Similar results were evident from the crystal structure analysis of daunomycin-DNA d (CpGpTpApCpG) complexes (**Figure 4**) [10]. The specificity for the GC base pair is due to the hydrogen bonds formed during the interaction. The hydroxyl group on C9 of daunorubicin interact with N2 and N3 of guanine with two hydrogen bonds. This preference to GC base pair also explains the increase in binding affinity of the drug with an increase in GC content of DNA [10]. Similarly, crystal structures of anthracyclines like doxorubicin, epirubicin, and idarubicin show sequence-specific intercalative binding mode between DNA bases (**Figures 3** and 5).

Moreover, several experiments were done to study the intercalation mechanism of anthracyclines with DNA. A spectrofluorometric method was also developed for the estimation of anthracycline intercalation in living cells and DNA solutions [12]. Belloc et al. have done measurement of anthracyclines (daunorubicin and idarubicin) intercalation in the DNA of living cells by flow cytometry [13]. Ashley et al. has demonstrated the intercalative property of anthracyclines in nuclear as well as in mitochondrial DNA using picogreen (fluorescent DNA binding dye) [14]. The intercalation of anthracycline into mitochondrial DNA has a significant impact

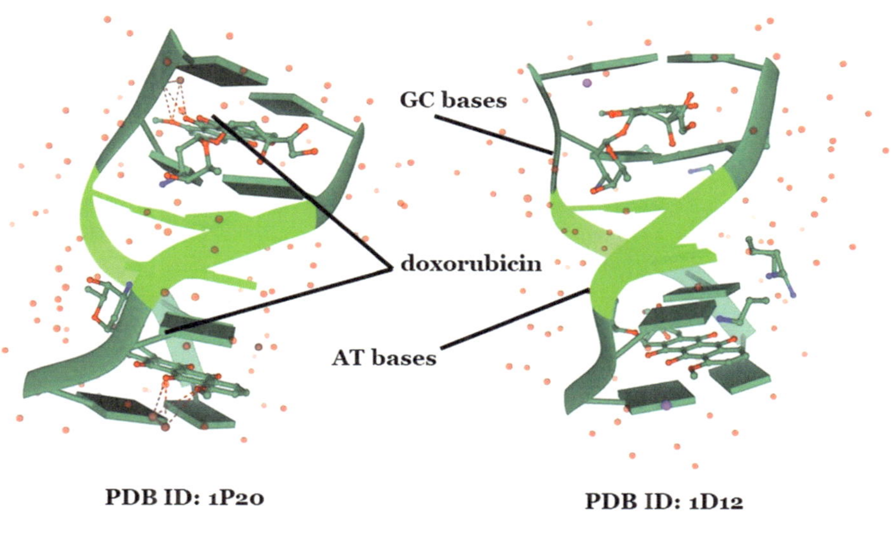

Figure 3.
Intercalation of doxorubicin between GC basepairs. Crystal structure of doxorubicin getting intercalated between GC bases. Structures are taken from protein data bank. Light green color depicts AT baseparing and dark green color shows GC bases. Red dots represent crystallized water molecules. Figure clearly depicts intercalation of doxorubicin in GC bases of DNA and preferential binding with nucleotide sequences.

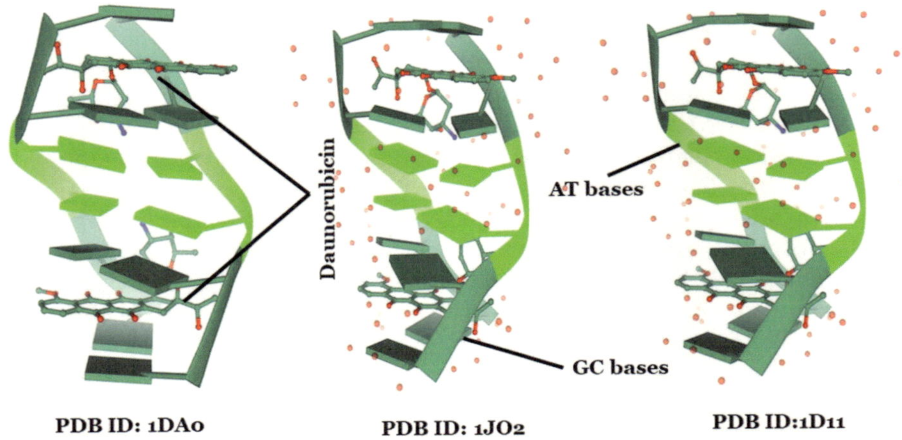

Figure 4.
Intercalation of daunorubicin between GC basepairs. Crystal structure of daunorubicin getting intercalated between GC bases. Structures are taken from protein data bank. Light green color depicts AT baseparing and dark green color shows GC bases. Red dots represent crystallized water molecules. Figure clearly depicts intercalation of doxorubicin in GC bases of DNA and preferential binding with nucleotide sequences.

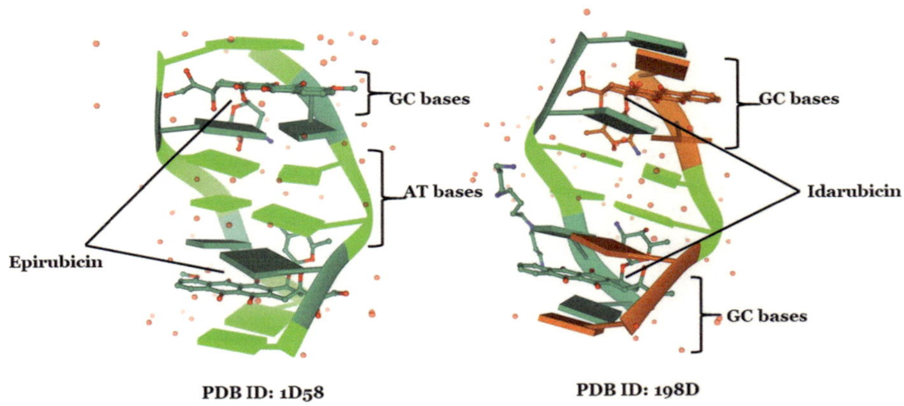

Figure 5.
Intercalation of epirubicin and idarubicin between GC basepairs. Crystal structure of epirubicin getting intercalated between AT and GC basepairs. Crystal structure of idarubicin getting intercalated between GC bases. Structures are taken from protein data bank. Red dots represent crystallized water molecules. Figure clearly depicts intercalation of epirubicin and idarubicin in GC bases of DNA and preferential binding with nucleotide sequences.

on mitochondrial toxicity. The effect of doxorubicin binding on the morphology of the single stranded DNA was further quantitatively analyzed using Atomic Force Microscopy (AFM). AFM studies strengthen the probable mechanism of intercalative binding mode as consequences of doxorubicin interaction with DNA [15].

Other studies found that B-DNA is preferred over Z-DNA by the daunorubicin for binding. Allosteric conversion of the Z form into B form has also been observed in some cases. Ionic concentration in which usually Z form of DNA is present changes to B form on the binding of daunorubicin to poly dGdC or resist to change from B form to Z form [16]. There are several pieces of evidence suggesting drug binding to DNA results in the inhibition of specific DNA function contributing towards their therapeutic effects.

2.2 How anthracyclines damage DNA?

Anthracyclines are known to damage DNA by several mechanisms which include topoisomerase-II poisoning, free radical formation, and DNA-anthracycline adduct formation. The semiquinone radical of anthracycline can intercalate between DNA base pair resulting in DNA damage by forming reactive oxygen species (ROS).

2.2.1 Via topoisomerase II poisoning

Along with DNA intercalation, topoisomerase II is also considered as the primary target of anthracyclines [17]. Topoisomerases help in solving the topological problems like supercoiling, knotting, and catenation of DNA during replication, transcription, and recombination by creating single and double stranded breaks and subsequently rejoining the breaks. Based on structure and function, mammalian cells have two types of topoisomerases which are topoisomerase I and II. Topoisomerase I is monomeric and forms single strand breaks in DNA whereas topoisomerase II is dimeric and introduces double stranded breaks in DNA. Anthracyclines interfere with the normal functioning of breaking and rejoining of DNA strands by topoisomerases, particularly topoisomerase II consequence in the formation of an abortive anthracycline- DNA-topoisomerase ternary complex, hence poisoning the enzyme action. This ternary complex impends the religation of breaks in the dsDNA. Hence, anthracyclines act on topoisomerase II and stabilize the DNA-topoisomerase II complex. Due to this topoisomerase II which otherwise is essential for the normal functioning of the cell now acts as a lethal toxin to the cell and leads the cell to apoptosis. During intercalation, the planar ring of the aglycone and sugar moiety remains in contact with DNA bases while the A ring and the substituents present the C9 which are present in the minor groove of DNA interact with the enzyme (**Figures 1** and **2**). Perhaps that's why modifying the C9 substituent changes the activity of the drug. Cleavage does not occur on all the sites recognized by the Topoisomerase II and depends on the specific base sequence where the drug interacts with the enzyme. An increase in drug activity is seen when the 4-methoxy group is removed and the sugar moiety is substituted on 3′. 3′ substitution also has a significant role in the determination of specific sites for anthracycline associated cleavage of DNA.

Several lines of evidence have shown that these anthracyclines induce irreversible DNA damage by forming a ternary complex with DNA topoisomerase which introduces permanent double stranded breaks which ultimately lead to apoptosis in rapidly dividing cells [18, 19].

2.2.2 Via oxidative stress

Anthracyclines also causes the production of free radicals inside the cell which are responsible for the cytotoxic effect of these drugs. Though the mechanism of this process is still unclear increased number of reactive oxygen species (ROS) and the presence of deoxyaglycone in the urine after the administration of drugs indicates the possibility of this mechanism [5]. Oxidative stress is the imbalance between the reactive nitrogen species and reactive oxygen species in the cell. Mitochondria are believed to take part in this process. Quinone ring of the anthracyline aglycone act as electron acceptor (**Figures 1** and **2**). In the electron transport chain (ETC), one electron is transferred from NADPH to flavoprotein and then to the aglycone due to which quinone gets reduced to form semiquinone free radical. This reaction is catalyzed by NADPH cytochrome P-450 reductase [20]. From the semiquinone, this electron gets transferred to oxygen and semiquinone gets converted into stable hydroquinone in this redox cycle. Due to this electron transfer oxygen gets reduced to superoxide which readily gets converted to other reactive oxygen species like hydroxyl radical which is harmful to cells. These reactive oxygen species can lead to DNA damage and lipid peroxidation which finally result in cell apoptosis.

When oxygen becomes limiting, semiquinone free radical transfer the electron to other electron acceptors, and rearrangement in anthracyclines takes place. The aglycone ring remains connected to sugar moiety by a glycosidic bond which is an ether containing linkage with oxygen in it which accepts the unpaired electron and due to this cleavage of glycosidic bond takes place. As a result, the formation of 7-deoxyaglycone takes place which either directly passes through urine or as conjugates in the bile [5]. There are several hypotheses explaining why superoxide dismutase (SOD), catalase, and antioxidants do not work effectively after the administration of anthracyclines. Studies have shown that anthracyclines can alter the glutathione (GSH) level and the enzymes involved in its redox pathway. According to another hypothesis free radicals are formed on the cell surface or internally in the cell and then get transferred to the cell surface due to which SOD and catalase fail to act upon these ROS [17].

2.2.3 Via forming DNA-anthracycline adduct

Formation of the anthracycline-DNA adduct in the presence of formaldehyde is another proposed mechanism of anthracycline action. There are studies that show the formation of doxorubicin-DNA at clinically relevant concentrations of drugs [21]. Anthracycline forms covalent bond with one DNA strand and hydrogen bond with other DNA strand resulting in DNA damage. The reaction between anthracycline and cellular formaldehyde is the foremost step to form activated Schiff base which then forms aminal linkage with the exocyclic amino group of guanosine. Formaldehyde in the cells is derived from the various carbon sources like lipids and spermine by iron mediated free radical reactions. In addition, Kato et al. have found increased formaldehyde levels in the cancer cells as compared to normal cells [22].

Phillips et al. using the bidirectional transcription footprinting technique demonstrate that adriamycin-DNA adduct formation induces transcription inhibition with alkylation at specific DNA sites [23]. However, Bilardi et al. have demonstrated that anthracycline-DNA adduct induces breaks in DNA via a mechanism independent of topoisomerase-II [24]. Moreover, DNA breaks formation occurs mainly due to the stalled or collapsed replication fork and these DNA breaks are repaired by homologous recombination dependent process. Forrest et al. investigated the activation of DNA damage response pathways after doxorubicin-DNA adduct formation and found that the downstream processing is dependent on various stages like recognition of adduct during replication, transcription, or any other stage of the cell cycle. Ataxia telangiectasia mutated (ATM) and ATM and Rad3 related protein kinase (ATR) are the DNA damage recognition proteins that get activated in response to double and single DNA strand breaks respectively. Forrest et al. demonstrate that both ATM and ATR proteins have the capability to react with intermediates produced as a result of doxorubicin-DNA adduct formation [25].

DNA-anthracycline adduct formation probably follows a similar pattern as followed by cisplatin-DNA adduct (**Figure 6**). The same process also takes place in presence of xanthine oxidase which is present in the living cells [23, 26]. Other studies revealed that formaldehyde is also an important factor for the DNA adduct formation which is formed in the reaction media due to oxidation of different components in media by hydrogen peroxide. Formaldehyde has the carbon through

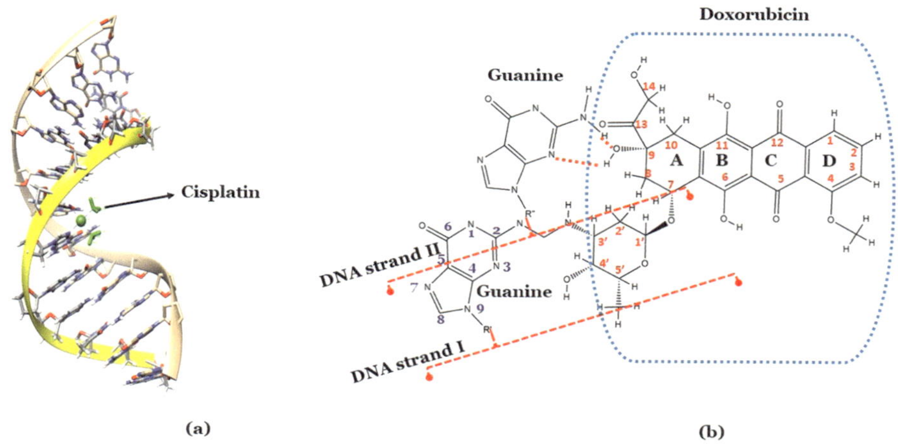

Figure 6.
DNA-drug adduct formation. DNA cisplatin structure was visualized and rendered using Chimera software. Chemical structures were rendered using ChemDraw software. (a) DNA-cisplatin adduct (PDB ID: 2NPW). (b) Schematic representation of doxorubicin-DNA adduct.

which N-C-N i.e. covalent bond forms between 3′ NH_2 of amino sugar of doxorubicin/daunorubicin and 2-NH_2 of guanosine residue of DNA backbone (**Figure 6**) [25]. Quinone methide 1 is present as a transient form in this reaction. Further, it is stabilized by the hydrogen bond formed between two strands of double helical DNA. Though the structure of the adduct is known but the mechanism by which it promotes cell death is not clear [27].

Doxorubicin forms DNA adduct with the assistance of formaldehyde and the concentration of formaldehyde in the cell is low. So, to overcome this, some pro-drugs are administered which gets converted to formaldehyde inside the cell for e.g. pivaloyloxymethyl butyrate give rise to formaldehyde inside the cell when cleaved by esterase. Due to DNA-anthracycline adduct formation cytotoxicity of anthracyclines readily increases [21].

3. Side effects

Cardiotoxicity is one of the main side effects caused by anthracyclines. Types of cardiotoxicity are Type I and Type II, Type I cardiotoxicity results irreversible cell death, while Type II cause reversible damage. At the beginning, cardiotoxicity thought to directly correlate with the cumulative drug dose, but later on, it was discovered that cardiotoxicity can occur even during the treatment [28, 29].

Increased ROS level in cardiac cells is considered as one of the factors contributing to anthracycline mediated cardiotoxicity. Administration of anthracyclines consequences in increased ROS involving the transfer of an electron to oxygen during the reduction of quinone to semiquinone which further gets converted to hydroquinone to complete the redox cycle. This process takes place in mitochondria and the number of mitochondria is mostly higher in cardiomyocytes as compared to other cells [30]. Moreover, enzymes such as SOD, catalase, glutathione transferase, and cytochrome P450 which can reduce the level of ROS in cells are comparatively less in cardiomyocytes resulting in an increased cardiotoxic effect [31]. According to some reports, doxorubicin also increases NADPH oxidase level and enzymes containing flavin like nitric oxide synthase, p450 reductase in cardiomyocytes. These enzymes increase the level of reactive oxygen species in the cell which leads to oxidative stress [31, 32].

Doxorubicin has a strong affinity for Fe^{+3} ions and the reaction of ferric ions with hydroxyl and ketone groups of doxorubicin results in a free radical complex of doxorubicin-Fe^{+2} [33]. The interaction between the negatively charged cell membranes and as this positively charged doxorubicin-Fe complex consequences in lipid peroxidation [33, 34]. Normally the level of iron is quite low in cells and usually, at this low level, doxorubicin cannot interact with iron [29]. The balance of iron is maintained by some transport proteins in the cell and according to some recent studies, doxorubicin disturbs this balance and as a result accumulation of iron occurs in mitochondria [34, 35]. Doxorubicin also interacts with the Fe/S group of iron regulatory protein IRP1 and affects its post-translational modification due to which function of IRP1 is affected and its binding affinity to IRE (iron response element) becomes low resulting in an increased amount of iron in the cell [33]. Mitoferrin, a mitochondrial carrier protein that helps in the entry of iron into the mitochondria and another transfer protein mABC1 export out the iron from mitochondria. Doxorubicin affects the functioning of mABC1 protein due to which it stops the export of iron out of the mitochondria while mitoferrin functions normally and as a result amount of free iron increases inside mitochondria [36].

4. Anthracycline resistance

Along with cardiotoxicity, anthracyclines treatment also induce anthracycline resistance even at the desired cumulative dose [37]. Resistance to drugs can be either natural or can be acquired. Natural resistance is detected in some cells even before the administration of the drug. While the acquired one occurs after the administration of the drug. Several mechanics of drug resistance responsible for the incidence of drug-resistance which are: change in ATP- binding cassette [ABC] related drug efflux and accumulation, qualitative and quantitative changes in topoisomerase II, p53 activity, overexpression of ROS scavenging enzymes, etc. ABC (ATP- binding cassette) transporter proteins are considered as the primary cause of anthracycline related drug resistance [R]. P-glycoprotein (Pgp) is one of the ABC proteins believed to induce anthracycline resistance by drug efflux, inhibition of influx, and drug accumulation inside the cell [38]. Anthracycline interacts with Pgp which causes the active efflux of anthracycline from the cell through its transmembrane domain. Pgp is encoded by the mdr1 gene which becomes active in case of cell differentiation under any chemical or environmental effect. As the anthracycline interacts with the plasma membrane, Pgp recognizes it and exports it out. So, the increased level of Pgp creates an imbalance between the export and import of the drug.

Moreover, alteration in topoisomerase II activity either quantitative i.e. decrease in the number of enzyme or qualitative i.e. alteration in the normal activity of enzyme due to mutation or other reason can give resistance to cell against further doses of anthracyclines. Anthracycline mediated cell apoptosis also depends on the expression of p53. So, inactivation or down regulation of p53 can give rise to drug resistance [38]. SOD, GSH, catalase are the scavengers of ROS and their over expression can also impart anthracycline resistance during cytotoxicity [39]. An increase in the repair of the DNA damage caused by anthracyclines also contributes towards anthracyclines resistance in cells.

5. Anthracycline analogs

Several studies were conducted to understand the effect of structural changes in anthracyclines on their antitumor efficacy. Modification of anthracyclines has a significant impact on their antitumor activity as well as on their side effects. Therefore, a comprehensive study on understanding the effect of specific structural modifications in anthracyclines to its antitumor potential and efficacy leads to the development of better analogs. Subtle modifications in the chemical structure of anthracyclines had a significant impact on the rate of drug penetration into the nucleus [40]. Doxorubicin and it semisynthetic analog epirubicin prepared by epimerization at C-4′ sugar display different antitumor potential (**Figures 1** and **2**). Moreover, epirubicin causes less cardiac damage as compared to its parent compound. Similarly, the removal of the methoxy group in the anthraquinone structure of daunorubicin results in the formation of idarubicin, considered to a better analog with a broad spectrum of antitumor potential as compared to daunorubicin (**Figures 1** and **2**).

Numerous studies were undertaken in preparation for better analogs. One such study was done with the aim of preparing a better daunorubicin analog that was prepared and their level of cytotoxicity, DNA damaging property, cellular uptake of daunorubicin analogs was investigated to find an anthracycline that can overcome drug resistance. Anthracycline derivatives display different action mechanisms in causing DNA lesions in various human cancer cell lines as well as in their resistant sublines [41]. It was hypothesized that the replacing primary amino group at the C3 position of the daunosamine moiety by a trisubstituted amidino group might help in overcoming drug resistance [41].

Shaul et al. investigated the subcellular localization as well as their cytotoxic effect of anthracyclines and their analogs in various cell lines [42]. Association between the chemical structure of different anthracyclines and their subcellular distribution and their function was investigated in cancer cell lines. Confocal microscopy experiments were done to study subcellular localization of anthracyclines and their analogs. Fluorescent DNA intercalator displacement experiments conducted for studying the intercalative properties demonstrated that the DNA intercalation property of anthracycline was not related to their cytotoxic effect. Structural information on the binding of anthracycline drugs with the target molecule helps in the development of effective drugs.

X-ray crystallographic and NMR (nuclear magnetic resonance) spectroscopic studies on anthracyclines-target complex have been conducted in the past and provide significant information that helps in the rational designing of drugs. Proceeding in similar lines, Yan et al. investigated the interactions of doxorubicin and its derivatives with DNA using resonance Raman and surface-enhanced resonance Raman scattering spectroscopy and provide significant details on anthracycline binding with DNA [43]. Spectroscopic techniques like Fourier transform infrared spectroscopy (FTIR), circular dichroism, fluorescence provided significant information binding properties of anthracyclines with nucleic acid [44–48]. Conformational studies on anthracycline-nucleic acid complex using computational methods like molecular dynamics (MD) simulations also contributes significantly to the development of the better anthracycline alternative.

6. Conclusion

Anthracyclines are widely used as antineoplastic agents owing to their great anticancer potential. There are several mechanisms proposed by which anthracyclines exert their cytotoxic effect. These drugs mostly act as DNA intercalators and halt vital functions like transcription and replication of cells. DNA damage by topoisomerase II poisoning, oxidative stress, and by forming anthracycline-DNA adduct are other proposed mechanism of anthracycline action. Despite their widespread usage in cancer treatment, their administration consequences in certain adverse side effects including cardiotoxicity that limits their clinical use. Therefore, further elucidation of the mechanism by which anthracycline drugs exert their cytotoxic effect becomes extremely important. Structural, *in silico* molecular docking/MD simulations studies and their correlation with the cytotoxic effect provide significant information for the development of structure-based analogs. The synthesis of novel structure-based anthracycline analogs should be continued to get an analog with better efficacy and minimum side effects. The development of an analog that can reverse the effect of drug resistance as well as reduce dose-dependent toxicity is essential.

Acknowledgements

Manish Shandilya and Shrutika Sharma would like to acknowledge the support provided under the DST-FIST grant no. SR/FST/PS-I/2019/68 of Government of India. Sonika Charak is thankful to National Brain Research Centre for providing financial assistance.

Conflict of interest

The authors declare no conflict of interest.

Author details

Manish Shandilya[1], Shrutika Sharma[1], Prabhu Prasad Das[2] and Sonika Charak[3*]

1 Amity School of Applied Sciences, Amity University Haryana, Gurugram, Haryana, India

2 ACOAST, Amity University Haryana, Gurugram, Haryana, India

3 National Brain Research Centre, Manesar, Gurugram, Haryana, India

*Address all correspondence to: sonu.mbhu@gmail.com

References

[1] Fujiwara A, Hoshino T, Westley JW. Anthracycline antibiotics. Critical Reviews in Biotechnology. 1985;3(2):133-57.

[2] Bhagat A, Kleinerman ES. Anthracycline-Induced Cardiotoxicity: Causes, Mechanisms, and Prevention. Current Advances in Osteosarcoma: Springer; 2020. p. 181-92.

[3] Doroshow JH. Mechanisms of Anthracycline-Enhanced Reactive Oxygen Metabolism in Tumor Cells. Oxidative medicine and cellular longevity. 2019;2019.

[4] Krohn K. Anthracycline Chemistry and Biology I: Biological Occurence and Biosynthesis, Synthesis and Chemistry: Springer; 2009.

[5] Bachur NR. Anthracycline antibiotic pharmacology and metabolism. Cancer Treat Rep. 1979;63(8):7-820.

[6] Beretta GL, Zunino F. Molecular mechanisms of anthracycline activity. Anthracycline Chemistry and Biology II: Springer; 2007. p. 1-19.

[7] Organization WH. The selection and use of essential medicines: report of the WHO Expert Committee on Selection and Use of Essential Medicines, 2019 (including the 21st WHO Model List of Essential Medicines and the 7th WHO Model List of Essential Medicines for Children). 2019.

[8] Nadas J, Sun D. Anthracyclines as effective anticancer drugs. Expert Opinion on Drug Discovery. 2006;1(6):549-68.

[9] Chaires JB. Biophysical chemistry of the daunomycin-DNA interaction. Biophysical chemistry. 1990;35(2-3):191-202.

[10] Wang AH, Ughetto G, Quigley GJ, Rich A. Interactions between an anthracycline antibiotic and DNA: molecular structure of daunomycin complexed to d (CpGpTpApCpG) at 1.2-. ANG. resolution. Biochemistry. 1987;26(4):1152-63.

[11] Chaires JB, Fox KR, Herrera JE, Britt M, Waring MJ. Site and sequence specificity of the daunomycin-DNA interaction. Biochemistry. 1987;26(25):8227-36.

[12] Tarasiuk J, Frézard F, Garnier-Suillerot A, Gattegno L. Anthracycline incorporation in human lymphocytes. Kinetics of uptake and nuclear concentration. Biochimica et Biophysica Acta (BBA)-Molecular Cell Research. 1989;1013(2):109-17.

[13] Belloc F, Lacombe F, Domain P, Lopez F, Bernard P, Boisseau MR, et al. Intercalation of anthracyclines into living cell DNA analyzed by flow cytometry. Cytometry. 1992;13(8):880-5.

[14] Ashley N, Poulton J. Mitochondrial DNA is a direct target of anti-cancer anthracycline drugs. Biochemical and biophysical research communications. 2009;378(3):450-5.

[15] Cassina V, Seruggia D, Beretta GL, Salerno D, Brogioli D, Manzini S, et al. Atomic force microscopy study of DNA conformation in the presence of drugs. European Biophysics Journal. 2011;40(1):59-68.

[16] Chaires JB. Long-range allosteric effects on the B to Z equilibrium by daunomycin. Biochemistry. 1985;24(25):7479-86.

[17] Gewirtz D. A critical evaluation of the mechanisms of action proposed for the antitumor effects of the anthracycline antibiotics adriamycin and daunorubicin. Biochemical pharmacology. 1999;57(7):727-41.

[18] Pommier Y, Leo E, Zhang H, Marchand C. DNA topoisomerases and their poisoning by anticancer and antibacterial drugs. Chemistry & biology. 2010;17(5):421-33.

[19] Visone V, Szabó I, Perugino G, Hudecz F, Bánóczi Z, Valenti A. Topoisomerases inhibition and DNA binding mode of daunomycin–oligoarginine conjugate. Journal of enzyme inhibition and medicinal chemistry. 2020;35(1):1363-71.

[20] Murabito A, Hirsch E, Ghigo A. Mechanisms of anthracycline-induced cardiotoxicity: is mitochondrial dysfunction the answer? Frontiers in Cardiovascular Medicine. 2020;7.

[21] Coldwell KE, Cutts SM, Ognibene TJ, Henderson PT, Phillips DR. Detection of Adriamycin–DNA adducts by accelerator mass spectrometry at clinically relevant Adriamycin concentrations. Nucleic acids research. 2008;36(16):e100.

[22] Kato S, Burke PJ, Koch TH, Bierbaum VM. Formaldehyde in human cancer cells: detection by preconcentration-chemical ionization mass spectrometry. Analytical chemistry. 2001;73(13):2992-7.

[23] Cullinane C, Phillips DR. Induction of stable transcriptional blockage sites by adriamycin: GpC specificity of apparent adriamycin-DNA adducts and dependence on iron (III) ions. Biochemistry. 1990;29(23):5638-46.

[24] Bilardi R, Kimura K-I, Phillips D, Cutts S. Processing of anthracycline-DNA adducts via DNA replication and interstrand crosslink repair pathways. Biochemical pharmacology. 2012;83(9):1241-50.

[25] Forrest RA, Swift LP, Rephaeli A, Nudelman A, Kimura K-I, Phillips DR, et al. Activation of DNA damage response pathways as a consequence of anthracycline-DNA adduct formation. Biochemical pharmacology. 2012;83(12):1602-12.

[26] Cutts SM, Nudelman A, Rephaeli A, Phillips DR. The power and potential of doxorubicin-DNA adducts. IUBMB life. 2005;57(2):73-81.

[27] Taatjes DJ, Gaudiano G, Resing K, Koch TH. Alkylation of DNA by the anthracycline, antitumor drugs adriamycin and daunomycin. Journal of medicinal chemistry. 1996;39(21):4135-8.

[28] Smith LA, Cornelius VR, Plummer CJ, Levitt G, Verrill M, Canney P, et al. Cardiotoxicity of anthracycline agents for the treatment of cancer: systematic review and meta-analysis of randomised controlled trials. BMC cancer. 2010;10(1):1-14.

[29] Salazar-Mendiguchía J, González-Costello J, Roca J, Ariza-Solé A, Manito N, Cequier Á. Anthracycline-mediated cardiomyopathy: basic molecular knowledge for the cardiologist. Arch Cardiol Mex. 2014;84(3):218-23.

[30] Pai VB, Nahata MC. Cardiotoxicity of chemotherapeutic agents. Drug safety. 2000;22(4):263-302.

[31] Octavia Y, Tocchetti CG, Gabrielson KL, Janssens S, Crijns HJ, Moens AL. Doxorubicin-induced cardiomyopathy: from molecular mechanisms to therapeutic strategies. Journal of molecular and cellular cardiology. 2012;52(6):1213-25.

[32] Aviello G, Knaus UG. NADPH oxidases and ROS signaling in the gastrointestinal tract. Mucosal Immunology. 2018;11(4):1011-23.

[33] Renu K, Abilash V, PB TP, Arunachalam S. Molecular mechanism of doxorubicin-induced cardiomyopathy–An update.

European journal of pharmacology. 2018;818:241-53.

[34] Gammella E, Maccarinelli F, Buratti P, Recalcati S, Cairo G. The role of iron in anthracycline cardiotoxicity. Frontiers in pharmacology. 2014;5:25.

[35] Xu X, Persson H, Richardson D. Molecular pharmacology of the interaction of anthracyclines with iron. Molecular pharmacology. 2005;68(2):261-71.

[36] Ichikawa Y, Ghanefar M, Bayeva M, Wu R, Khechaduri A, Prasad SVN, et al. Cardiotoxicity of doxorubicin is mediated through mitochondrial iron accumulation. The Journal of clinical investigation. 2014;124(2):617-30.

[37] Kaye S, Merry S. Tumour cell resistance to anthracyclines—a review. Cancer chemotherapy and pharmacology. 1985;14(2):96-103.

[38] Lam V. p53 gene status and chemosensitivity of childhood acute lymphoblastic leukemia cells to antinoneoplastic agents: National Library of Canada= Bibliothèque nationale du Canada; 2001.

[39] Harbottle A, Daly AK, Atherton K, Campbell FC. Role of glutathione S-transferase P1, P-glycoprotein and multidrug resistance-associated protein 1 in acquired doxorubicin resistance. International journal of cancer. 2001;92(6):777-83.

[40] Kerr D, Kaye S. Aspects of cytotoxic drug penetration, with particular reference to anthracyclines. Cancer chemotherapy and pharmacology. 1987;19(1):1-5.

[41] Ciesielska E, Studzian K, Wąsowska M, Oszczapowicz I, Szmigiero L. Cytotoxicity, cellular uptake and DNA damage by daunorubicin and its new analogues with modified daunosamine moiety. Cell biology and toxicology. 2005;21(3-4):139-47.

[42] Shaul P, Frenkel M, Goldstein EB, Mittelman L, Grunwald A, Ebenstein Y, et al. The structure of anthracycline derivatives determines their subcellular localization and cytotoxic activity. ACS medicinal chemistry letters. 2013;4(3):323-8.

[43] Yan Q, Priebe W, Chaires JB, Czernuszewicz RS. Interaction of doxorubicin and its derivatives with DNA: Elucidation by resonance Raman and surface-enhanced resonance Raman spectroscopy. Biospectroscopy. 1997;3(4):307-16.

[44] Ray B, Agarwal S, Kadian H, Gambhir K, Sharma P, Mehrotra R. Deciphering molecular aspects of interaction between anticancer drug mitoxantrone and tRNA. Journal of Biomolecular Structure and Dynamics. 2017;35(10):2090-102.

[45] Li N, Ma Y, Yang C, Guo L, Yang X. Interaction of anticancer drug mitoxantrone with DNA analyzed by electrochemical and spectroscopic methods. Biophysical chemistry. 2005;116(3):199-205.

[46] Charak S, Shandilya M, Mehrotra R. RNA targeting by an anthracycline drug: spectroscopic and in silico evaluation of epirubicin interaction with tRNA. Journal of Biomolecular Structure and Dynamics. 2020;38(6):1761-71.

[47] Charak S, Jangir DK, Tyagi G, Mehrotra R. Interaction studies of Epirubicin with DNA using spectroscopic techniques. Journal of Molecular Structure. 2011;1000(1-3):150-4.

[48] Charak S, Mehrotra R. Structural investigation of idarubicin–DNA interaction: Spectroscopic and molecular docking study. International journal of biological macromolecules. 2013;60:213-8.

Chapter 10

Overview on the Side Effects of Doxorubicin

Chittipolu Ajaykumar

Abstract

Doxorubicin is an anthracycline antibiotic extracted from the bacterium Streptomyces peucetius. Its cytotoxic effect produced by intercalating with DNA causing breakdown of DNA strand which causes cancer cell apoptosis. Despite being an effective anticancer agent it causes several crucial side effects like carditoxicity, neuropathy, hepatotoxicity, nephrotoxicity, alopecia, typhlitis, myelosuppression, neutropenia, anaemia, thrombocytopenia, nausea, and diarrhoea were caused mainly due to the inability to distinguish between cancer cells and normal cells. This chapter mainly focuses on doxorubicin's side effects, current understanding of the molecular mechanisms, and management and preventive strategies of doxorubicin's cardiotoxicity during the treatment of various type of cancer.

Keywords: doxorubicin, nephrotoxicity, neurotoxicity, hepatotoxicity, cardiotoxicity

1. Introduction

1.1 Historical background

In the 1950s Italian based company; Farmitalia research laboratory began a research program in finding the anticancer compounds from soil-based microbes. In the process of research collected a soil sample from the castle named as castle Del monte, which was built in the 13th century. The collected soil sample contains new strains of bacterial species and isolated from it. The separated microbe recognised with the name Streptomyces peucetius which is typically produces a significant red pigment. The antibiotic produced from this bacterium discovered to be efficient in treating the tumours especially solid tumours while researching on mice. Since a group of French scientists found the same compound about at the same time, they agreed to call the antibiotic daunorubicin, referring to the two nations. In which, Dauni refers to the pre-Roman tribe who inhabited the position in Italy where the species of bacteria were isolated and ruby represents the colour in Italy. The clinical trials of daunorubicin were began in 1960s and confirmed as successful in treating the lymphoma and acute leukaemia [1, 2]. After a short note of the time, in 1967 daunorubicin was discovered to be cause fatal cardiotoxicity. Then, by using nitroso-N-methyl urethane, the Italian research company mutated the strains of Streptomyces peucetius and developed a new strain of bacterial species that produces 14-hydroxylated daunorubicin, also known as Adriamycin (named after the Adriatic Sea), then changed its name to doxorubicin, which has a strong therapeutic index, but cardiac toxicity remains [3].

IntechOpen

1.2 Doxorubicin chemical structure and properties

Doxorubicin (DOX) is an anthracycline antibiotic structurally similar to Daunorubicin as natural anti-cancer antibiotic used in cancer treatment. Its anti-cancer effect produced intercalating with DNA and this will inhibit DNA transcription and replication; and by binding to the topoisomerase II enzyme and inhibit the resealing of the DNA fragments. The presence of sugar moiety attached to the anthracycline ring further enhances the binding to phosphate and sugar moieties in to DNA. This led to stops the proliferation of cancer cells in the host [4]. Besides, the presence of quinone moiety apart from contributing the cytolytic ability by generating the intermediate radicals, which further react with the oxygen and forms superoxide ions and these ions also shows a high tendency towards the damaging the cell membranes causes a dose-dependent the cardiac myopathy [5, 6].

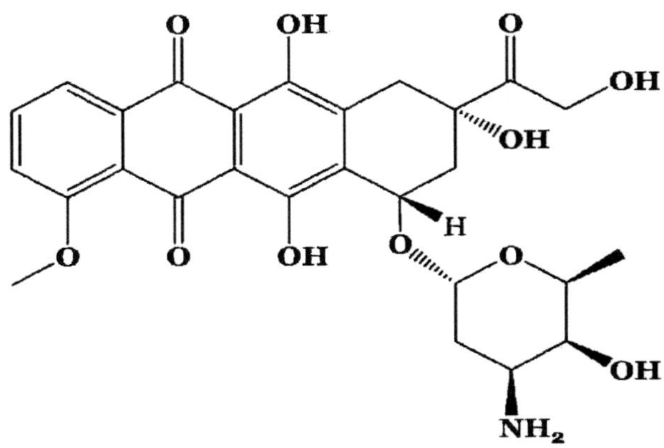

The Doxorubicin is mainly used in case of patients suffering from Breast cancer, ovarian cancers, lung cancers, bladder cancers, leukaemia (acute lymphoblastic leukaemia, acute myeloid leukaemia) and AIDS-related Kaposi's sarcoma and various solid tumours. DOX also used in combination with other agents in case of bone sarcomas, soft tissue sarcomas, uterus cancer, endoblastoma cancer, cervix cancer, pancreatic cancer, Ewing's sarcoma, mesothelioma, multiple myeloma, Wilms tumour and in neuroblastoma [7, 8].

2. Doxorubicin side effects

2.1 Hepatotoxicity

Liver is one of the essential organs of the body; it plays a major role in metabolism and detoxification of several drugs. This can explains why liver is the primary body organ affected by chemotherapy. Despite being cytostatic and cytotoxic effects on cancer cells DOX documented to accumulate in the various tissues include liver cells. In humans, it is estimated as 50% of DOX eliminated in un-exchanged form, the remainder dose metabolised through hydroxylation, semiquinone formation [9]. The major pathway for biotransformation of DOX is catalysed by the NADPH-dependent carbonyl reductase, Nitric oxide synthase, cytochrome P-450 reductase, aldo-keto reductase enzymes. The hydroxylation occurs at C-13 carbon in group commonly reaction referred as electron reduction forms the secondary alcohol metabolites [10–13].

The metabolized intermediates in the presence of oxygen converted to carbonyl moieties resulting in generation of Superoxide anions and hydrogen peroxides causes peroxidation of lipids in membranes of cell, aggregation of proteins (**Figure 1**) [13–15].

The regenerative capacity of liver is more can cure the damage caused by various agents such as DOX, which causes damage and decreases the regeneration of liver cells by increasing the oxidative stress due to the radical generation by oxidation in hepatocytes. The generated radical causes decrease in GSH levels, damages in DNA and also act as secondary metabolites in in many metabolic pathways which includes in cell proliferation and cell death [16–18]. To overcome such situations liver employs the efflux mechanisms, the efflux of DOX is achieved through from liver by ATP dependent ABC proteins (P-glycoprotein) which increase the efflux of the intracellular DOX and maintain the homeostasis. The mechanism uses large quantity of energy but with the presence of the DOX in liver cells decreases the ATP production and increases the ADP and Pi within the cells [19–21]. Due to this effect sometimes liver cells can't able to regenerate from DOX induced effects and causes hepatotoxicity.

2.2 Nephropathy

Besides maintaining the homeostasis by regulating the body fluids, kidneys work to reabsorb the low concentrations general constituents in the body and also remove the foreign substances like drugs or other kinds of agents. For this kind of reasons kidneys considered as metastatic organs of human beings [22]. The regenerative capacity of the kidneys is low when compared to the liver and highly susceptible to

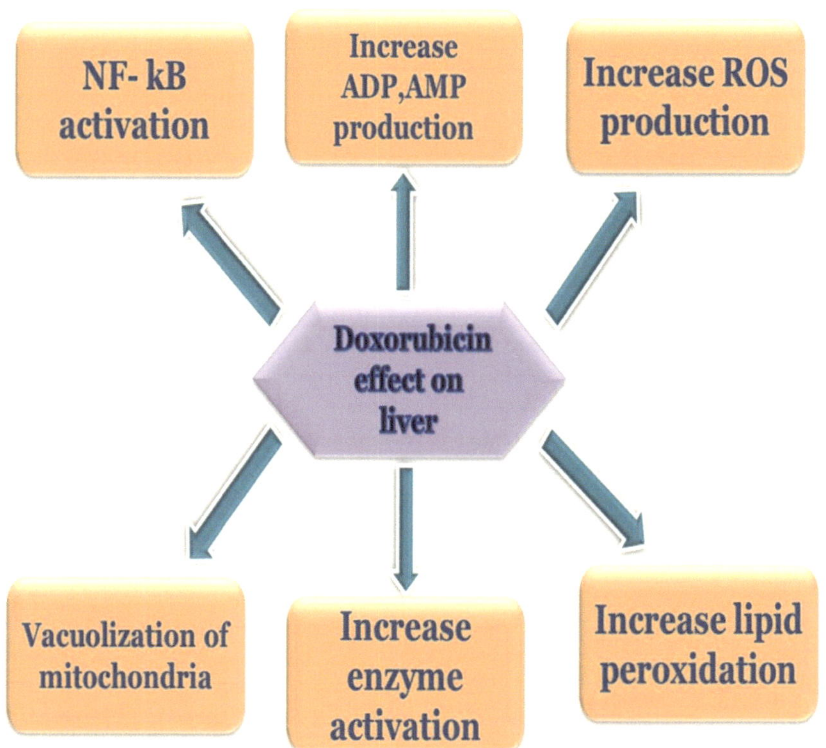

Figure 1.
DOX mediated effects on the liver.

epithelial degeneration occurs at renal glomerulus where the filtration occurs may lead to the glomerulosclerosis [23].

DOX interferes with the glandular podocytes of the kidney and cause nephropathy the most accepted mechanism behind the nephropathy is an accumulation of proteinuria in the kidney by the local passage of leaked proteins [23]. Increase in the structural changes in nephrons causes hypertension, steroid resistance, high incidents of renal failure and glomerular vacuolization, inflammation, tubular dilation, intestinal fibrosis, permeability differences in the glomerulus, and certain conditions like hypoalbuminemia, dyslipidemia, hypercoagulation, size differences in kidney most likely observed [24]. A study conducted on the DOX effect on the mitochondria by the Lebrecht suggested that DOX interfere the mitochondrial mtDNA in the kidney with ROS produced from it and accelerating the damaging of the nephron. Another study reports suggesting that DOX forming an iron-mediated anthracycline complex, which produces the ROS led to an increase in the oxidative lesions in the cells causing damage to the critical cellular components [25, 26].

The decreasing the levels of the GSH (Glutathione), vitamin E levels and other natural oxidant levels production from the liver cells enhances the nephropathic conditions which may initially affect the Bowman's capsule thickness and the glomerular tuft of the nephron. The study conducted by Rook et al. [26] Reported as Angiotensin-converting enzyme is said to be one of the responsible factors for tissue damage triggered by the DOX therapy. The ACE is causing the pro-inflammatory, pro-fibrotic effects which make interference in the kidney and nephrons to maintain the glomerular pressure and filtration rate of blood [27, 28]. The cases of nephropathy and proteinuria are rare in humans susceptibility towards such condition based on the genetic makeup of the individual.

2.3 Neurotoxicity

The brain is the largest and most complex organ in the human body contains about 100 billion neurons with 1 trillion established connections throughout the body. DOX is not able to transfer through the blood–brain barrier (BBB), therefore DOX effects against the brain via indirect way [29, 30]. These effects include: depression, anxiety, decrease in motor functions, haemoglobin levels, perception skills affected, and menopausal status, visuospatial skills are affected through cancer chemotherapy. The recovery of the cognitive functions may take up to a year [31]. The DOX mediate increase TNF-α level (inflammatory cytokines produced by the macrophages/monocytes during the acute inflammation involved in many signalling pathways) in the brain at cortex and hippocampus of mice [32–34]. The mitochondrial activity, glutathione-S-transferase, GSH levels, and MnSOD levels in the brain are decreased and increase in levels of 4-hydroxynoneal (HNA), thiobarbituric acid reactive substances (TBARS), malondialdehyde (MDA) and increase in levels of protein carbonyl groups [35–38], which causes increase the oxidative stress in the brain cells and further led to cause cell damage.

The MnSOD levels in the brain generally detoxify the oxygen free radicals, inactivated by the Nitric oxide (NO). The DOX indirectly increased the concentration of NO by overexpressing the Nitric oxide synthase enzyme [37]. A study conducted on the NOS dependent brain injury with DOC reinforcing the nitric oxide tissue damage [38]. The mitochondrial activity is very important in the brain because it is a powerhouse of cells (energy production) brain uses 20% of body glucose for energy production to conduct and maintain the regular activities [39]. The DOX induces generation of MDA, TBARS, and HNA which cause the decrease the mitochondrial activities. A study conducted on the DOX-induced toxicity on rats with 10 mg/kg dose, the rats died between 10 and 50 days with observed light microscopic studies reveals that specific changes in the ganglionic cells of the peripheral nervous system [40].

2.4 Cardiomyopathy

This side effect found to be a dose-dependent on DOX. The DOX-induced cardiotoxicity occurs acutely and chronically. The acute effects occur within one week period the patient may experience arrhythmia, hypotension, and super ventricular tachycardia. These abnormalities are generally reversible in a noticeable period [41]. The chronic effects are shown in only 1.7% of patients with a 50% mortality rate [42, 43]. The chronic effect of DOX such as congestive heart failure reported in a study, when the patients are treated with dose 500–550 mg/m^2 in more than 4% of patients when treated with the dose is 551–600 mg/m^2 18% of patients cause the CHF, and almost 35% of patients observed with CHF when treated with >601 mg/m^2 [44, 45].

A study conducted by the Zordosky and EI-kadi on DOX-induced toxicity reported as the induction of Brain natriuretic peptides, atrial natriuretic peptides genes, monooxygenases, cytochrome P genes and hypertrophy markers responsible for the xenobiotics and certain endogenous substances [46]. The inductions of these genes are cause cardiac hypertrophy leading to heart failure and altered the arachidonic acid mechanisms. A study reported the DOX effects based on the concentrations, at low concentrations DOX dose (0.5–1 μM) causes the alterations in structural proteins (includes sarcomeric myosin, nuclear lamina), plasma membrane blebbing (causes change in cell shape), and mitochondrial depolarization and fragmentation. At high concentration causes (5–50 μM) causes the cytoplasm vacuolization, swelling of mitochondrial cells, promote the cellular alterations (**Figure 2**) at the cellular and nuclear membranes [47]. The DOX reportedly binds

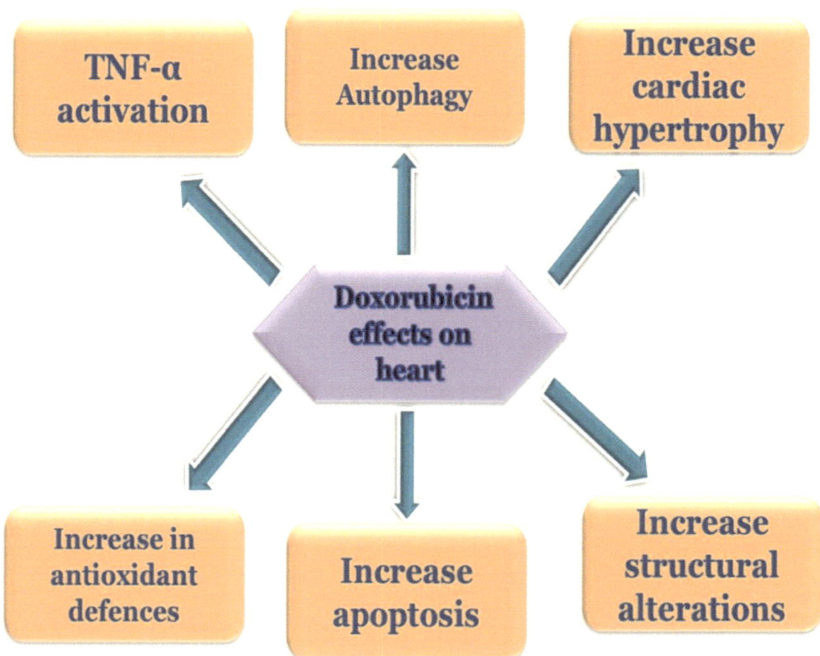

Figure 2.
DOX-mediated effects on the Heart.

to the cardiolipin (a mitochondrial inner membrane component), which raises the accumulation of the DOX inside the mycoplasma when compared to the other body cells. The high concentration existence of the NADPH dehydrogenase inside the mitochondria initiates the redox reaction in the complex and promotes the production of the Reactive oxygen species. Myocytes are generally having low levels of anti-oxidants when compared to the other tissue cells, considerably DOX shows enhanced effects on the heart and cause toxicity [48–50].

The antioxidant level differences were observed in rats under DOX treatment based on the age differences, younger Fischer rats contain more levels of antioxidants when compared to old Fischer rats. A recent study stated the involvement of the Toll-like receptor TLR-4 (a specific receptor in the immune system generally recognise the multiple bacterial antigens and plays a major role in the maturation of the phagosomes) [51]. The increase in TLR-4 expression in the DOX-induced Cardiomyocytes, when studied the cardiomyopathic cells in humans and animals. The deficiency of TLR shows decreased in lipid peroxidation and nitrotyrosine levels in cardiomyopathic cells. The other study on the glutathione peroxidase 1 (GPx) enzyme is present in both cytosol and mitochondria play a major role in the detoxification. The study conducted with the insertion of DOX on non-GPx and wild type mice, the results showed based on the study on myocytes of the non-GPx mice having the high concentration of the DOX deposits in cells, when compared to wild type mice [52–54].

The oxidative stress is a major cause for the exhibiting the cardiotoxicity, involved the generation of higher amounts of ROS cause the cellar alterations and damage are referred to as oxidative stress. The ROS is countered by the anti-oxidant system in the body, in cancer patients under the DOX chemotherapy observed the decreased the levels of GSH, TRAP levels in the body. The ROS is generation is catalysed by NADPH oxidase enzyme [55, 56].

$$\begin{gathered} O_2 + e^- \rightarrow \dot{\bar{O_2}} \\ 2O_2 + NADPH \rightarrow 2O_2^{\cdot -} + NADP^+ + H^+ \end{gathered} \tag{1}$$

In mitochondrial cells, the same reaction is mediated by NADH –ubiquinone oxidoreductase enzyme.

$$2O_2 + NADH + H^+ \rightarrow O_2^{\cdot -} + NAD^+ + 2H^+ \tag{2}$$

The generated oxygen radical undergo dimutation with hydrohen molecules and forms hydrogen peroxide reaction is mediated by the SOD enzyme [55].

$$2O_2^{\cdot -} + 2H \xrightarrow{SOD} H2O2 + O_2 \tag{3}$$

The generated less active hydrogen peroxide is removed by the enzymes like catalase, glutathione peroxidase.

$$\begin{gathered} H2O2 \xrightarrow{Catalase} 2H2O + O2 \\ 2GSH + H2O2 \xrightarrow{GPx} GSSG + 2H2O \end{gathered} \tag{4}$$

The generated oxygen radicals combine with the H2O2 and form the highly active hydroxyl radicals. The H2O2 also reacted with the ferrous ions resulting in the formation of ferric ions and reactive hydroxyl radicals [55].

$$\begin{gathered} O_2^{\cdot -} + \mathbf{H2O2} \rightarrow OH^- + OH^{\cdot} + O_2 \\ Fe^{2+} + H2O2 \rightarrow Fe^{3+} + OH^- + OH^{\cdot} \\ Fe^{3+} + O_2^{\cdot -} \rightarrow Fe^{2+} + O_2 \end{gathered} \tag{5}$$

Under stress conditions, oxygen radical facilitates the ferrous iron from the ferric ion. The iron, under normal conditions sequestered within the ferritin (a globular protein and forms the nanocage with the metal-protein complexes) but with regards to DOX when converted to its semi-quinone form complexes with iron-free radical and converted to DOX forms while generating the oxygen free radical. The generated complexes block the iron-free regulating proteins (IRP), and then these IRPs bound to the iron-responsive elements in mRNA ferritin. The tremendous amounts of free iron releases and gain complexes with the DOX. This specific condition magnifies the production of ROS in cells [57–59].

The ROS acts as secondary signalling molecules shows direct effects on the lipids, proteins, DNA, and RNA in various pathways involved in cell proliferation, cell death and maintain the homeostasis. It is domineering to maintain the levels of ROS in the body, in case of the heart the effect is maximum by ROS due to lack of efficient levels of anti-oxidants in myocytes. The conditions such as cellular hypertrophy, alterations in the gene expressions, ventricular remodelling, the extracellular matrix of the mitochondria transformation, calcium transient perturbation and cell death activation such kinds of pathological changes may be observed in myocytes lead the death of cells.

2.5 Mechanisms involved at different levels of cardio toxicity

2.5.1 Cellular hypertrophy

A particular disorder marked by an increase in cell size and volume. The abnormality shows an improvement in the degree of protein synthesis, increased in the organisation of sarcomere (contractile muscle fibre unit). At molecular level induction of hypertrophy associated genes are triggered by the DOX treatment which are alpha myosin heavy chain, ventricular myosin light chain-2, and atrial natriuretic peptide genes [60]. The main signalling cascades of the hypertrophy are tyrosine kinases, PI3K/Akt [61], and NF-κB [62, 63], protein kinase C (PKC), mitogen-activated protein kinases (AMPK [64]; ERK1/2 [65], p38 [66], and JNK) which are increased in DOX therapy induce cellular hypertrophic conditions [67].

2.5.2 ECM remodelling

Extra cellular matrix is a molecular network consisting of glycol conjugates, proteins, glycosaminoglycans and adhesive receptors that associate with each other and forms frame network, where cells reside on them [68]. The ECM frame work is present in all tissues it continuously shifts in quantitative and qualitative terms on a daily basis. In case of myocytes ECM is essential for attachment, alignment and orientation facilities the cellular contractions in myocytes. Changes in the ECM of the heart found in DOX treatments, the symptoms of DOX are related to the activation of the Membrane Metalloproteinase enzymes MMP-2 & 9 in 4 weeks of treatment [69]. Changes in MMP-2 activate the Akt channels; suppress the superoxide dismutase enzyme, which raises the amount of superoxide levels, and induce caspase-3 and all other agents together promote remodelling and apoptosis [70].

2.5.3 Impaired cardiac contraction

The heart cells (cardiomyocytes) composed of myofibrils with typical contraction and relaxation. Pump and propel the blood to systemic circulation. Myofibrils contain multiple contractile units called sarcomere, which have actin and myosin filaments. In a calm state, actin is coated in tropomyosin and protects the myosin-binding sites. The troponin and tropomyosin are attached when the calcium enters into the cytosol from the sarcoplasmic reticulum; calcium binds to the troponin and the position of the tropomyosin and troponin changes resulting in shortening of the sarcomere. That specific condition termed as cardiac contraction controlled by calcium influx and myofilaments. DOX could affect the transcription and expression of the specific proteins [71]. Transcription factor-like GATA4 for the regulation of sarcomeric synthesis and cardiac differentiation and survival of myocytes. DOX-induced ROS decreases binding function, disrupts sarcomere structure, contractile reduction and myofibrillar deterioration [72]. DOX is believed to interact with calcium homeostasis by modifying the ion pump and modifying the ion channel movement, resulting in lipid peroxidation. ROS quickly targets the fatty acids of the membrane lipids and disrupts the mitochondrial calcium channels by increasing the activity of the voltage-sensitive L-type calcium channels on the cell membrane resulting in accumulation of calcium [73]. Calcium overload throughout cytosol, Causes the disruption in the contraction and relaxing of cardiomyocytes.

2.5.4 Cell death

The general apoptosis is a process where a cell commits to suicide, damage to genetic material, protein, cellular organelles that beyond the repair would trigger the suicide to save the energy and resources. Apoptosis firmly regulated process involves intrinsic mitochondrial apoptosis, extrinsic death receptor pathways [74]. The mitochondrial pathway relays on the Trans membrane potential is a key indicator of membrane permeability. It is assumed that permeability can be either permeability-dependent or independent of the pore transition [PT]. The PT pore consists of the adenine nucleotide translocator, matrix protein cyclophilin D, and voltage-dependent anion channel. The opening of the PT pore activates the dissipation of the proton gradient produced by electron transport, resulting in the uncoupling of oxidative phosphorylation. The opening of the PT pore also allows water to penetrate the mitochondrial matrix, resulting in the swelling of the intermembrane space and the rupturing of the outer membrane allowing the release of apoptogenic proteins. Released proteins include cytochrome c, apoptosis-inducing factor and endonuclease G. Cytochrome c in conjunction with apoptosis protease activating factor (APAF-1) and pro-caspase 9 forms an apoptosome, which in turn activates effector caspases that collectively facilitate the execution of apoptosis. Due to decrease in the number of normal cardiomyocytes is significantly reduced, the heart failed to pump the blood sequentially ventricular remodelling and death of myocytes [75].

The death receptor pathway involves the binding of death ligands such as FasL, TNF-α to their respective membrane-bound receptors. The bonded ligands signals to various proteins mediate the cascade, which leads to apoptosis of the cell [76]. In cancer therapy, DOX-induced ROS activates the p^{38}, p^{53} and NF-kB pathways resulting in the differences in pro- and anti-apaptonic signalling imbalance, such imbalance cause release of cytochrome C from mitochondrial membrane proteins, subsequently lead to apoptosis of cell [77, 78].

2.5.5 Autophagy

Autophagy is a method of restoring or repairing the destroyed cells. It is a self-degrading mechanism (survival mechanism) to maintain a balance of life in response to dietary stress, energy depletion. Autophagy destroys malformed proteins, weakened organelles, and other cell infections, which can be unique or non-specific, but processes are not completely thought out. Under diseased environments, autophagy either facilitates cell death or induces cell death depending on the demands of different people [79, 80]. In DOX-based therapy toxicity mediated autophagy by suppressing GTAT4 expression and activating S6K1, this plays a direct and indirect role in autophagy control. Autophagy varies due to species differences; autophagy dependent on DOX is increased in mice but decreased in autophagy has been seen in mouse cases [81–84]. The autophagy achieved in DOX therapy via several mechanisms, such as ATG 5 & 12 is the inhibitors of the Bcl-2 family, which regulate the cytochrome release from the mitochondria. Cytochrome C releases the caspase-9 lead to the autophagosome, can regulate the apoptosis. In some other studies, autophagy reduces the DOX-induced cardiotoxicity by decreasing mitochondrial ROS formation.

2.6 Diagnosis

The DOX-induced cardiomyopathy consists of a complete examination of the cardiovascular system for detecting the symptoms, such as S3 gallop and elevated jugular vapour pressure, T wave impairments; low voltage QRS complexes are measured.

- Electrocardiography combined with Doopler studies used to study early diagnostic symptoms of the cardiac myopathy through the measure of latero-ventricular dysfunction.

- Radionuclide ventriculography used to access the latero-ventricular systolic and diastolic function. Observes the cardiac adrenergic denervation occurs in case of doxorubicin induced cardiomyopathy.

- Metaiodobenzylguanidine based nuclear imaging can be employed to assess cardiac adrenergic denervation occurred trough the DOX based cardiomyopathy.

- The DOX treated patients are sensitive to the indium labelled monoclonal antimyosin antibodies (myosin an ATP dependent superfamily of motor proteins major role in muscle contraction and motility) used to detect the cardiac myopathy, myocarditis, chagas heart disease ischemic myocardium, and kawasaki heart disease [85].

- The measurement of the cardiac enzymes and neurohormones are used for detecting the heart failure but not a characteristic feature of the DOX-induced cardiomyopathy [86].

- The presence of endomyocardial biopsy is the best route for detecting the DOX-induced diseases, according to the grade of biopsy severity of the disease is measured [87, 88]. It is invasive and requires experience for recognising the results become a disadvantage for this technique.

3. Management & preventive strategies for doxorubicin cardiotoxicity

The DOX has an extreme side effect like cardiotoxicity, but is still in use because of its efficacy in the treatment of cancers. Toxicity can be avoided in several ways. Many studies have shown that cardioprotective agents can achieve a reduction in cardiotoxicity. A recent research on HSP-20 (heat-shock protein) has shown that the protection of Akt activity prevents the cardiotoxic effect caused by DOX [89–92]. Different kind of agents is used to control the DOX effects such as Dexrazoxane (DZR); it contains bisdioxopiperazine rings falling under alpha-amino acid and the derivative compound also known as cardioxane or Totect or Zincard. A promising compound that activates after hydrolysis and resembles the EDTA structure after conversion makes complexes with Iron and reduces the incidence of anthracycline-iron complexes, thus preventing ROS generation in myocytes. Dexrazoxane has also been known to contain the Topoisomerase II enzyme function and inhibit the tumour cell growth. Used mainly for the activities of iron-chelating agent, cardiac protection, anti-neoplastic activities, and chemo protection. Indirectly active in chromatin remodelling complexes by activating vitamin D receptors. DZR is often known to provide up-regulation of the ERK and Akt pathways to guard against cardiomyopathy [93–96] but DZR is not approved for routine use in patients with metastatic cancer and other forms of cancer, as stated by the American Clinical Oncology Society [97, 98]. DOX was analysed in association with DZR for 10 years in women with breast cancer [99]. No, people suffer from heart disease over the time and there are no records of adverse effects with respect to the heart.

Diuretics are used to avoid signs of systemic and pulmonary ventricular obstruction, and medications dependent on β-adrenergic receptors are used depending on the type of systolic heart problem [100]. Metoprolol is safe and effective in the treatment of cardiac myopathy [97], angiotensin II is also recommended for advanced heart disease cases, and low-dose isosorbide dinitrate substituted angiotensin inhibitor medication is favoured and hydralazine is favoured for cardiomyopathic myopathy.

The successful release of DOX at a particular site of operation is another form of preventive step. Like liposomal dosage formulations, the specified delivery mechanism passively decreases the impact caused by non-cancerous cells. For liposomes drug interaction with blood and cancer cells, structural characteristics such as vesicle size, pharmacokinetic characteristics such as stability and pharmacodynamic characteristics such as plasma clearance are important. Tumour cells have conditions that favour high-level depositions, because newly developed cells have microvasculature-permeable vessels, which contain poor lymphatic drainage, low levels of lipase enzymes and other oxidising agents. Due to these features of cancer cells shows aggregation. Once liposomes enter the tumour cells the differences in the intestinal pH favours the release of drugs constituents. The pH of cancer cells is differ from other normal cells because of this the drug is preferentially released in tumour cells and avoid the toxicity in non-cancer cells. The recently reported formulation of polyethylene glycol-coated liposomal doxorubicin (PLD) shows better pharmacokinetics relative to general formulations and has fewer side effects [101]. A phase clinical trial of 50 mg/m2 PLD administration in patients with carcinoma with a demonstrated history of platinum-based chemotherapy at intervals of 4 weeks reported low toxicity. The other formulation like poly (ethylene oxide)-b-poly (e-caprolactone-DOX) [PEO-b- P(CL-DOX)] prevents the premature release outside of the tumor cells [102].

The development of analogues is another possible strategy for reducing the toxicity [96], in the case of anthracyclines nuclear targeted and Non-nuclear targeted are two kinds of strategies concerned in the development of non-toxic chemotherapeutic agents. Analogues such as Methoxymorpholinyl doxorubicin (MMDX), sabarubicin and *N*-Benzyladriamycin-14-valerate now under development to reduce the toxicity caused by DOX. In which, MMDX is nuclear-targeted analogue activated by the liver enzyme cytochrome P450 3A and metabolize into a cytotoxic metabolite and degrades slowly [103]. Based on gene therapy expression of cytochrome enzyme activity increased, cytochrome increases the therapeutic potency of the DOX. The sabarubicin (disaccharide analogue) is also another nuclear targeted molecule that has improved efficiency especially used in case of lung and gynaecological cancer [104]. This stimulates the NF-kB transcription factor, which happens earlier as DNA is involved with multiple tumorogenesis, regulating the expressions of differentiation, variations, cell adhesion and apoptosis [105]. N-Benzyladriamycin-14-valerate is a non-nuclear target molecule obtained by modification of the C-3 amino group and the C-14 position [106]. The compound has comparable activity to DOX but is theoretically more effective than DOX by activating the protein kinase enzyme resulting in cardio-protective activity.

4. Conclusion

Even DOX used for treating several types of cancers as a result of its wide range of pharmacological activities, but at the same time it causes a wide range of side effects. The major side effects caused by DOX are: carditoxicity, neuropathy, hepatotoxicity, nephrotoxicity, alopecia, typhlitis, myelosuppression, neutropenia, anaemia, and thrombocytopenia. DOX increasing the oxidative stress, decrease the GSH, vitamin E levels, and activates the NF-kB levels causes' hepatotoxicity. Besides, it interferes with the glandular podocytes of the kidney and cause nephropathy. Also, it induces generation of MDA, TBARS, and HNA which decrease the mitochondrial activities and increase in ROS generation causes cell necrosis. Moreover, it causes induction of brain natriuretic peptides, atrial natriuretic peptides genes, mono oxygenases, cytochrome P genes; binds to the cardiolipin, the increase in TLR-4 expression, generation of ROS led to several pathological changes in myocytes causes cardiomyopathy. Several strategies are made to manage and decrease DOX's cardiotoxicity effects, includes a change in the dosage forms for efficacious delivery systems, administration along with anti-oxidants, DZR, diuretics and β-adrenergic agents, and development of different analogues for increasing the efficiency of DOX.

Acknowledgements

The author is grateful to Prof. M. Sarangapani, Principal of University College of pharmaceutical sciences, Kakatiya University, Warangal.

Conflict of interest

The author declares no conflict of interest.

Author details

Chittipolu Ajaykumar
Vision College of Pharmaceutical Sciences and Research, Hyderabad, India

*Address all correspondence to: ajay239172@gmail.com

References

[1] Carvalho C, Santos RX, Cardoso S, Correia S, Oliveira PJ, Santos MS, et al. Doxorubicin: the good, the bad and the ugly effect. Current medicinal chemistry. 2009 Sep 1;**16**(25):3267-3285

[2] Wani SH. Lone SA. Cancer: Diseases. Educreation Publishing; 2018 Nov 10

[3] Danesi R, Fogli S, Gennari A, Conte P, Del Tacca M. Pharmacokinetic-pharmacodynamic relationships of the anthracycline anticancer drugs. Clinical Pharmacokinetics. 2002 May 1;**41**(6):431-444

[4] Danesi R, Fogli S, Gennari A, Conte P, Del Tacca M. Pharmacokinetic-pharmacodynamic relationships of the anthracycline anticancer drugs. Clinical Pharmacokinetics. 2002 May 1;**41**(6):431-444

[5] Song Y, Buettner GR. Thermodynamic and kinetic considerations for the reaction of semiquinone radicals to form superoxide and hydrogen peroxide. Free Radical Biology and Medicine. 2010 Sep 15;**49**(6):919-962

[6] Chatterjee K, Zhang J, Tao R, Honbo N, Karliner JS. Vincristine attenuates doxorubicin cardiotoxicity. Biochemical and biophysical research communications. 2008 Sep 5;**373**(4):555-560

[7] Available from: http://chemocare.com/chemotherapy/drug-info/doxorubicin.aspx [accessed on 2020-10-11].

[8] Alghorabi AA, Kabel AM, Elmaaboud MA. Doxorubicin: Insights into Dynamics, Clinical Uses and Adverse Effects. J. Cancer Res. 2019;**7**:17-20

[9] Hanna AD, Lam A, Tham S, Dulhunty AF, Beard NA. Adverse effects of doxorubicin and its metabolic product on cardiac RyR2 and SERCA2A. Molecular Pharmacology. 2014 Oct 1;**86**(4):438-449

[10] Maton A, Hopkins J, McLaughlin CW, Johnson S, Warner MQ, LaHart D, et al. Human biology and health. Englewood Cliffs, New Jersey, US: Prentice Hall; 1993

[11] Shirani K, Yousefsani BS, Shirani M, Karimi G. Protective effects of naringin against drugs and chemical toxins induced hepatotoxicity: A review. Phytotherapy Research. 2020 Feb;**17**

[12] Zhao X, Jin Y, Li L, Xu L, Tang Z, Qi Y, et al. MicroRNA-128-3p aggravates doxorubicin-induced liver injury by promoting oxidative stress via targeting Sirtuin-1. Pharmacological Research. 2019 Aug 1;**146**:104276

[13] Yang XL, Fan CH, Zhu HS. Photo-induced cytotoxicity of malonic acid [C60] fullerene derivatives and its mechanism. Toxicology in vitro. 2002 Feb 1;**16**(1):41-46

[14] Forrest GL, Gonzalez B, Tseng W, Li X, Mann J. Human carbonyl reductase overexpression in the heart advances the development of doxorubicin-induced cardiotoxicity in transgenic mice. Cancer research. 2000 Sep 15;**60**(18):5158-5164

[15] Gavelová M, Hladíková J, Vildová L, Novotná R, Vondráček J, Krčmář P, et al. Reduction of doxorubicin and oracin and induction of carbonyl reductase in human breast carcinoma MCF-7 cells. Chemico-biological interactions. 2008 Oct 22;**176**(1):9-18

[16] Ahmed OM, Abdul-Hamid MM, El-Bakry AM, Mohamed HM, Abdel Rahman ES. Camellia sinensis and epicatechin abate doxorubicin-induced hepatotoxicity in male Wistar rats via

their modulatory effects on oxidative stress, inflammation, and apoptosis. J Appl Pharm Sci. 2019 Apr;**9**:30-44

[17] Injac R, Perse M, Obermajer N, Djordjevic-Milic V, Prijatelj M, Djordjevic A, et al. Potential hepatoprotective effects of fullerenol C60 (OH) 24 in doxorubicin-induced hepatotoxicity in rats with mammary carcinomas. Biomaterials. 2008 Aug 1;**29**(24-25):3451-3460

[18] Lu H, Zhu ZG, Yao XX, Zhao R, Yan C, Zhang Y, et al. Hepatic preconditioning of doxorubicin in stop-flow chemotherapy: NF-κB/IκB-α pathway and expression of HSP72. World Journal of Gastroenterology: WJG. 2005 Apr 14;**11**(14):2136

[19] Smuder AJ. Exercise stimulates beneficial adaptations to diminish doxorubicin-induced cellular toxicity. American Journal of Physiology-Regulatory, Integrative and Comparative Physiology. 2019 Nov 1;**317**(5):R662-R672

[20] Songbo M, Lang H, Xinyong C, Bin X, Ping Z, Liang S. Oxidative stress injury in doxorubicin-induced cardiotoxicity. Toxicology letters. 2019 Jun 1;**307**:41-48

[21] Pisoschi AM, Pop A. The role of antioxidants in the chemistry of oxidative stress: A review. European journal of medicinal chemistry. 2015 Jun 5;**97**:55-74

[22] S Lahoti T, Patel D, Thekkemadom V, Beckett R, D Ray S. Doxorubicin-induced in vivo nephrotoxicity involves oxidative stress-mediated multiple pro-and anti-apoptotic signaling pathways. Current neurovascular research. 2012 Nov 1;9(4):282-295.

[23] Okuda S, Oh Y, Tsuruda H, Onoyama K, Fujimi S, Fujishima M. Adriamycin-induced nephropathy as a model of chronic progressive glomerular disease. Kidney international. 1986 Feb 1;**29**(2):502-510

[24] Fogo AB. Mechanisms of progression of chronic kidney disease. Pediatric nephrology. 2007 Dec 1;**22**(12):2011-2022

[25] Wang Y, Wang YP, Tay YC, Harris DC. Progressive adriamycin nephropathy in mice: sequence of histologic and immunohistochemical events. Kidney international. 2000 Oct 1;**58**(4):1797-1804

[26] Rook M, Lely AT, Kramer AB, van Goor H, Navis G. Individual differences in renal ACE activity in healthy rats predict susceptibility to adriamycin-induced renal damage. Nephrology Dialysis Transplantation. 2005 Jan 1;**20**(1):59-64

[27] Khames A, Khalaf MM, Gad AM, Abd El-raouf OM, Kandeil MA. Nicorandil combats doxorubicin–induced nephrotoxicity via amendment of TLR4/P38 MAPK/NFκ-B signaling pathway. Chemico-biological interactions. 2019 Sep 25;**311**:108777

[28] Korbet SM, Schwartz MM, Lewis EJ. Primary focal segmental glomerulosclerosis: clinical course and response to therapy. American journal of kidney diseases. 1994 Jun 1;**23**(6):773-783

[29] Jansen C, Miaskowski C, Dodd M, Dowling G, Kramer J. Potential mechanisms for chemotherapy-induced impairments in cognitive function. InOncology nursing forum 2005 Nov 1 (Vol. 32, No. 6, p. 1151). Oncology Nursing Society.

[30] Ferreira A, Neves P, Gozzelino R. Multilevel impacts of Iron in the brain: the cross talk between neurophysiological mechanisms, cognition, and social behavior. Pharmaceuticals. 2019 Sep;**12**(3):126

[31] Tangpong J, Cole MP, Sultana R, Joshi G, Estus S, Vore M, et al. Adriamycin-induced, TNF-α-mediated central nervous system toxicity. Neurobiology of Disease. 2006 Jul 1;**23**(1):127-139

[32] Brezden CB, Phillips KA, Abdolell M, Bunston T, Tannock IF. Cognitive function in breast cancer patients receiving adjuvant chemotherapy. Journal of Clinical Oncology. 2000 Jul 14;**18**(14):2695-2701

[33] Ahles TA, Saykin AJ, Furstenberg CT, Cole B, Mott LA, Skalla K, et al. Neuropsychologic impact of standard-dose systemic chemotherapy in long-term survivors of breast cancer and lymphoma. Journal of Clinical Oncology. 2002 Jan 15;**20**(2):485-493

[34] Tangpong J, Cole MP, Sultana R, Estus S, Vore M. St. Clair W, Ratanachaiyavong S, St. Clair DK, Butterfield DA. Adriamycin-mediated nitration of manganese superoxide dismutase in the central nervous system: insight into the mechanism of chemobrain. Journal of Neurochemistry. 2007 Jan;**100**(1):191-201

[35] Park ES, Kim SD, Lee MH, Lee HS, Lee IS, Sung JK, et al. Protective effects of N-acetylcysteine and selenium against doxorubicin toxicity in rats. Journal of veterinary science. 2003 Aug 1;**4**(2):129-136

[36] Joshi G, Sultana R, Tangpong J, Cole MP, St Clair DK, Vore M, et al. Free radical mediated oxidative stress and toxic side effects in brain induced by the anticancer drug adriamycin: insight into chemobrain. Free radical research. 2005 Jan 1;**39**(11):1147-1154

[37] Joshi G, Hardas S, Sultana R. St. Clair DK, Vore M, Butterfield DA. Glutathione elevation by γ-glutamyl cysteine ethyl ester as a potential therapeutic strategy for preventing oxidative stress in brain mediated by in vivo administration of adriamycin: Implication for chemobrain. Journal of Neuroscience Research. 2007 Feb 15;**85**(3):497-503

[38] Öz E, İlhan MN. Effects of melatonin in reducing the toxic effects of doxorubicin. Molecular and Cellular Biochemistry. 2006 Jun 1;**286**(1-2):11-15

[39] Mohanty A, Tiwari-Pandey R, Pandey NR. Mitochondria: the indispensable players in innate immunity and guardians of the inflammatory response. Journal of Cell Communication and Signaling. 2019 Sep;**1**:1-6

[40] Gorini S, De Angelis A, Berrino L, Malara N, Rosano G, Ferraro E. Chemotherapeutic drugs and mitochondrial dysfunction: focus on doxorubicin, trastuzumab, and sunitinib. Oxidative medicine and cellular longevity. 2018 Oct;**2018**

[41] Mancilla TR, Iskra B, Aune GJ. Doxorubicin-Induced Cardiomyopathy in Children. Comprehensive Physiology. 2011 Jan 17;**9**(3):905-931

[42] Arcamone F, Franceschi G, Penco S, Selva A. Adriamycin (14-hydroxydaunomycin), a novel antitumor antibiotic. Tetrahedron letters. 1969 Jan 1;**10**(13):1007-1010

[43] Singal PK, Iliskovic N. Doxorubicin-induced cardiomyopathy. New England Journal of Medicine. 1998 Sep 24;**339**(13):900-905

[44] Von Hoff DD, Layard MW, Basa P, DAVIS Jr HL, Von Hoff AL, Rozencweig M, Muggia FM. Risk factors for doxorubicin-lnduced congestive heart failure. Annals of internal medicine. 1979 Nov 1;**91**(5):710-717

[45] Swain SM, Whaley FS, Ewer MS. Congestive heart failure in patients treated with doxorubicin: a

retrospective analysis of three trials. Cancer: Interdisciplinary International Journal of the American Cancer Society. 2003 Jun 1;**97**(11):2869-2879

[46] Zordoky BN, El-Kadi AO. Induction of several cytochrome P450 genes by doxorubicin in H9c2 cells. Vascular pharmacology. 2008 Oct 1;**49**(4-6):166-172

[47] Sardão VA, Oliveira PJ, Holy J, Oliveira CR, Wallace KB. Morphological alterations induced by doxorubicin on H9c2 myoblasts: nuclear, mitochondrial, and cytoskeletal targets. Cell biology and toxicology. 2009 Jun 1;**25**(3):227-243

[48] Goormaghtigh E, Huart P, Praet M, Brasseur R, Ruysschaert JM. Structure of the adriamycin-cardiolipin complex: role in mitochondrial toxicity. Biophysical Chemistry. 1990 Apr 1;**35**(2-3):247-257

[49] Childs AC, Phaneuf SL, Dirks AJ, Phillips T, Leeuwenburgh C. Doxorubicin treatment in vivo causes cytochrome C release and cardiomyocyte apoptosis, as well as increased mitochondrial efficiency, superoxide dismutase activity, and Bcl-2: Bax ratio. Cancer research. 2002 Aug 15;**62**(16):4592-4598

[50] Odom AL, Hatwig CA, Stanley JS, Benson AM. Biochemical determinants of adriamycin® toxicity in mouse liver, heart and intestine. Biochemical Pharmacology. 1992 Feb 18;**43**(4):831-836

[51] Riad A, Bien S, Gratz M, Escher F, Heimesaat MM, Bereswill S, et al. Toll-like receptor-4 deficiency attenuates doxorubicin-induced cardiomyopathy in mice. European journal of heart failure. 2008 Mar;**10**(3):233-243

[52] Esworthy RS, Ho YS, Chu FF. TheGpx1Gene encodes mitochondrial glutathione peroxidase in the mouse liver. Archives of biochemistry and biophysics. 1997 Apr 1;**340**(1):59-63

[53] Li T, Singal PK. Adriamycin-induced early changes in myocardial antioxidant enzymes and their modulation by probucol. Circulation. 2000 Oct 24;**102**(17):2105-2110

[54] Sazuka Y, Tanizawa H, Takino Y. Effect of adriamycin on the activities of superoxide dismutase, glutathione peroxidase and catalase in tissues of mice. Japanese journal of cancer research. 1989 Jan;**80**(1):89-94

[55] Angsutararux P, Luanpitpong S, Issaragrisil S. Chemotherapy-induced cardiotoxicity: overview of the roles of oxidative stress. Oxidative medicine and cellular longevity. 2015 Oct;**2015**

[56] Thorn CF, Oshiro C, Marsh S, Hernandez-Boussard T, McLeod H, Klein TE, et al. Doxorubicin pathways: pharmacodynamics and adverse effects. Pharmacogenetics and genomics. 2011 Jul;**21**(7):440

[57] Hirotani S, Otsu K, Nishida K, Higuchi Y, Morita T, Nakayama H, et al. Involvement of nuclear factor-κB and apoptosis signal-regulating kinase 1 in G-protein–coupled receptor agonist–induced cardiomyocyte hypertrophy. Circulation. 2002 Jan 29;**105**(4):509-515

[58] Minotti G, Recalcati S, Mordente A, Liberi G, Calafiore AM, Mancuso C, et al. The secondary alcohol metabolite of doxorubicin irreversibly inactivates aconitase/iron regulatory protein-1 in cytosolic fractions from human myocardium. The FASEB Journal. 1998 May;**12**(7):541-552

[59] Minotti G, Mancuso C, Frustaci A, Mordente A, Santini SA, Calafiore AM, et al. Paradoxical inhibition of cardiac lipid peroxidation in cancer patients treated with doxorubicin. Pharmacologic and molecular reappraisal of anthracycline

cardiotoxicity. The Journal of clinical investigation. 1996 Aug 1;**98**(3):650-661

[60] Izumiya Y, Kim S, Izumi Y, Yoshida K, Yoshiyama M, Matsuzawa A, et al. Apoptosis signal-regulating kinase 1 plays a pivotal role in angiotensin II–induced cardiac hypertrophy and remodeling. Circulation Research. 2003 Oct 31;**93**(9):874-883

[61] Xin Y, Bai Y, Jiang X, Zhou S, Wang Y, Wintergerst KA, et al. Sulforaphane prevents angiotensin II-induced cardiomyopathy by activation of Nrf2 via stimulating the Akt/GSK-3ss/Fyn pathway. Redox Biology. 2018 May 1;**15**:405-417

[62] Hirotani S, Otsu K, Nishida K, Higuchi Y, Morita T, Nakayama H, et al. Involvement of nuclear factor-κB and apoptosis signal-regulating kinase 1 in G-protein–coupled receptor agonist–induced cardiomyocyte hypertrophy. Circulation. 2002 Jan 29;**105**(4):509-515

[63] Izumiya Y, Kim S, Izumi Y, Yoshida K, Yoshiyama M, Matsuzawa A, et al. Apoptosis signal-regulating kinase 1 plays a pivotal role in angiotensin II–induced cardiac hypertrophy and remodeling. Circulation Research. 2003 Oct 31;**93**(9):874-883

[64] Lue Y, Gao C, Swerdloff R, Hoang J, Avetisyan R, Jia Y, et al. Humanin analog enhances the protective effect of dexrazoxane against doxorubicin-induced cardiotoxicity. American Journal of Physiology-Heart and Circulatory Physiology. 2018 Sep 1;**315**(3):H634-H643

[65] Wu W, Chordia MD, Hart BP, Kumarasinghe ES, Ji MK, Bhargava A, et al. Macrocyclic MEK1/2 inhibitor with efficacy in a mouse model of cardiomyopathy caused by lamin A/C gene mutation. Bioorganic & medicinal chemistry. 2017 Feb 1;**25**(3):1004-1013

[66] Zuo G, Ren X, Qian X, Ye P, Luo J, Gao X, et al. Inhibition of JNK and p38 MAPK-mediated inflammation and apoptosis by ivabradine improves cardiac function in streptozotocin-induced diabetic cardiomyopathy. Journal of Cellular Physiology. 2019 Feb;**234**(2):1925-1936

[67] Zhen J, Yu H, Ji H, Cai L, Leng J, Keller BB. Neonatal murine engineered cardiac tissue toxicology model: Impact of dexrazoxane on doxorubicin induced injury. Life Sciences. 2019 Dec 15;**239**:117070

[68] Kwon SH, Pimentel DR, Remondino A, Sawyer DB, Colucci WS. H2O2 regulates cardiac myocyte phenotype via concentration-dependent activation of distinct kinase pathways. Journal of molecular and cellular cardiology. 2003 Jun 1;**35**(6):615-621

[69] Rabinovich-Nikitin I, Love M. Kirshenbaum LA. Cardiovascular Research: Inhibition of MMP prevents doxorubicin-induced cardiotoxicity by attenuating cardiac intracellular and extracellular matrix remodelling; 2020 Jul 10

[70] Zhao Y, McLaughlin D, Robinson E, Harvey AP, Hookham MB, Shah AM, et al. Nox2 NADPH oxidase promotes pathologic cardiac remodeling associated with Doxorubicin chemotherapy. Cancer research. 2010 Nov 15;**70**(22):9287-9297

[71] Jeyaseelan R, Poizat C, Wu HY, Kedes L. Molecular Mechanisms of Doxorubicin-induced Cardiomyopathy Selective suppression of reiske iron-sulfur protein, adp/atp translocase, and phosphofructokinase genes is associated with atp depletion in rat cardiomyocytes. Journal of Biological Chemistry. 1997 Feb 28;**272**(9):5828-5832

[72] Aries A, Paradis P, Lefebvre C, Schwartz RJ, Nemer M. Essential role

of GATA-4 in cell survival and drug-induced cardiotoxicity. Proceedings of the National Academy of Sciences. 2004 May 4;**101**(18):6975-6980

[73] Arai M, Yoguchi A, Takizawa T, Yokoyama T, Kanda T, Kurabayashi M, et al. Mechanism of doxorubicin-induced inhibition of sarcoplasmic reticulum Ca2+-ATPase gene transcription. Circulation Research. 2000 Jan 7;**86**(1):8-14

[74] Lavrik IN, Krammer PH. Regulation of CD95/Fas signaling at the DISC. Cell Death & Differentiation. 2012 Jan;**19**(1):36-41

[75] Sawyer DB, Peng X, Chen B, Pentassuglia L, Lim CC. Mechanisms of anthracycline cardiac injury: can we identify strategies for cardioprotection? Progress in cardiovascular diseases. 2010 Sep 1;**53**(2):105-113

[76] Kotamraju S, Konorev EA, Joseph J, Kalyanaraman B. Doxorubicin-induced apoptosis in endothelial cells and cardiomyocytes is ameliorated by nitrone spin traps and ebselen role of reactive oxygen and nitrogen species. Journal of Biological Chemistry. 2000 Oct 27;**275**(43):33585-33592

[77] Nitobe J, Yamaguchi S, Okuyama M, Nozaki N, Sata M, Miyamoto T, et al. Reactive oxygen species regulate FLICE inhibitory protein (FLIP) and susceptibility to Fas-mediated apoptosis in cardiac myocytes. Cardiovascular Research. 2003 Jan 1;**57**(1):119-128

[78] Lien YC, Noel T, Liu H, Stromberg AJ, Chen KC, Clair DK. Phospholipase C-δ1 Is a Critical Target for Tumor Necrosis Factor Receptor–Mediated Protection against Adriamycin-Induced Cardiac Injury. Cancer research. 2006 Apr 15;**66**(8):4329-4338

[79] Lu L, Wu W, Yan J, Li X, Yu H, Yu X. Adriamycin-induced autophagic cardiomyocyte death plays a pathogenic role in a rat model of heart failure. International journal of cardiology. 2009 May 1;**134**(1):82-90

[80] Dimitrakis P, Romay-Ogando MI, Timolati F, Suter TM, Zuppinger C. Effects of doxorubicin cancer therapy on autophagy and the ubiquitin-proteasome system in long-term cultured adult rat cardiomyocytes. Cell and tissue research. 2012 Nov 1;**350**(2):361-372

[81] Kawaguchi T, Takemura G, Kanamori H, Takeyama T, Watanabe T, Morishita K, et al. Prior starvation mitigates acute doxorubicin cardiotoxicity through restoration of autophagy in affected cardiomyocytes. Cardiovascular Research. 2012 Dec 1;**96**(3):456-465

[82] Smuder AJ, Kavazis AN, Min K, Powers SK. Doxorubicin-induced markers of myocardial autophagic signaling in sedentary and exercise trained animals. Journal of Applied Physiology. 2013 Jul 15;**115**(2):176-185

[83] Zhang YY, Meng C, Zhang XM, Yuan CH, Wen MD, Chen Z, et al. Ophiopogonin D attenuates doxorubicin-induced autophagic cell death by relieving mitochondrial damage in vitro and in vivo. Journal of Pharmacology and Experimental Therapeutics. 2015 Jan 1;**352**(1):166-174

[84] Shabalala S, Muller CJ, Louw J, Johnson R. Polyphenols, autophagy and doxorubicin-induced cardiotoxicity. Life Sciences. 2017 Jul 1;**180**:160-170

[85] Wakasugi S, Fischman AJ, Babich JW, Callahan RJ, Elmaleh DR, Wilkinson R, et al. Myocardial substrate utilization and left ventricular function in adriamycin cardiomyopathy. Journal of Nuclear Medicine. 1993 Sep 1;**34**(9):1529-1535

[86] Suzuki T, Hayashi D, Yamazaki T, Mizuno T, Kanda Y, Komuro I, et al. Elevated B-type natriuretic peptide levels after anthracycline administration. American heart journal. 1998 Aug 1;**136**(2):362-363

[87] Takemura G, Fujiwara H. Doxorubicin-induced cardiomyopathy: from the cardiotoxic mechanisms to management. Progress in cardiovascular diseases. 2007 Mar 1;**49**(5):330-352

[88] Bristow MR, Sageman WS, Scott RH, Billingham ME, Bowden RE, Kernoff RS, et al. Acute and chronic cardiovascular effects of doxorubicin in the dog: the cardiovascular pharmacology of drug-induced histamine release. Journal of cardiovascular pharmacology. 1980 Sep 1;**2**(5):487-516

[89] Takemura G, Fujiwara H. Doxorubicin-induced cardiomyopathy: from the cardiotoxic mechanisms to management. Progress in cardiovascular diseases. 2007 Mar 1;**49**(5):330-352

[90] ZHU YH, MA TM, Wang X. Gene transfer of heat-shock protein 20 protects against ischemia/ reperfusion injury in rat hearts 1. Acta Pharmacologica Sinica. 2005 Oct;**26**(10):1193-1200

[91] Fan GC, Zhou X, Wang X, Song G, Qian J, Nicolaou P, et al. Heat shock protein 20 interacting with phosphorylated Akt reduces doxorubicin-triggered oxidative stress and cardiotoxicity. Circulation research. 2008 Nov 21;**103**(11):1270-1279

[92] 87Kim KH, Oudit GY, Backx PH. Erythropoietin protects against doxorubicin-induced cardiomyopathy via a phosphatidylinositol 3-kinase-dependent pathway. Journal of Pharmacology and Experimental Therapeutics. 2008 Jan 1;**324**(1):160-169

[93] Marty M, Espie M, Llombart A, Monnier A, Rapoport BL, Stahalova V. Multicenter randomized phase III study of the cardioprotective effect of dexrazoxane (Cardioxane®) in advanced/metastatic breast cancer patients treated with anthracycline-based chemotherapy. Annals of Oncology. 2006 Apr 1;**17**(4):614-622

[94] van Dalen EC, Caron HN, Dickinson HO, Kremer LC. Cardioprotective interventions for cancer patients receiving anthracyclines. Cochrane database of systematic reviews. 2011;**6**

[95] In U, Hensley LM, Hagerty KL, Kewalramani T, Green DM, Meropol NJ, et al. American Society of Clinical Oncology 2008 clinical practice guideline update: use of chemotherapy and radiation therapy protectants. Journal of Clinical Oncology. 2008;**27**:127-132

[96] Testore F, Milanese S, Ceste M, de Conciliis E, Parello G, Lanfranco C, et al. Cardioprotective effect of dexrazoxane in patients with breast cancer treated with anthracyclines in adjuvant setting. American journal of cardiovascular drugs. 2008 Jul 1;**8**(4):257-263

[97] Shaddy RE, Olsen SL, Bristow MR, Taylor DO, Bullock EA, Tani LY, et al. Efficacy and safety of metoprolol in the treatment of doxorubicin-induced cardiomyopathy in pediatric patients. American heart journal. 1995 Jan 1;**129**(1):197-199

[98] Lotrionte M, Palazzoni G, Natali R, Comerci G, Abbate A, Di Persio S, et al. Appraising cardiotoxicity associated with liposomal doxorubicin by means of tissue Doppler echocardiography end-points: Rationale and design of the LITE (Liposomal doxorubicin–Investigational chemotherapy–Tissue Doppler imaging Evaluation) randomized pilot study. International journal of cardiology. 2009 Jun 12;**135**(1):72-77

[99] Wildiers H, Jurcut R, Ganame J, Herbots L, Neven P, De Backer J, et al. A pilot study to investigate the feasibility and cardiac effects of pegylated liposomal doxorubicin (PL-DOX) as adjuvant therapy in medically fit elderly breast cancer patients. Critical reviews in oncology/hematology. 2008 Aug 1;**67**(2):133-138

[100] Arnold JM, Howlett JG, Ducharme A, Ezekowitz JA, Gardner MJ, Giannetti N, et al. Canadian Cardiovascular Society Consensus Conference guidelines on heart failure–2008 update: best practices for the transition of care of heart failure patients, and the recognition, investigation and treatment of cardiomyopathies. Canadian Journal of Cardiology. 2008 Jan 1;**24**(1):21-40

[101] Culty M, Nguyen HA, Underhill CB. The hyaluronan receptor (CD44) participates in the uptake and degradation of hyaluronan. The Journal of cell biology. 1992 Feb 15;**116**(4):1055-1062

[102] Lewis AD, Lau DH, Durán GE, Wolf CR, Sikic BI. Role of cytochrome P-450 from the human CYP3A gene family in the potentiation of morpholino doxorubicin by human liver microsomes. Cancer research. 1992 Aug 15;**52**(16):4379-4384

[103] Baldwin A, Huang Z, Jounaidi Y, Waxman DJ. Identification of novel enzyme–prodrug combinations for use in cytochrome P450-based gene therapy for cancer. Archives of biochemistry and biophysics. 2003 Jan 1;**409**(1):197-206

[104] Michael JB, Tannock IF. Lysosomes, lysosomal enzymes and cancer. Advances in Cancer Research. 1993;**60**:269-291

[105] Roca-Alonso L, Castellano L, Mills A, Dabrowska AF, Sikkel MB, Pellegrino L, Jacob J, Frampton AE, Krell J, Coombes RC, Harding SE. Myocardial MiR-30 downregulation triggered by doxorubicin drives alterations in β-adrenergic signaling and enhances apoptosis. Cell death & disease. 2015 May;6(5):e1754-.

[106] Ma ZG, Dai J, Yuan YP, Bian ZY, Xu SC, Jin YG, et al. T-bet deficiency attenuates cardiac remodelling in rats. Basic Research in Cardiology. 2018 May 1;**113**(3):19

Chapter 11

Overcoming P-Glycoprotein-Mediated Doxorubicin Resistance

Suree Jianmongkol

Abstract

Intracellular concentration of doxorubicin in target cancer cells is a major determinant of therapeutic success of doxorubicin-based regimens. As known, doxorubicin is a substrate of P-glycoprotein (P-gp), the drug efflux transporter in the ABC superfamily. High expression level of P-gp in cancer cells can prevent intracellular accumulation of doxorubicin up to its effective level, leading to doxorubicin resistance and treatment failure. Moreover, these P-gp-overexpressed cells display multi-drug resistance (MDR) phenotype. Regarding this, application of P-gp modulators (suppressor of P-gp activity and expression) is likely to reverse MDR and restore cell sensitivity to doxorubicin treatment. In searching for potential chemo-sensitizer against resistant cancer, a number of phytochemicals or dietary compounds have been studied extensively for their P-gp modulating effects. Furthermore, combination between doxorubicin and P-gp modulators (e.g., plant-derived compounds, siRNA) given through specific target delivery platforms have been an effective strategic approach for MDR reversal and restore doxorubicin effectiveness for cancer treatment.

Keywords: P-glycoprotein, doxorubicin-resistance, P-gp modulators

1. Introduction

Multidrug resistance (MDR) is one of the major factors contributing to a failure of doxorubicin for cancer treatment. Typically, the loss of cell sensitivity to chemotherapy is not limit to only doxorubicin and anthracycline derivatives. The MDR phenomenon evidently extends across various structurally-unrelated anticancer drugs, regardless of their molecular targets [1–3]. Hence, MDR development in cancer cells can simultaneously reduce the effectiveness of several cytotoxic drugs, leading to chemotherapeutic failure. Consequently, patients need higher doses of the anticancer agents to achieve therapeutic success. Either intrinsic or acquired resistance to doxorubicin-based chemotherapy has been attributed to various mechanisms including high expression of the drug efflux transporters, alteration of cell cycle checkpoints and apoptotic signals, increased drug detoxification and DNA repair processes [4–6]. Regarding this, MDR reversal can be one of the strategic approaches to enhance the efficacy, without increased adverse events, of doxorubicin.

This chapter focused on the most studied drug efflux transporter P-glycoprotein (P-gp) and its role in doxorubicin resistance in chemotherapy. In addition, some strategic approaches to conquer P-gp-based MDR in cancer treatment were also described.

2. The drug efflux transporter: P-glycoprotein

Drug transporters can be grouped, according to their transport direction, into uptake and efflux pumps. Most of the known efflux transporters particularly P-glycoprotein (P-gp or MDR1; encoded by *ABCB1*), multidrug resistance protein 1 (MRP1, encoded by *ABCC1*), multidrug resistance protein 2 (MRP2, encoded by *ABCC2*) and breast cancer resistance protein (BCRP; encoded by *ABCG2*) are members of the adenosine triphosphate (ATP)-binding cassette (ABC) superfamily. The ABC transporters require ATP hydrolysis for their transport activity across plasma membrane in the secretive direction. These efflux transporters share similar structural assembly across plasma membrane, composing of a membrane-spanning α-helix structure as a transmembrane domain (TMD) and a relatively hydrophilic ATP-binding site in nucleotide binding domain (NBD). High activity and expression of these ABC drug efflux pumps is a major contributing factor for development of MDR phenomenon in cancer cells [1, 4].

Among the ABC efflux transporters, P-gp is the first and most studied transporter for MDR development in chemotherapy and drug-transporter-related interaction issues. This transporter was first identified from its involvement with multidrug-resistance in cancer cells. Particularly, overexpression of P-gp in cancer cells, either intrinsic or acquired, has been strongly associated with MDR occurrence, thereby P-gp becomes a promising target for development of chemosensitizers.

2.1 Overview of P-gp (structure, function, location, expression, and MDR)

P-gp (MW approximately 170 kDa) is a single polypeptide with 1280 amino acids arranging in two duplicated units of a 6 α-helix structure hydrophobic TMD with linkage to a hydrophilic NBD (**Figure 1**) [1, 2, 7]. These two TMD with the total of 12 helices forms together into one channel as the membrane crossing passage. A substrate binds to the drug-binding site in the TMD whereas an ATP binds to the NBD. After ATP binding, ATP undergoes hydrolysis into ADP for energy to activate P-gp action through protein conformational alteration [7, 8]. This transporter, then, is able to move its substrates across lipid bilayer structure of plasma membrane to extracellular environment.

2.1.1 P-gp and its normal physiological functions

P-gp is constitutively located in the apical surface of either epithelial or endothelial linings of various normal tissues/organs such as adrenal glands, intestine, liver, kidney, pancreas, placenta, capillary vessels in the brain and testes [2, 7–10]. Some organs such as prostate, skin, heart and skeletal muscle have low constitutive expression of P-gp. It should be noting that expression level of P-gp varies in each organ. For example, the numbers of P-gp in colon and ileum are higher than those in jejunum, duodenum and stomach [11, 12]. The tissue distribution of P-gp indicates that this transporter normally serves as an intrinsic determinant of oral drug bioavailability and drug disposition [13–18]. Intestinal P-gp can influence the absorptive amount of its drug substrates, except those in BCS class I (i.e., high permeability and high solubility drugs such as verapamil), into the body after orally taken [13, 19–21]. The constitutive expression of P-gp at the mucosal surface in the lower gastrointestinal (GI) tract (i.e. jejunum, ileum, and colon) may prevent an uptake of its substrate, and perhaps also facilitate GI excretion. Moreover, the interplay between P-gp and the major phase I drug metabolizing enzymes (e.g. cytochrome P450, CYP450) can be anticipated due to their substrate similarity [22].

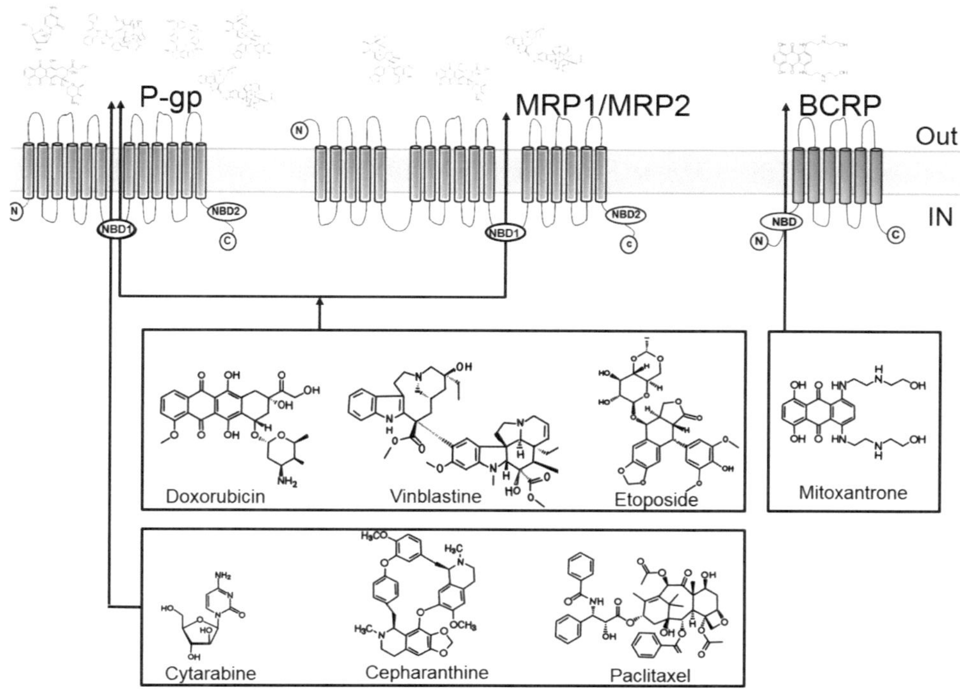

Figure 1.
The key ABC drug efflux transporters and their selected anticancer drug substrates.

As such, P-gp and CYP3A4 act in concert to affect metabolic biotransformation of their substrates such as paclitaxel in intestine and liver, influencing the oral drug bioavailability [22–24]. Localization of P-gp in the blood-organ barriers such as brain or testis prevents drug penetration into such organ systems such as brain, testes [13, 23, 25, 26]. The presence of P-gp on the brush border of nephron proximal tubule and hepatocytes involve with excretion of drugs and endogenous substrates into the urine and bile [13, 27]. To this end, P-gp can be considered as the protective mechanism against xenobiotics as well as pharmacokinetic influencer particularly on absorption, distribution and disposition.

2.1.2 P-gp expression and signaling pathways

Expression of P-gp at plasma membrane involves several cellular processes that linking to P-gp mRNA and protein expression. The regulatory mechanisms have been largely associated with (1) activation or inactivation of oncogenes (e.g., Ras, c-Raf) and transcriptional process, (2) MDR1 translation into P-gp and post translational modification, protein trafficking, and (3) P-gp turn over. It has been reported that the dysregulated microRNA levels (e.g., miR-21, -27a, -451, -130a, -298) could cause MDR development in various cancer cells [28–34]. For example, miR-130 was correlated to MDR1/P-gp overexpression, and cisplatin resistance in SKOV3/CIS cells [32]. Overexpression of miR-27a and miR-451 was linked to increased MDR1 expression and MDR phenotype in resistant cancer cells A2780DX5 and KB-V1 [28].

Overexpression of P-gp particularly in MDR phenomenon has been evidently connected to up-regulation of MDR1 gene through alteration of various signaling pathways and transcription factors. Example of the transcriptional factors involving in MDR1 transcription are nuclear factor-κB (NF-κB) [35, 36], Y-box binding protein-1 (YB-1) [37, 38], activator protein-1 (AP-1) [39], and hypoxia-inducible factor-1 (HIF-1) [38, 40]. The activities of these transcription factors have been linked to various signal transduction pathways, particularly the two major cell survival signaling cascades i.e. (1) the mitogen-activated protein kinase (MAPK) [37, 41], and (2) the phosphatidylinositol 3-kinase (PI3K) pathways [42, 43]. It has been shown that hyperactivation of either MAPK/ERK1/2 or PI3K/Akt/NF-κB signaling pathways results in overexpression of P-gp in doxorubicin-resistant cells such as lung, breast and ovarian cancer cells [44–49]. An up-regulation of P-gp expression in vincristine-resistant human gastric cancer cells was associated with activation of the p-38/MAPK pathway [50].

After activation and translocation into nucleus, transcription factors such as NF-kB and YB-1 (Y-box binding protein) bind to MDR1 promoter region, leading to initiation of MDR1 transcription. Increase in YB-1 nuclear activity is related to P-gp-mediated development of MDR in several cancers including breast cancer, lung cancer, ovarian cancer, colorectal cancer, prostate cancer and osteosarcoma [38]. In response to cell stress such as hyperthermia, viral infection and chemical assault, the survival Akt and MAPKs signaling would be activated, and subsequently increase YB-1 expression and translocation into nucleus for its MDR1-transcription activity [51]. Doxorubicin is a known P-gp inducer in various cancer cells. Doxorubicin up-regulates MDR1 gene expression via the MAPK/ERK1/2 signaling that linked to activation of YB-1 in B-cell lymphoma [37]. Moreover, upregulation of P-gp has been reported after prolonged exposure to various functional unrelated compounds, leading to the loss of drug efficacy and safety [52]. Examples of the known P-gp inducers include anticancer (e.g., cisplatin, doxorubicin, etoposide vinblastine), antidepressants (e.g., trazodone, St. John's Wort), anticonvulsants (e.g., carbamazepine, phenytoin), anti-HIV (e.g., saquinavir, indinarvir, tenofovir), immunosuppressants (e.g., cyclosporine, tacrolimus), steroids (e.g., dexamethasone) [52–54]. It is worth noting that certain CYP450 inducers such as rifampin and St. John's Wort are able to up-regulate P-gp expression, possible sharing through the PXR regulation [55, 56]. Prolonged exposure to rifampin and St. John's Wort in human led to increased intestinal P-gp level, and increased digoxin absorption [57, 58]. Since, P-gp-mediated MDR in cancer is largely due to up-regulation of P-gp expression, better understanding of the signaling proteins and transcription factors will provide a promising targets in overcoming MDR for anticancer chemotherapy.

2.1.3 P-gp and multi-drug resistance in cancer

Overexpression of P-gp has been strongly correlated with chemo-resistance and cancer relapses in several cancer patients such as breast cancer, adult acute myeloid leukemia, pheochromocytoma patients, leading to poor prognosis from therapeutic failure in patients receiving chemotherapy [1, 59–62]. Accordingly, P-gp is intrinsically expressed in various cancer types, particularly those derived from tissues with high basal MDR1 expression levels such as colon, kidney and liver tissues. Being a transmembrane efflux pump, P-gp serves as a cellular defense mechanism against drug assault by limiting intracellular drug accumulation up to toxic threshold level. Regarding this, the susceptibility of cancer to anticancer drugs being P-gp substrate varies, depending on intrinsic expressed P-gp levels. Certain types of cancers may be classified as poor responder showing their unresponsiveness to chemotherapy regimens containing P-gp substrates. For example, prostate cancer appears to be better responder to chemotherapy, as compared to colorectal or renal cancers [63, 64]. Moreover, some cancers such as leukemia, lymphoma and breast cancer having low levels of intrinsic P-gp expression, and thus initially respond well to chemotherapy. Later, after repeated treatment, the expression level of P-gp markedly increases, and those cancers display multi-drug resistance (MDR) phenotype [1, 65, 66]. This acquired MDR phenomenon can be viewed as cellular adaptive survival response to cytotoxic challenge.

2.2 Substrates and modulators

Examples of substrates and modulators of P-gp are listed in **Table 1**.

2.2.1 Substrates

Human ABC efflux transporters demonstrate their broad substrate specificity toward structurally diverse lipophilic compounds. Most of their substrates are weakly amphipathic and hydrophobic planar structure with aromatic ring and positively charged nitrogen atom [52, 54, 67, 68]. Examples of P-gp substrates are anticancer drugs (vinca alkaloids, anthracyclines, and epipodophyllotoxins), cardiovascular drugs (e.g., digoxin, quinidine, talinolol, diltiazem, losartan, verapamil), anti-microbial agents (e.g., doxycycline, erythromycin, itraconazole, rifampin), anti-viral drugs (e.g., indinavir), anticonvulsants (e.g., phenytoin), acid blockers (e.g., cimetidine), immunosuppressants (e.g., cyclosporine, tacrolimus), steroids (e.g., aldosterone, cortisol, dexamethasone), opioids (loperamide, morphine).

Substrates (Anti-cancer drugs)	**Inducers (Anti-cancer drugs)**	**P-gp modulators**	
		Direct inhibitors	**Suppressors of expression**
Actinomycin D	Daunorubicin	Small molecule inhibitors	Small molecule inhibitors
Colchicine	Docetaxel	*First generation*	Curcumin
Docetaxel	Doxorubicin	Cyclosporin A	Dasatinib
Doxorubicin	Flutamide	Verapamil	Dexverapamil
Daunorubicin	Paclitaxel	*Second generation*	Reserpine
Epirubicin	Vinblastine	VX-710 (Biricodar)	Imatinib
Etoposide	Vincristine	Dexverapamil	Nilotinib
Idarubicin		PSC833 (Valspodar)	Sorafenib
Imatinib		*Third generation*	Trifluoperazine
Methotrexate		GF120918 (Elacridar)	Toremifene
Paclitaxel		XR9576 (Tariquidar)	PSC833 (Valspodar)
Teniposide		LY335979 (Zosuquidar)	RNA interference
Topotecan		*Fourth generation*	*MDR1* small-interfering RNA (siRNA)
Vinblastine		Capsaisin	Antisense oligonucleotides
Vincristine		Curcumin	*MDR1* antisense oligonucleotides delivered via lysosomes
		Limonin	
		Piperine	
		Quercetin	
		Monoclonal antibodies	
		MRK 16	
		MRK 17	
		UIC 2	

Table 1.
Selected substrates, inducers and modulators of P-gp.

2.2.2 Modulators

Modulators suppress P-gp activity through either (1) direct inhibition of P-gp function by either competitive or non-competitive inhibitors; or (2) suppression of P-gp expression levels by interferences with either transcription, translation/post-translation, and degradation processes.

2.2.2.1 Direct inhibition of functionally active P-gp

The direct inhibition of active P-gp can be attributed to the interaction between chemicals and P-gp at either TMB or NBD [67–69]. Any compound such as tyrosine Kinase Inhibitors interferes with ATP binding or hydrolysis in NBD site can reduce P-gp transport action [70]. Chemicals identified as small molecule P-gp inhibitors such as amiodarone, diltiazem, verapamil bind to substrate binding sites or allosteric sites in TMB, resulting in interference on substrate binding and transport. It has been reported that certain compounds such as cyclosporine A could exert their inhibitory action by interfering with substrate recognition and ATP hydrolysis [8, 67–69]. It is not surprising that these TMB type inhibitors and substrates share many common molecular features such as hydrophobic planar structure. In addition, due to the diversity in chemical structure of P-gp inhibitors, establishment of the structure activity relationship (SAR) of P-gp inhibitors is very challenging. The structure pattern of the inhibitors contains planar rings and basic nitrogen atom within an extended side chain of the aromatic ring. The presence of tertiary amino groups, in comparison with primary and secondary amine, increases the anti-MDR potency considerably. Furthermore, the presence of nitrogen atom in non-aromatic ring apparently increases inhibitory action of the compounds [71]. Examples of P-gp inhibitors are calcium channel blockers (verapamil, diltiazem), and various phytochemicals such as flavonoid and steroidal compounds (e.g., quercetin, resveratrol), indole alkaloids and polycyclic compounds (e.g., capsaicin, piperine, rhinacanthin C) [66, 72–74].

Ideally, the P-gp inhibitors should be potent and selective to P-gp function at target cells/tissues, with no systemic side effects. To date, there are four generations of small molecule inhibitors. The first generation inhibitors are known drug substrates of the ABC transporters such as verapamil, cyclosporine A, tamoxifen and quinidine [75]. They were not specifically designed to be P-gp inhibitors, and could not display good clinical outcomes in their MDR reversal activity. The clinical disappointment could be due to their weak inhibitory potency against the MDR transporters including P-gp, and their pharmacokinetic interactions with chemotherapeutic agents, leading to the need of high doses and intolerable adverse effects [1, 76]. Next, the second generation inhibitors such as valspodar (cyclosporine A derivative) were developed, based on structure activity relationships of the first generation compounds, in order to improve potency, specificity, and to reduce systemic toxicity. Although this group of inhibitors demonstrated their improvement in inhibitory potency, their clinical outcomes were still unsatisfied due to their pharmacokinetic interaction with the anti-cancer drugs via inhibition of cytochrome P450, and their severe toxicity [75, 77]. Subsequently, the third generation P-gp inhibitors such as elacridar, tariquidar and zosuquidar were developed in order to address the limitations of the second generation compounds. These inhibitors elicit no effect on CYP P450 metabolism, therefore they are unlikely to affect the plasma concentrations of anti-cancer drugs. They were also more potent and selective P-gp inhibitors, effectively working in nanomolar concentration range. However, the potent P-gp inhibitor tariquidar can be either substrate or inhibitor of P-gp depending on its given dose [78]. To date, the clinical efficacy for MDR reversal of this generation has yet completely satisfied, its effectiveness possibly also depends on given dosage and intrinsic tumor properties.

Currently, phytochemicals or natural compounds with MDR reversal activity have been subject of interest in searching for new effective chemo-sensitizer against cancer. This group of inhibitors obtained from natural sources is classified as the fourth generation inhibitor. Numerous phytochemical researches on pharmacological activities and pharmacokinetics have revealed that plant-based compounds elicit a broad spectrum of pharmacological actions such as anti-cancer, anti-oxidant, anti-microbial, anti-inflammation, etc. In addition, these plant-based compounds, depending upon its molecular structure, may interfere with P-gp and metabolizing enzymes, leading to the concerning issues in drug bioavailability and pharmacokinetic drug interactions. The advantages of the fourth generation inhibitors in part rely on their natural origin with long history of uses in dietary or health supplements and in traditional medicine. It may be able to presume that this group of inhibitors derived from known edible products possessed less toxicity and more tolerable than those of the previous generation compounds. Evidently, even vegetables (e.g., bitter melon), spices (e.g., black pepper, turmeric) or fruits (e.g., orange, grapefruit) also contain substances that could inhibit P-gp and other efflux transporters in the ABC superfamily [72–75, 77, 79–82]. Their competitive inhibition against the efflux transporters enhance cytotoxicity of anticancer drugs such as doxorubicin and vinblastine, leading to potential MDR reversal in various cancer cells. However, the inhibitory potency of these plant-based compounds against P-gp activity might be low. Their IC50 values obtained from the in vitro cell culture models appear to be in micromolar range. Thus, this group of inhibitors is unlikely a good MDR reversing agent through direct P-gp inhibition at MDR cancer cells in clinical setting. In addition, the interference of P-gp activity of these compounds in pharmacokinetic aspect may influence on P-gp-related ADME and bioavailability of chemotherapeutic drugs that concomitantly given. Nevertheless, the opportunities of further development into effective chemosensitizers cannot be excluded. Better understanding of QSAR may enable to facilitate chemical modification of these identified plant-based P-gp inhibitors to generate more potent and high selective P-gp inhibitors. Furthermore, several plant-based compounds (e.g, curcumin, resveratrol, quercetin) have been demonstrated their potential in down-regulation of P-gp and other key regulators in transporter-independent MDR mechanisms [75, 82–86].

In addition to small molecule inhibitors, monoclonal antibodies can be another alternative approach in inhibiting P-gp activity. Theoretically, any agents that specifically affect lipid-protein interactions or protein structure of targeted P-gp can be developed into P-gp inhibitor. Typically, monoclonal antibody can be developed to specifically recognize and bind to its target protein, leading to inhibition of changes in protein conformation. Regarding this, human P-gp-specific antibodies UIC2, MRK-16 and 4E3 reacted specifically to the extracellular loop of both halves of P-gp, and disabled P-gp transport activity [87]. Consequently, treatment cancer cells with these antibodies resulted in increased concentrations of anticancer drugs (e.g., vincristine, actinomycin D, doxorubicin, paclitaxel) within the cells, and improve drug effectiveness [87–91]. In athymic mice model, MRK16 was demonstrated its ability to significantly reduce tumor mass [92]. Further clinical studies of human P-gp-specific antibodies are needed to conduct in terms of safety and efficacy.

2.2.2.2 Suppressor of P-gp expression

In addition to direct inhibition, reduction of P-gp activity can arise from decrease of protein expression at plasma membrane. Interference on transcription and translation of MDR1 gene, resulting in reduction of P-gp expression, can be another approach to overcome MDR in cancer. Several innovative tools targeting at MDR transcription or mRNA including small molecules, antisense oligonucleotides, hammerhead ribozymes and RNA interference strategies have been employed.

2.2.2.2.1 MicroRNA and RNA interference (RNAi) technologies

Application of microRNA and RNAi technologies with either small-interfering RNA (siRNA) or small hairpin RNA (shRNA) to specific silence MDR1 expression in cancer cells with MDR phenotype has been demonstrated their effectiveness in down-regulation of MDR1 and P gp expression with paralleled increases drug accumulation and improved sensitivity to treatment. MicroRNAs (miRNAs) are small non-coding RNA molecules that can inhibit ABCB1 mRNA translation processes [93, 94]. A number of miRNAs have been studied on their ability to down-regulate P-gp expression and restore cell sensitivity to P-gp drug substrates in drug resistant cells [34]. For example, miRNA-4539 could increase doxorubicin-mediated cell death in MDA-MB-231 breast cancer cells [93, 94].

The RNAi technologies involve either transient gene-silencing by siRNA or stable inhibition by MDR1 shRNA-transfected on plasmid DNA of MDR cancer cells. Treatment with siRNA against MDR1 increases drug-mediated cytotoxicity in various MDR cancer cells such as paclitaxel in MDR1 ovarian cancer cells and doxorubicin in doxorubicin-resistant breast cancer cells [95]. In addition, siRNA was able to significant reduced size of doxorubicin-resistant xenograft in a mouse model [96]. MDR1 ShRNA transfected in taxol-resistant human ovarian cancer cell line A2780 effectively down-regulated P-gp expression, and enhanced paclitaxel-mediated toxicity in this cells [97].

Selective suppression of P-gp/MDR1 expression with either microRNA or RNAi technologies offers the novel approach to specifically combat P-gp-based MDR in cancer, and re-sensitize the MDR cells to chemotherapeutic agents. However, for their therapeutic applications, there are several challenges required especially the effective miR/RNAi delivery to target cancer cells, design of expression vectors for shRNA, systemic stability and degradation, and safety of patients.

2.2.2.2.2 Small molecules as P-gp down-regulator

Numerous small molecules particularly those in the fourth generation of P-gp inhibitors such as curcumin, ginsenoside, quercetin and resveratrol have been demonstrated their ability to reduce P-gp function in the MDR cancer cells via down-regulation of P-gp expression [83–85]. By targeting at the signaling pathways related to transcription process of MDR1, several plant-based compounds suppress P-gp expression in the resistance cells and improve chemo-sensitivity to anticancer drugs. For instance, the P-gp modulating effect of asiatic acid, ginsenoside, isoquinoline alkaloids (e.g. cepharantine, tetrandine) resulted from their blockade of MAPK/ERK1/2 or PI3K/Akt pathways in MDR cancer cells [86, 98–101]. Another isoquinoline alkaloid berberine inhibited P-gp expression and enhanced doxorubicin-mediated toxicity in MCF-7 cells through down-regulation of AMPK-HIF1α signaling cascade [102]. Anti-MDR property of natural curcuminoids (e.g., curcumin, bisdemethoxycurcumin) involved with inhibition of human MDR1 gene expression in MDR cervical carcinoma KB-V1 cells [103]. In addition, certain compounds such as a natural marine product Et743 inhibit MDR1 transcription via blocking its promoter activation [104].

3. Doxorubicin and P-gp

Doxorubicin is one of the most effective cytotoxic anticancer drugs. This drug has been used for combating various types of cancers such as cancers of breast, ovary, prostate, stomach, thyroid; small cell cancer of lung; squamous cell cancer of head and neck; multiple myeloma; Hodgkin's disease; lymphomas; acute lymphoblastic leukemia (ALL) and acute myeloblastic leukemia (AML). Unfortunately, the uses of doxorubicin can be limited because of its dose-related toxicity (e.g., nausea, vomiting, hair loss, leucopenia, cardiomyopathy, heart failure) and high MDR incidence [105, 106]. Despite the good clinical therapeutic responses are seen in patients receiving doxorubicin in the earliest stage of treatment, multi-drug resistance may later develop and lead to treatment failure.

One of the major mechanisms responsible for doxorubicin-induced MDR is up-regulation of MDR1/P-gp expression. Doxorubicin is an anthracycline derivative with a four-membered ring system containing an anthraquinone chromophore, and an aminoglycoside (**Figure 1**). This molecular structure accommodates its interaction with major MDR efflux transporters in the ABC superfamily proteins. It has been well established that doxorubicin and other anthracycline derivatives are P-gp substrates with ability to up-regulate P-gp/MDR1 expression after repeated exposure in various cancer cells such as breast and lung cancers as well as in vivo and in clinical settings [66, 107, 108]. For instance, lung perfusion with doxorubicin resulted in an increase of MDR1 RNA in patients with sarcoma pulmonary metastases [18]. The P-gp-overexpressed cancer cells would have intracellular doxorubicin concentration below its effective threshold level. Consequently, cancer cells increasingly survive from doxorubicin-mediated cytotoxity. In this circumstance, titrating dose up to overcome MDR may not enable to achieve a successful outcome due to dose-limiting toxicity. Because the adverse effects of doxorubicin and other anti-cancer drugs are mostly concentration-dependent, increasing doses can produce higher degree of severity and unendurable adverse events, leading to patient's intolerability and even fatal outcome. Addition of other cytotoxic drugs into doxorubicin-based regimens may not also enable to obtain a chemotherapeutic success, if those drugs are also substrates of the MDR transporters.

Generally, clinical efficacy of doxorubicin depends on its pharmacokinetics after systemic exposure influencing (1) the therapeutic concentration at target organs, and (2) the homogeneity of drug distribution in the cancerous tissues particularly solid tumor. In addition, it is very critical that doxorubicin accumulates within the targeted cancer cells at the level greater than its cytotoxic threshold to elicit its pharmacological actions.

3.1 P-gp effects on doxorubicin's Pharmacokinetics aspect

Doxorubicin is poorly absorbed through GI with low bioavailability (approximately 5%) after orally taken, due to its instability in stomach acidic pH and CYP450 biotransformation in liver. In addition, doxorubicin can induce cytotoxicity in normal tissue. Currently, doxorubicin is commercially available for cancer treatment in injection dosage form. Due to its lipophilicity, doxorubicin moves through plasma membrane into the cells via passive diffusion, and its extent of tissues/cellular permeation and cellular retention can be limit by the existence of efflux transporters particularly P-gp. Apparently, doxorubicin is extensively distributed to several organs such as liver, heart, kidney after injection. Being the efflux transporters, P-gp has a significant impact on doxorubicin distribution to certain target tissues such as brain, testes [109, 110]. Certain P-gp inhibitors such as PSC-833, piperine capsaicin, resveratrol, silymarin and quercetin were reported their influence on the pharmacokinetics and tissue distribution of doxorubicin in animal models [85, 110]. Capsaicin was reported to significantly increase the extent of doxorubicin accumulation in mice brain after iv injection probably through inhibition of P-gp at blood brain barrier [110]. In addition, piperine and capsaincin, through P-gp inhibition, reduced drug excretion into bile and urine, leading to increased drug levels in liver and kidney [110].

3.2 P-gp effects on doxorubicin's Pharmacodynamic aspects

Critically, overexpression of P-gp on the plasma membrane of cancer cells is a major determinant in preventing intracellular doxorubicin accumulation up to its cytotoxic level. Doxorubicin resistant cancer cells clearly display significant lower intracellular doxorubicin retention with more tolerable to doxorubicin exposure than their parental sensitive cells [65, 66]. Thus, P-gp can be a potential therapeutic target for either MDR reversal or bio-enhancing effect in cancer therapy. The presence of P-gp modulators clearly demonstrates their abilities to restore doxorubicin-mediated killing effect in various cancer cells by increasing intracellular level of doxorubicin [66, 111]. Several plant-based compounds such as limonin, quercetin, resveratrol, curcumin and rhinacanthin-C at their non-cytotoxic concentration have been reported to significantly enhance doxorubicin-mediated cytotoxicity in various cancer resistance cells through modulation of P-gp function [66, 112]. These phytochemical P-gp modulators may suppress P-gp function either by direct inhibition of activity or down-regulation of protein expression.

Moreover, the influence of P-gp on clinical resistance to doxorubicin-based treatment has been reported in cancer patients [113–116]. In order to improve drug efficacy and patient tolerability, several approaches targeting at the P-gp function and expression have been introduced to increase cellular doxorubicin drug level and restore drug sensitivity without the need of higher concentration or additional chemotherapeutic drugs in the therapeutic regimen.

4. Strategic approaches to overcome P-gp mediated resistance to doxorubicin

Taken that doxorubicin is a known substrate of P-gp, the drug efflux transporters in the ATP binding cassette (ABC) family. Hence, any approaches target at the function of these transporters can be presumed to increase therapeutic success for doxorubicin-based chemotherapeutic regimens. Regarding this, the strategies are as follows:

- Increases in dose of doxorubicin or number of cytotoxic drugs to achieve therapeutic success. This has not been a satisfactory approach due to drug toxicity and patients' intolerability.

- Utilization of P-gp modulators to inhibit either function or expression.

- Development of better drug delivery platforms to bypass P-gp activity, leading to increase intracellular retention of doxorubicin within target cells.

The current MDR reversal strategy has been exploited P-gp modulators that either directly inhibit P-gp activity or down-regulate P-gp expression in order to restore cell chemo-sensitivity to doxorubicin [107]. With the encapsulation technology, P-gp modulators can be co-administered with doxorubicin in the same drug delivery platform, and enhance intracellular doxorubicin accumulation. This approach can be accomplished if the potent, non-cytotoxic P-gp modulators that specifically target at cancer cells are implemented. In addition, the P-gp modulators that also target at non-transporter based resistance such as activation of cellular survival pathways can exert potentially synergistic impact on MDR reversal effect and better response to doxorubicin treatment. Collectively, the combined doxorubicin and P-gp modulators with multiple-hit targets is a promising strategy to achieve chemotherapeutic efficacy without the need of high dose or additional cytotoxic drugs in the therapeutic regimen.

4.1 Synergy with P-gp modulators

This approach aims to suppress P-gp activity at plasma membrane of target cancer cells. Several P-gp modulators in combination with anti-cancer drugs have been evaluated for safety and efficacy in clinical trials. The clinical outcomes from the first three generations of ABC inhibitors such as quinine, verapamil, cyclosporine-A, tariquitor, PSC 833, LY335979, and GF120918 were quite disappointed, partly because of their dose-limiting adverse events. Most of the P-gp inhibitors required high doses for their clinical MDR reversal effects. In addition, their interference on the P-gp or other ABC transporters at non-target tissues such as brain and kidney could adversely increase accumulation of cytotoxic drugs in these tissues.

The fourth generation of P-gp modulators which are mostly natural products have gained a great interest as potential chemosensitizers in MDR cancer treatment. The advantages of being natural products with long history of use are inclined to the known safety profiles in human and potential hit multiple targets that can restore cell sensitivity to doxorubicin. In addition to direct inhibition of P-gp activity, a number of the natural compounds at non-cytotoxic concentration elicit their chemo sensitizing effects through down-regulation of MDR1 and signaling proteins in cell adaptive survival mechanisms. The higher degree of synergism between doxorubicin and a P-gp modulator can be anticipated with potential therapeutic success. Synergistic outcomes between doxorubicin and natural compounds such as resveratrol, quercetin, silymarin, gallic acid, curcumin, epigallocatechin-3-gallate have been demonstrated in various cancer cell models [82, 83, 103, 111, 117–120]. In addition to P-gp modulatory activity (inhibiting both P-gp function and expression), these natural compounds have a broad spectrum of pharmacological activities such as antioxidant, anticancer, anti-inflammation, possible through multiple signaling pathways. For example, the biological effects of curcumin have been related to multiple signaling pathways including NF-kB, Akt, MAPK, Nrf2, AMPK, JAK/STAT that involve in MDR1 expression, cell inflammation, and apoptosis [121]. Co-administration of doxorubicin and curcumin significantly improved doxorubicin-mediated cytotoxicity in vitro cell models and in vivo hepatic xenograft mice model, compared with doxorubicin alone [121–125].

In addition to chemical-based modulators, the uses of specific antibody against P-gp or RNA interference (RNAi) technology to silence P-gp expression may be effective approach to suppress P-gp activity and restore chemo-sensitivity to doxorubicin treatment. Clinical studies on these MDR reversing methods should be extensively conducted to support their uses and benefits in cancer patients.

4.2 Drug delivery system and formulation

This approach aims to develop targeted delivery platforms for improving the permeation of doxorubicin/P-gp modulators/ chemo-sensitizers (e.g., antibodies against ABCB1, siRNA) into target cancer cells, leading to an increased intracellular doxorubicin concentration [3, 89, 96, 126–128]. Various nano-drug delivery platforms such as polymeric and solid lipid nanoparticle (SLNs), liposomes, micelles, mesoporous silica nanoparticles, nanostructured lipid carriers, dendrimers have been constructed to better targeting drug delivery to site of action. This approach in couple with utilization of P-gp modulators can overcome MDR and enhance therapeutic efficacy of doxorubicin. Furthermore, with cancer-targeting ability, this target specific delivery would limit the adverse effect to normal tissues. With the encapsulation technology, nanoparticles (NPs) loaded with doxorubicin and P-gp modulators or other molecules (e.g., siRNAs) has been reported their effectiveness in target delivery into the cells. For examples, aerosol OT (AOT)-alginate NPs enhanced cellular delivery of doxorubicin in MCF-7 cells [129]. Lipid-modified dextran-based NPs loaded with doxorubicin and MDR1 siRNA significantly increased intracellular doxorubicin and reduced P-gp expression levels in osteosarcoma cell line, as compared to doxorubicin alone [130]. Doxorubicin-curcumin composite NPs (e.g., NanoDoxCurc, pegylated-DOX-CUR NPs) could enhance effects of doxorubicin both in vitro and in vivo models of DOX-resistant cancers (e.g., multiple myeloma, acute leukemia, prostate and ovarian cancers). In addition, doxorubicin-curcumin NPs did not cause cardiac toxicity and bone marrow suppression in mice model [131].

5. Conclusion

Doxorubicin is an effective anti-cancer drug that has high MDR incidence. High expression of an efflux transporter P-gp is one established mechanism responsible for the loss of drug effectiveness and MDR development. This can be due to the P-gp function in preventing intracellular accumulation of doxorubicin up to its effective level. Several approaches have been introduced in order to increase the efficacy of doxorubicin-based chemotherapy and overcome MDR. The combination of doxorubicin and non-cytotoxic P-gp modulators, particularly when given to the specific target cancer can be a promising approach to increase cancer sensitivity to doxorubicin through suppression of P-gp function. With the novel encapsulation technologies, it is very possible to develop the drug delivery platforms with specific targeted cancer cells as well as improvement of doxorubicin delivery into the cells. By these means, enhancement of doxorubicin-mediated cytotoxicity can be achieved with minimal dosing of the anti-cancer drugs. After clinically approval, it will provide a great benefit to patients receiving doxorubicin-based chemotherapy.

Acknowledgements

The author gratefully thanks IntechOpen Limited for the sponsorship program in publishing this work.

Conflict of interest

The Author declares no conflicts of interest.

Author details

Suree Jianmongkol
Department of Pharmacology and Physiology, Faculty of Pharmaceutical Sciences, Chulalongkorn University, Bangkok, Thailand

*Address all correspondence to: suree.j@pharm.chula.ac.th

References

[1] Robey RW, Pluchino KM, Hall MD, Fojo AT, Bates SE. and Gottesman MM. (2018). Revisiting the role of ABC transporters in multidrug-resistant cancer. Nature reviews Cancer 18(7): 452-464.

[2] Liu X. (2019). ABC Family Transporters. Adv Exp Med Biol. 1141: 13-100.

[3] Li W, Zhang H, Assaraf YG, Zhao K, Xu X, Xie J, Yang DH, and Chen ZS. (2016). Overcoming ABC transporter-mediated multidrug resistance: Molecular mechanisms and novel therapeutic drug strategies. Drug Resist Updat 27:14-29.

[4] Ji X, Lu Y, Tian H, Meng A, Wei M, and Cho WC. (2019). Chemoresistance mechanisms of breast cancer and their countermeasures, Biomedicine & Pharmacotherapy. 114: 108800.

[5] Mansoori B, Mohammadi A, Davudian S, Shirjang S, and Baradaran B. (2017). The Different Mechanisms of Cancer Drug Resistance: A Brief Review. Adv Pharm Bull. 7(3): 339-348.

[6] Kartal-Yandim M, Adan-Gokbulut A, and Baran Y. (2016). Molecular mechanisms of drug resistance and its reversal in cancer, Crit Rev Biotechnol. 36 716-726.

[7] Li Y, Yuan H, Yang K, Xu W, Tang W, Li X. (2010). The structure and functions of P-glycoprotein. Curr Med Chem. 17(8):786-800.

[8] Zhou SF. (2008). Structure, function and regulation of P-glycoprotein and its clinical relevance in drug disposition. Xenobiotica 38(7-8):802-832.

[9] Müller J, Keiser M, Drozdzik M, Oswald S. (2017). Expression, regulation and function of intestinal drug transporters: an update. Biol Chem. 398(2):175-192.

[10] Staud F, Ceckova M, Micuda S, and Pavek P. (2010). Expression and function of p-glycoprotein in normal tissues: effect on pharmacokinetics. Methods Mol Biol 596:199-222.

[11] Takano M, Yumoto R, and Murakami T. (2006). Expression and function of efflux drug transporters in the intestine. Pharmacology & Therapeutics. 109 (1-2): 137-161.

[12] Mouly S, and Paine MF. (2003). P-glycoprotein increases from proximal to distal regions of human small intestine. Pharm Res. 20(10):1595-1599.

[13] Schinkel AH. (1998). Pharmacological insights from P-glycoprotein knockout mice. Int J Clin Pharmacol Ther. 36(1):9-13.

[14] Murakami T. and Takano M. (2008). Intestinal efflux transporters and drug absorption. Expert Opin Drug Metab Toxicol. 4(7): 923-939.

[15] Ipar VS, Dsouza A, Devarajan PV. (2019). Enhancing curcumin oral bioavailability through nanoformulations. Eur J Drug Metab Pharmacokinet. 44(4):459-480.

[16] Mathur P, Rawal S, Patel B, Patel MM. (2019). Oral delivery of anticancer agents using nanoparticulate drug delivery system. Curr Drug Metab 20(14):1132-1140.

[17] Jain AK, Jain S. (2016). Advances in oral delivery of anti-cancer prodrugs. Expert Opin Drug Deliv. 13(12):1759-1775.

[18] Price DF, Luscombe CN, Eddershaw PJ, Edwards, CD, and Gumbleton M. (2017). The differential absorption of a series of P-glycoprotein

substrates in isolated perfused lungs from Mdr1a/1b genetic knockout mice can be attributed to distinct physico-chemical properties: an insight into predicting transporter-mediated, pulmonary specific disposition. Pharm Res. 34:2498-2516.

[19] Yasir M., Asif M., Kumar A. and Aggarval A. (2010). Biopharmaceutical classification system : an account. International Journal of PharmTech Research. 2(3): 1681-1690.

[20] Wu C.Y. and Benet L.Z. (2005). Predicting drug disposition via application of BCS: transport/ absorption/ elimination interplay and development of a biopharmaceutics drug disposition classification system. Pharm Res. 22(1): 11-23.

[21] B Shekhawat P, B Pokharkar V. (2017). Understanding peroral absorption: regulatory aspects and contemporary approaches to tackling solubility and permeability hurdles. Acta Pharm Sin B. 7(3):260-280.

[22] Domínguez-AvilaJA,Wall-MedranoA, Velderrain-Rodríguez GR, Chen CO, Salazar-López NJ, Robles-Sánchez M, González-Aguilar GA. (2017). Gastrointestinal interactions, absorption, splanchnic metabolism and pharmacokinetics of orally ingested phenolic compounds. Food Funct 8(1):15-38.

[23] van Waterschoot RAB, and Schinkel AH. (2011). A Critical Analysis of the Interplay between Cytochrome P450 3A and P-Glycoprotein: Recent Insights from Knockout and Transgenic Mice. Pharmacol Rev 63:390-410.

[24] Hendrikx J, Lagas J, Rosing H, Schellens J, Beijnen J, and Schinke AH. (2013). P-glycoprotein and cytochrome P450 3A act together in restricting the oral bioavailability of paclitaxel. Int J of Cancer 132(10): 2439-2447.

[25] Villanueva S, Zhang W, Zecchinati F, Mottino A, Vore M. (2019). ABC transporters in extrahepatic tissues: pharmacological regulation in heart and intestine. Curr Med Chem. 26(7):1155-1184.

[26] Abdullahi W, Davis TP, Ronaldson PT. (2017). Functional expression of p-glycoprotein and organic anion transporting polypeptides at the blood-brain barrier: understanding transport mechanisms for improved CNS drug delivery? AAPS J. 19(4):931-939.

[27] König J, Müller F, Fromm MF. (2013). Transporters and drug-drug interactions: important determinants of drug disposition and effects. Pharmacol Rev 65(3):944-966.

[28] An X, Sarmiento C, Tan T, and Zhu H. (2017). Regulation of multidrug resistance by microRNAs in anti-cancer therapy. Acta Pharmaceutica Sinica B. 7(1): 38-51

[29] Zhu H, Wu H, Liu X, Evans BR, Medina DJ, Liu CG, Yang JM. (2008). Role of microRNA miR-27a and miR-451 in the regulation of MDR1/ Pglycoprotein expression in human cancer cells. Biochem Pharmacol. 76:582-588.

[30] Dong WH, Li Q, Zhang XY, Guo Q, Li H, Wang TY. (2015). Deep sequencing identifies deregulation of microRNAs involved with vincristine drug-resistance of colon cancer cells. Int J Clin Exp Pathol, 8(9): 11524-11530.

[31] Bao L, Hazari S, Mehra S, Kaushal D, Moroz K, and Dash S. (2012). Increased expression of P-glycoprotein and doxorubicin chemoresistance of metastatic breast cancer is regulated by miR-298. Am J Pathol 180(6): 2490-2503.

[32] Yang L., Li N., Wang H., Jia X., Wang X., Luo J. (2012). Altered

microRNA expression in cisplatin-resistant ovarian cancer cells and upregulation of miR-130a associated with MDR1/P-glycoprotein-mediated drug resistance. Oncol. Rep. 28:592-600.

[33] Lopes-Rodrigues V, Seca H, Sousa D, Sousa E, Lima RT, and Vasconcelos MH. (2014). The network of P-glycoprotein and microRNAs interactions. Int J of Cancer 135(2): 253-263.

[34] Xie Y, Shaap Y, Deng X, Wang M, and Chen Y. (2018). MicroRNA-298 Reverses Multidrug Resistance to Antiepileptic Drugs by Suppressing MDR1/P-gp Expression in vitro. Front Neurosci 12: 602.

[35] Ronaldson, P. T., Ashraf, T., Bendayan, R. (2010). Regulation of multidrug resistance protein 1 by tumor necrosis factor alpha in cultured glial cells: involvement of nuclear factor-kappaB and c-Jun N-terminal kinase signaling pathways. Mol Pharmacol. 77: 644-659.

[36] Kuo MT, Liu Z, Wei Y, Lin-Lee YC, Tatebe S, Mills GB, and Unate H. (2002). Induction of human MDR1 gene expression by 2-acetylaminofluorene is mediated by effectors of the phosphoinositide 3-kinase pathway that activate NF-kappaB signaling. Oncogene. 27: 1945-1954.

[37] Shen H, Xu W, Luo W, Zhou L, Yong W, Chen F, and Han X. (2011). Upregulation of mdr1 gene is related to activation of the MAPK/ERK signal transduction pathway and YB-1 nuclear translocation in B-cell lymphoma. Exp Hematol. 39: 558-569.

[38] Maurya PK, Mishra A, Yadav BS, Singh S, Kumar P, Chaudhary A, and Mani A. (2017). Role of Y Box Protein-1 in cancer: As potential biomarker and novel therapeutic target. J Cancer. 8: 1900-1907.

[39] Chen Q, Bian Y, and Zeng S. (2014). Involvement of AP-1 and NF-κB in the Up-regulation of P-gp in Vinblastine Resistant Caco-2 Cells. Drug Metab. Pharmacokinet. 29(2): 223-226.

[40] Doublier S, Belisario DC, Polimeni M, Annaratone L, Riganti L, Allia E, Ghigo D, Bosia A, and Sapino A. (2012). HIF-1 activation induces doxorubicin resistance in MCF7 3-D spheroids via P-glycoprotein expression: a potential model of the chemo-resistance of invasive micropapillary carcinoma of the breast. BMC Cancer 12:4.

[41] Winder M, and Virós A. (2018). Mechanisms of drug resistance in melanoma. Handb Exp Pharmacol. 249:91-108.

[42] Shariati M, and Meric-Bernstam F. (2019). Targeting AKT for cancer therapy. Expert Opin Investig Drugs. 28(11):977-988.

[43] Sharma VR, Gupta GK, Sharma AK, Batra N, Sharma DK, Joshi A, and Sharma AK. (2017). PI3K/Akt/mTOR Intracellular Pathway and Breast Cancer: Factors, Mechanism and Regulation. Curr Pharm Des. 23(11):1633-1638.

[44] Christowitz C, Davis T, Isaacs A, van Niekerk G, Hattingh S, and Engelbrecht AM. (2019). Mechanisms of doxorubicin-induced drug resistance and drug resistant tumour growth in a murine breast tumour model. BMC Cancer 19(1):757.

[45] Fang XJ, Jiang H, Zhu YQ, Zhang LY, Fan QH, and Tian Y. (2014). Doxorubicin induces drug resistance and expression of the novel CD44st via NF-κB in human breast cancer MCF-7 cells. Oncol Rep. 31(6):2735-2742.

[46] Zheng HC. (2017). The molecular mechanisms of chemoresistance in cancers. Oncotarget. 6: 59950-59964.

[47] Yang SY, Miah A, Sales KM, Fuller B, Seifalian AM, and Winslet M.

(2011). Inhibition of the p38 MAPK pathway sensitises human colon cancer cells to 5-fluorouracil treatment. Int J Oncol. 38: 1695-1702.

[48] Liu S, Chen S, Yuan W, Wang H, Chen K, Li D, and Li D. (2017). PD-1/PD-L1 interaction up-regulates MDR1/P-gp expression in breast cancer cells via PI3K/AKT and MAPK/ERK pathways. Oncotarget 8(59):99901-99912.

[49] Liu Z, Zhu G, Getzenberg RH, and Veltri RW. (2015). The upregulation of PI3K/Akt and MAP kinase pathways is associated with resistance of microtubule-targeting drugs in prostate cancer. J Cell Biochem 116(7):1341-1349.

[50] Guo X, Ma N, Wang J, Song J, Bu X, Cheng Y, and Wei L. (2008). Increased p38-MAPK is responsible for chemotherapy resistance in human gastric cancer cells. BMC Cancer. 8: 375.

[51] Li S, Zhao Q, Wang B, Yuan S, Wang X, and Li K. (2018). Quercetin reversed MDR in breast cancer cells through down-regulating P-gp expression and eliminating cancer stem cells mediated by YB-1 nuclear translocation. Phytother Res. 32: 1530-1536.

[52] Elmeliegy M, Vourvahis M, Guo C, and Wang DD. (2020). Effect of P-glycoprotein (P-gp) Inducers on Exposure of P-gp Substrates: Review of Clinical Drug-Drug Interaction Studies. Clin Pharmacokinet 59(6):699-714.

[53] Lund M, Petersen TS, and Dalhoff KP. (2017). Clinical Implications of P-Glycoprotein Modulation in Drug-Drug Interactions. Drugs. 77(8):859-883.

[54] Colabufo N, Berardi F, Perrone MG,Capparelli E, Cantore M, Inglese C, and Perrone R. (2010). Substrates, inhibitors and activators of P-glycoprotein: candidates for radiolabeling and imaging perspectives. Curr Top Med Chem 17:1703-1714.

[55] Hennessy M, Kelleher D, Spiers JP, Barry M, Kavanagh P, Back D, Mulcahy F, and Feely J. (2002). St John's Wort increases expression of P-glycoprotein: Implications for drug interactions. Br J Clin Pharmacol. 3(1): 75-82.

[56] Kota BP, Tran VH, Allen J, Bebawy M, and Roufogalis BD. (2010). Characterization of PXR mediated P-glycoprotein regulation in intestinal LS174T cells. Pharmacological Research 62: 426-431.

[57] Greiner B, Eichelbaum M, Fritz P, Kreichgauer HP, von Richter O, Zundler J, and Kroemer HK. (1999). The role of intestinal P-glycoprotein in the interaction of digoxin and rifampin. J Clin Invest 104(2):147-153.

[58] Dürr D, Stieger B, Kullak-Ublick GA, Rentsch KM, Steinert HC, Meier PJ, and Fattinger K. (2000). St John's Wort induces intestinal P-glycoprotein/MDR1 and intestinal and hepatic CYP3A4. Clin Pharmacol Ther. 68(6):598-604.

[59] Lili X, and Xiaoyu T. (2015). Expression of PKCα, PKCε, and P-gp in epithelial ovarian carcinoma and the clinical significance. Eur J Gynaecol Oncol. 36(2):181-185.

[60] Nam YS, Im KI, Kim N, Song Y, Lee JS, Jeon YW, Cho SG. (2019). Down-regulation of intracellular reactive oxygen species attenuates P-glycoprotein-associated chemoresistance in Epstein-Barr virus-positive NK/T-cell lymphoma. Am J Transl Res 11(3):1359-1373.

[61] Tong XZ, Wang F, Liang S, Zhang X, He JH, Chen XG, Liang YJ, Mi YJ, To KK, Fu LW. (2012). Apatinib (YN968D1) enhances the efficacy of conventional chemotherapeutical drugs in side population cells and

ABCB1-overexpressing leukemia cells. Biochem Pharmacol. 83(5):586-597.

[62] Lee TB, Park JH, Min YD, Kim KJ, and Choi CH. (2008). Epigenetic mechanisms involved in differential MDR1 mRNA expression between gastric and colon cancer cell lines and rationales for clinical chemotherapy. BMC Gastroenterol, 8: 33

[63] Linn SC, and Giaccone G. (1995). MDR1/P-glycoprotein expression in colorectal cancer. Eur J Cancer. 31(7-8): 1291-1294.

[64] Henrique R, Oliveira AI, Costa VL, Baptista T, Martins AT, Morais A, Oliveira AI, and Jeronimo C. (2013). Epigenetic regulation of MDR1 gene through post-translational histone modifications in prostate cancer. BMC Genomics. 14(898): 1-12.

[65] Mealey KL, Barhoumi R, Burghardt RC, Safe S, and Kochevar DT. (2002). Doxycycline induces expression of P-glycoprotein in MCF-7 breast carcinoma cells. Antimicrob. Agents Chemother. 46, 755-761.

[66] Chaisit. T., Siripong. P., Jianmongkol. S. (2017). Rhinacanthin-C enhances doxorubicin cytotoxicity via inhibiting the functions of P-glycoprotein and MRP2 in breast cancer cells. Eur J Pharmacol. 15, 50-57.

[67] Cantore M, Leopoldo M, Berardi F, Perrone R, and Colabufo NA. (2016). Design and Synthesis of New Selective P-gp Substrates and Inhibitors. Curr Pharm Des. 22(38):5774-5778.

[68] Kadioglu O, Saeed ME, Valoti M, Frosini M, Sgaragli G, and Efferth T. (2016). Interactions of human P-glycoprotein transport substrates and inhibitors at the drug binding domain: Functional and molecular docking analyses. Biochem Pharmacol. 104:42-51.

[69] Leopoldo M, Nardulli P, Contino M, Leonetti F, Luurtsema G, Colabufo NA. (2019). An updated patent review on P-glycoprotein inhibitors (2011-2018). Expert Opin Ther Pat. 29(6):455-461.

[70] He M, Wei MJ. (2012). Reversing multidrug resistance by tyrosine kinase inhibitors. Chin J Cancer. 31(3):126-133.

[71] Wiese M, and Pajeva IK. (2001). Structure-Activity Relationships of Multidrug Resistance Reversers. Current Medicinal Chemistry 8(6):685-713.

[72] Dewanjee S, Dua TK, Bhattacharjee N, Das A, Gangopadhyay M, Khanra R, Joardar S, Riaz M, Feo V, and Zia-Ul-Haq M. (2017). Natural Products as Alternative Choices for P-Glycoprotein (P-gp) Inhibition. Molecules. 25;22(6):871.

[73] Joshi P, Vishwakarma, and Bharate S. (2017). Natural alkaloids as P-gp inhibitors for multidrug resistance reversal in cancer. Eur J of Med Chem 138:273-292.

[74] Tinoush B, Shirdel I, and Wink M. (2020). Phytochemicals: Potential Lead Molecules for MDR Reversal. Front. Pharmacol. 11: 832.

[75] Srivalli KMR, and Lakshmi PK. (2012). Overview of P-glycoprotein inhibitors: a rational outlook. Braz J of Pharm Sci. 48(3): 353-363.

[76] Chung FS, Santiago JS, Jesus MF, Trinidad CV, and See MF. (2016). Disrupting P-glycoprotein function in clinical settings: what can we learn from the fundamental aspects of this transporter? Am J Cancer Res 6(8):1583-1598.

[77] Darby RA, Callaghan R, and Mcmahon RM. (2011). P-Glycoprotein inhibition; the past, the present and the future. Curr. Drug Metab. 12: 722-731.

[78] Kannan P, Telu S, Shukla S, Ambudkar S, Pike V, Halldin C, Gottesman MM, Innis RB and Hall MD. (2011). The "specific" P-glycoprotein inhibitor Tariquidar is also a substrate and an inhibitor for breast cancer resistance protein (BCRP/ABCG2). ACS Chem Neurosci. 2(2):82-89.

[79] Karthikeyan S, and Hoti SL. (2015). Development of Fourth Generation ABC Inhibitors from Natural Products: A Novel Approach to Overcome Cancer Multidrug Resistance. Anticancer Agents Med Chem.15(5):605-615.

[80] Bansal T, Jaggi M, Khar RK, and Talegaonkar S. (2009). Emerging Significance of Flavonoids as P-Glycoprotein Inhibitors in Cancer Chemotherapy. J. Pharm. Pharm. Sci. 12: 46-78.

[81] Bhardwaj RK, Glaeser H, Becquemont L, Klotz U, Gupta SK, and Fromm MF. (2002). Piperine, a major constituent of black pepper, inhibits human P-glycoprotein and CYP3A4, J. Pharmacol. Exp. Ther. 302: 645-650.

[82] Zhang W, Han Y, Lim SL, and Lim L. (2009). Dietary regulation of P-gp function and expression. Expert Opinion on Drug Metabolism & Toxicology 5(7):789-801.

[83] Aires V, Colin DJ, Doreau A, Di Pietro A, Heydel JM, Artur Y, Latruffe N, and Delmas D. (2019). P-Glycoprotein affects chemoactivities of resveratrol against human colorectal cancer cells. Nutrients 11(9): 2098.

[84] Huang C, Cai T, Bai L, Huang Y, Li Q, Wang Q, Chiba P, and Cai Y. (2019). State of the art of overcoming efflux transporter mediated multidrug resistance of breast cancer. Transl Cancer Res 8(1):319-329.

[85] Reddy DR, Khurana A, Bale S, Ravirala R, Reddy VSS, Mohankumar M, and Godugu C. (2016). Natural flavonoids silymarin and quercetin improve the brain distribution of co-administered P-gp substrate drugs. SpringerPlus 5:1618

[86] Choi BH, Kim CG, Lim Y, Shin SY, and Lee YH. (2008). Curcumin down-regulates the multidrug-resistance mdr1b gene by inhibiting the PI3K/Akt/NF kappa B pathway. Cancer Lett. 259: 111-118.

[87] Vahedi S, Lusvarghi S, Pluchino K, Shafrir Y, Durell SR, Gottesman MM, and Ambudkar SV. (2018). Mapping discontinuous epitopes for MRK-16, UIC2 and 4E3 antibodies to extracellular loops 1 and 4 of human P-glycoprotein. Sci Rep 8(1):12716

[88] Ma X, Zhao Z, Wang H, Liu Y, Xu Y, Zhang J, Chen B, Li L, and Zhao Y. (2019). P-glycoprotein antibody decorated porous hydrogel particles for capture and release of drug-resistant tumor cells. Adv Healthc Mater 8(13):e1900136.

[89] De Vera AA, Gupta P, Lei Z, Liao D, Narayanan S, Teng Q, Reznik SE, and Chen ZS. (2019). Immuno-oncology agent IPI-549 is a modulator of P-glycoprotein (P-gp, MDR1, ABCB1)-mediated multidrug resistance (MDR) in cancer: In vitro and in vivo. Cancer Lett. 442:91-103.

[90] Naito M, Tsuge H, Kuroko, Koyama T, Tomida A, Tatsuta T, Heike Y, and Tsuruo T. (1993). Enhancement of cellular accumulation of cyclosporine by anti-P-glycoprotein monoclonal antibody MRK-16 and synergistic modulation of multidrug resistance. J Natl Cancer Inst 85(4):311-316.

[91] Esser L, Shukla S, Zhou F, Ambudkar SV, and Xia D. (2016). Crystal structure of the antigen-binding fragment of a monoclonal antibody specific for the multidrug-resistance-linked ABC transporter human

P-glycoprotein. Acta Crystallogr F Struct Biol Commun 72(Pt 8):636-641.

[92] Iwahashi T, Okochi E, Ariyoshi K, Watabe H, Amann E, Mori S, Tsuruo T, and Ono K. (1993). Specific targeting and killing activities of anti-p-glycoprotein monoclonal antibody mrk16 directed against intrinsically multidrug-resistant human colorectal carcinoma cell lines in the nude mouse model. Cancer research 53: 5475-5482.

[93] Medarova A, Pantazopoulos P, and Yoo B. (2020). Screening of potential miRNA therapeutics for the prevention of multi-drug resistance in cancer cells. Sci Repo 10: 1970.

[94] Tormo E, Ballester S, Adam-Artigues A, Burgués O, Alonso E, Bermejo B, Menéndez S, Zazo S, Madoz-Gúrpide J, Rovira A, Albanell J, Rojo F, Lluch A, and Eroles P. (2019). The miRNA-449 family mediates doxorubicin resistance in triplenegative breast cancer by regulating cell cycle factors. Sci Repo 9: 5316.

[95] Wang Z, Lu B, Wang H, Cheng Z, and Yin Y. (2011). MicroRNA-21 modulates chemosensitivity of breast cancer cells to doxorubicin by targeting PTEN. Archives of medical research 42: 281-290.

[96] Nourbakhsh M, Jaafari MR, Lage H, Abnous K, Mosaffa F, Badiee A, and Behravan J. (2015). Nanolipoparticles-mediated MDR1 siRNA delivery reduces doxorubicin resistance in breast cancer cells and silences MDR1 expression in xenograft model of human breast cancer. Iran J Basic Med Sci 18:385-392

[97] Xu H, Hong F, Li S, and Zhang P. (2012). Short hairpin RNA-mediated MDR1 gene silencing increases apoptosis of human ovarian cancer cell line A2780/Taxol. Chinese Journal of cancer research 24(2): 138-142.

[98] Wang P, Yang H L, Yang YJ, Wang L, and Lee SC. (2015). Overcome cancer cell drug resistance using natural products. Evid Based Complement Alternat Med. 2015, 767136.

[99] Cheng Q, Liao M, Hu H, Li H, and Wu L. (2018). Asiatic Acid (AA) Sensitizes multidrug-resistant human lung adenocarcinoma A549/DDP cells to cisplatin (DDP) via downregulation of P-Glycoprotein (MDR1) and its targets. Cellular Physiology and Biochemistry, 47(1), 279-292.

[100] Huang CZ, Wang YF, Zhang Y, Peng YM, Liu YX, Ma F, Jiang JH, and Wang QD. (2017). Cepharanthine hydrochloride reverses P-glycoprotein-mediated multidrug resistance in human ovarian carcinoma A2780/Taxol cells by inhibiting the PI3K/Akt signaling pathway. Oncology Reports, 38(4), 2558-2564

[101] Zhao BX, Sun YB, Wang SQ, Duan L, Huo QL, Ren F, and Li GF. (2013). Grape seed procyanidin reversal of P-glycoprotein associated multi-drug resistance via downregulation of NF-κB and MAPK/ERK mediated YB-1 activity in A2780/T cells. PLoS ONE, 8(8), e71071.

[102] Pan Y, Shao D, Zhao Y, Zhang F, Zheng X, Tan Y, He Km Li J, and Chen L. (2017). Berberine Reverses Hypoxia-induced Chemoresistance in Breast Cancer through the Inhibition of AMPK- HIF-1α. Int J Biol Sci. 13(6): 794-803.

[103] Limtrakul P, Anuchapreeda S, and Buddhasukh D. (2004). Modulation of human multidrug-resistance MDR-1 gene by natural curcuminoids. BMC Cancer. 4:13.

[104] Jin S, Gorfajn B, Faircloth G, Scotto KW. (2000). Ecteinascidin 743, a transcription-targeted chemotherapeutic that inhibits MDR1

activation. 1.Proc Natl Acad Sci U S A. 97(12):6775-6779.

[105] AbuHammad S, and Zihlif M. (2013). Gene expression alterations in doxorubicin resistant MCF-7 breast cancer cell line. Genomics. 101: 213-220.

[106] Ichikawa Y, Ghanefar M, Bayeva M, Wu R, Khechaduri A, Naga Prasad SV, Mutharasan RK, Naik TJ, and Ardehali H. (2014). Cardiotoxicity of doxorubicin is mediated through mitochondrial iron accumulation. J. Clin. Invest. 124: 617-630.

[107] Kumar, S, Kushwaha PP, and Gupta S. (2019). Emerging targets in cancer drug resistance. Cancer Drug Resistance, 2, 161-177.

[108] Xu F, Wang F, Yang T, Sheng Y, Zhong T, and Chen. Y. (2014). Differential drug resistance acquisition to doxorubicin and paclitaxel in breast cancer cells. Cancer Cell Int. 21, 142.

[109] Patel KJ, and Tannock I. (2009). The influence of P-glycoprotein in expression and its inhibitors on the distribution of doxorubicin in breast tumors. BMC Cancer 9:356.

[110] Kim TH, Shin S, Yoo SD, and Shin BS. (2018). Effects of phytomedical P-glycoprotein modulators on the pharmacokinetics and tissue distribution of doxorubicin in mice. Molecules 23:349.

[111] Eid, S.Y., El-Readi, M.Z., Fatani, S.H., Mohamed Nour Eldin, E.E., Wink, M., 2015. Natural products modulate the multifactorial multidrug resistance of cancer. Pharmacology and Pharmacy. 6, 146-176.

[112] El-Readi M Z, Hamdan D, Farrag N, El-Shazly, A., Wink, M. (2010). Inhibition of P-glycoprotein activity by limonin and other secondary metabolites from Citrus species in human colon and leukaemia cell lines. Eur J Pharmacol. 626: 139-145.

[113] Kato T, Mizutani K, Kameyama K, Kawakami K, Fujita Y, Nakane K, Kanimoto Y, Ehara H, Ito H, Seishima M, Deguchi T, Ito M. (2015). Serum exosomal P-glycoprotein is a potential marker to diagnose docetaxel resistance and select a taxoid for patients with prostate cancer. Urol Oncol. 33(9):385.e15-20.

[114] Lili X, and Xiaoyu T. (2015). Expression of PKCalpha, PKCepsilon, and P-gp in epithelial ovarian carcinoma and the clinical significance. Eur J Gynaecol Oncol. 36(2):181-185.

[115] Han L, Guo X, Bian H, Zhou Y, Li T, and Yang J. (2015). Changed expression and function of P-gp in peripheral blood CD56 + cells predicting chemoresistance in non-Hodgkin lymphoma patients. Cancer Biomark. 15(3):289-297.

[116] Kim JW, Park Y, Roh JL, Cho KJ, Choi SH, Nam SY, Kim SY. (2016). Prognostic value of glucosylceramide synthase and P-glycoprotein expression in oral cavity cancer. Int J Clin Oncol. 21(5):883-889.

[117] Zhao Y, Huan ML, Liu M, Cheng Y, Sun Y, Cui H, Liu DZ, Mei QB, and Zhou SY. (2016). Doxorubicin and resveratrol co-delivery nanoparticle to overcome doxorubicin resistance. Sci Rep. 6:35267.

[118] El-Readi MZ, Eid S, Abdelghany AA, Al-Amoudi HS, Efferth T, and Wink M. (2019). Resveratrol mediated cancer cell apoptosis, and modulation of multidrug resistance proteins and metabolic enzymes. Phytomedicine. 55:269-281.

[119] Khan M, Maryam A, Mehmood T, Zhang Y, and Ma T. (2015). Enhancing Activity of Anticancer Drugs in Multidrug Resistant Tumors by Modulating P-Glycoprotein through

Dietary Nutraceuticals. Asian Pac J Cancer Prev. 16(16):6831-6839.

[120] Zhang S, and Morris ME. (2003). Effects of the flavonoids biochanin A, morin, phloretin, and silymarin on P-glycoprotein-mediated transport. J Pharmacol Exp Ther. 304(3):1258-1267.

[121] Satonaka H, Ishida K, Takai M, Koide R, Shigemasa R, Ueyama J, Ishikawa T, Hayashi K, Goto H, Wakusawa S. (2017). (−)-Epigallocatechin-3-gallate down-regulates doxorubicin-induced overexpression of p-glycoprotein through the coordinate inhibition of pi3k/akt and mek/erk signaling pathways. Anticancer Res 37(11):6071-6077.

[122] Lopes-Rodrigues V, Sousa E, and Vasconcelos MH. (2016). Curcumin as a Modulator of P-Glycoprotein in Cancer: Challenges and Perspectives. Pharmaceuticals 9: 71.

[123] Wang J, Ma W, and Tu P. (2015). Synergistically Improved Anti-tumor Efficacy by Co-delivery Doxorubicin and Curcumin Polymeric Micelles. Macromol Biosci. 15(9):1252-1261.

[124] Rastegar R, Akbari Javar H, Khoobi M, Dehghan Kelishadi P, Hossein Yousefi G, Doosti M, Hossien Ghahremani M, Shariftabrizi A, Imanparast F, Gholibeglu E, and Gholami M. (2018). Evaluation of a novel biocompatible magnetic nanomedicine based on beta-cyclodextrin, loaded doxorubicin-curcumin for overcoming chemoresistance in breast cancer. Artif Cells Nanomed Biotechnol. 46(sup2):207-216.

[125] Zhao X, Chen Q, Li Y, Tang H, Liu W, and Yang X. (2015). Doxorubicin and curcumin co-delivery by lipid nanoparticles for enhanced treatment of diethylnitrosamine-induced hepatocellular carcinoma in mice. Eur J Pharm Biopharm. 93:27-36.

[126] Zhang J, Du Z, Pan S, Shi M, Li J, Yang C, Hu H, Qiao M, Chen D, and Zhao X. (2018). Overcoming multidrug resistance by codelivery of mdr1-targeting sirna and doxorubicin using epha10-mediated ph-sensitive lipoplexes: in vitro and in vivo evaluation. ACS Appl Mater Interfaces. 10(25):21590-21600.

[127] Cavaco MC, Pereira C, Kreutzer B, Gouveia LF, Silva-Lima B, Brito AM, and Videira M. (2017). Evading P-glycoprotein mediated-efflux chemoresistance using Solid Lipid Nanoparticles. Eur J Pharm Biopharm 110:76-84.

[128] Yu J, Hu F, Zhu Q, Li X, Ren H, Fan S, Qian B, Zhai B, Yang D. (2020). PD-L1 monoclonal antibody-decorated nanoliposomes loaded with Paclitaxel and P-gp transport inhibitor for the synergistic chemotherapy against multidrug resistant gastric cancers. Nanoscale Res Lett 15(1):59.

[129] Chavanpatil MD, Khdair A, and Panyam J. (2007). Surfactant-polymer Nanoparticles: A Novel Platform for Sustained and Enhanced Cellular Delivery of Water-soluble Molecules. Pharmaceutical Research 24(4):8.3-810.

[130] Susa M, Iyer AK, Ryu K, Choy E, Hornicek FJ, Mankin H, Milane L, Amiji MM, and Duan Z. (2010). Inhibition of ABCB1 (MDR1) Expression by an siRNA Nanoparticulate Delivery System to Overcome Drug Resistance in Osteosarcoma. PLoS One. 5(5): e10764.

[131] Pramanik D, Campbell NR, Das S, Gupta S, Chenna V, Bisht S, Sysa-Shah P, Bedja D, Karikari C, Steenbergen C, Gabrielson KL, Maitra A, and Maitra A. (2012). A composite polymer nanoparticle overcomes multidrug resistance and ameliorates doxorubicin-associated cardiomyopathy. Oncotarget 3(6):640-650.

Chapter 12

Improving the Antitumor Effect of Doxorubicin in the Treatment of Eyeball and Orbital Tumors

Anatoliy Parfentievich Maletskyy, Yuriy Markovich Samchenko and Natalia Mikhailivna Bigun

Abstract

Malignant tumors of the orbit are the main cause for 41–45.9% of orbital tumor, and they will threaten both the organ of vision and the life of the patient. In our opinion, improving the effectiveness of treatment of malignant tumors can be implemented in the following areas: a) immobilization of doxorubicin in synthetic polymeric materials, which will fill the tissue structures that were resected and reduce the percentage of tumor recurrence. b) the use of nanomaterials for the delivery of doxorubicin to tumor cells. To develop a hydrogel implant and nanoparticles, to study the diffusion kinetics of doxorubicin in a hydrogel implant and the ability of nanoparticles to transport doxorubicin. The developed gels based on acrylic acid (AAc) were obtained by radical polymerization of an aqueous solution of monomers (AAc and N, N-methylenebisacrylamide (MBA)) at a temperature of 70°C. Matrices based on polyvinyl formal (PVF) were obtained by treatment of polyvinyl alcohol (PVA) with formaldehyde in the presence of a strong acid. Experimental studies were performed on rabbits of the Chinchilla breed, weighing 2–3 kg, aged 5–6 months, which during the study were in the same conditions. We implanted the hybrid gel in the scleral sac; orbital tissue and in the ear tissue of rabbits: Evaluation of the response of soft tissues and bone structures to implant materials was carried out on the basis of analysis of changes in clinical and pathomorphological parameters was performed after 10, 30 and 60 days. Diffusion of doxorubicin was examined by using UV spectroscopy [spectrophotometer-fluorimeter DS-11 FX + (DeNovix, USA)], analyzing samples at regular intervals during the day at a temperature of 25° C. The concentration of active substances was determined by the normalized peak absorption of doxorubicin at 480 nm. The release kinetics of the antitumor drug doxorubicin were investigated by using a UV spectrometer “Specord M 40” (maximum absorption 480 nm). The developed hydrogel implant has good biocompatibility and germination of surrounding tissues in the structure of the implant, as well as the formation of a massive fibrous capsule around it. An important advantage of the implant is also the lack of its tendency to resorption. Moreover, the results showed that the diffusion kinetics of doxorubicin from a liquid-crosslinked hydrogel reaches a minimum therapeutic level within a few minutes, while in the case of a tightly crosslinked - after a few hours. It was also found that the liquid-crosslinked hydrogel adsorbs twice as much as the cytostatic - doxorubicin. The analysis of the research results approved that

IntechOpen

the size of the nanoparticles is the main factor for improving drug delevary and penetration. Thus, nanoparticles with a diameter of less than 200 nm can penetrate into cells and are not removed from the circulatory system by macrophages, thereby prolonging their circulation in the body. About 10 nm. The developed hybrid hydrogel compositions have high mechanical strength, porosity, which provides 100% penetration of doxorubicin into experimental animal tissues. It was found that the kinetics of diffusion of drugs from liquid-crosslinked hydrogel reaches a minimum therapeutic level within a few minutes, whereas in the case of densely crosslinked hydrogel diffusion begins with a delay of several hours and the amount of drug released at equilibrium reaches much lower values (20–25%). The obtained preliminary experimental results allow us to conclude that our developed pathways for the delivery of drugs, in particular, doxorubicin to tumor cells will increase the effectiveness of antitumor therapy.

Keywords: eyeball and orbit tumors, doxorubicin, synthetic polymeric materials, nanomaterials

1. Introduction

Malignant tumors of the orbit represents the main cause for 41–45.9% of orbital tumors [1, 2] and they will threaten both the organ of vision and the life of the patient. According to some authors [2], recurrence of malignant tumors of the orbit within 5 years was observed in 36 of the 56 patients who were observed and recurrence of the tumor was observed in 64.3% of patients who died in subsequent years. As can be seen from the above data, the results of treatment of malignant tumors of the orbit are not satisfactory. In the analysis group of 56 patients with malignant tumors, only 36% had a 5-year survival.

The main method of treatment of orbit tumors is surgery, followed by radiotherapy and chemotherapy [3, 4].

However, surgical treatment of malignant tumors of the orbit leads to anatomical and functional damage. Independent use of radiation therapy does not lead to the desired result. In recent years, with the advent of new drugs and a deeper understanding of the theory of chemotherapy, the effectiveness of chemotherapy for malignant tumors has improved significantly. The clinician always has the task of creating a sufficient concentration of the drug in the tumor area in order to obtain a therapeutic result and at the same time minimize the load on healthy cells during the local tumor process.

In our opinion, increasing the effectiveness of treatment of such type of tumor can be detetcted by deleviring high concentration of doxorubicin in the tumor in the following ways;

a. Immobilization of doxorubicin in synthetic polymeric materials, which will fill the tissue structures that were resected, and long-term withdrawal of the drug will significantly reduce the recurrence rate of tumors.

b. Use of nanomaterials for delivery of doxorubicin to tumor cells.

To implement the first task, we needed to develop non-biological implants with a porous hollow structure that are capable of biointegration with the surrounding orbital tissues.

2. To develop non-biological implants and study the soft tissue response to it

Such capabilities are possessed by hydrogels - spatially crosslinked hydrophilic polymers that have been successfully used for several decades as materials for tissue engineering and plastic surgery, means for targeted transport of drugs, optical and analytical sensors, matrices for biological research [5], etc. Abnormally high compared with solid polymers, the biocompatibility of gels with high equilibrium water content, primarily due to the similarity of their 3D structure with the extracellular matrix [6]. Achieving a significant improvement in the physicochemical and operational parameters of gels seems to be possible by obtaining a hybrid hydrogel material based on polyvinyl alcohol and acrylic hydrogel, which was the subject of one of the studies performed by the authors [7].

Material and methods. Gels based on acrylic acid (AAc) were obtained by radical polymerization of an aqueous solution of monomers (AAc and N, N′-methylenebisacrylamide (MBA)) at a temperature of 70°C. Matrices based on polyvinylformal (PVF) were obtained by treating polyvinyl alcohol (PVA) with formaldehyde in the presence of a strong acid.

Experimental studies were conducted on the basis of the vivarium of the State Institution "The Filatov Institute of Eye Diseases and Tissue Therapy of the NAMS of Ukraine". Experimental studies were performed on rabbits of the Chinchilla breed, weighing 2–3 kg, aged 5–6 months, which during the study were in the same living conditions. All experimental studies were conducted in compliance with ethical standards provided by the international principles of the European Convention on the Protection of Vertebrate Animals Used for Experimental and Other Scientific Purposes (Strasbourg, 1986) and the norms of biomedical ethics approved by the First National Congress of Bioethics of Ukraine), as well as the law of Ukraine №3447-IV "On protection of animals from cruel treatment" (Kyiv, 2006).

To study the reaction of the soft tissues of the orbit and auricle, we used an implant hybrid hydrogel developed at the Ovcharenko Institute of Biocolloid Chemistry of the National Academy of Sciences of Ukraine in Kyiv. We implanted a hybrid hydrogel in a scleral sac; orbital tissue and in the ear tissue of rabbits.

We implanted a hybrid hydrogel implant into the scleral sac, parabulbar tissue of the eyeball and auricle of a rabbit/.

Surgical interventions were performed under general anesthesia (at the rate of 1 ml of 0.1% sodium thiopental solution per 1 kg of rabbit body weight intramuscularly). Evaluation of the response of soft tissues and bone structures to implant materials was carried out on the basis of analysis of changes in clinical and pathomorphological parameters was performed after 10, 30 and 60 days. Evaluation of the studied clinical signs (swelling of the tissues of the orbit, cheeks, auricle, the condition of the sutures, the presence of secretions) was performed on the 2nd, 5th, 10th and then every five days. Pathohistological evaluation of oculoorbital tissues, orbit and auricle tissue was performed after 10, 30 and 60 days.

Results and discussion. Analysis of scanning electron micrographs of the hybrid hydrogel material showed that its structure is characterized by a well-developed system of connected pores smaller than 1 mm, as well as the presence of pores with a diameter of several hundred micrometers. It should also be noted that the pore walls have a porous structure with an approximate pore diameter of 10 μm and a wall thickness of several micrometers. Thus, due to partial squeezing of the gel-forming composition from the pore space of the spongy polymer matrix based on the PVF, it was possible to prevent clogging of open and combined transport pores,

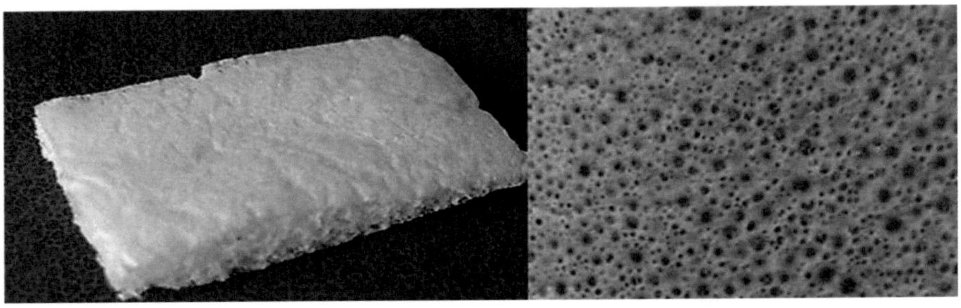

Figure 1.
Appearance of a hybrid hydrogel implant.

which allowed to ensure high permeability of hybrid material to gases, liquids and biological tissues (**Figure 1**).

In general modification of the PVF with acrylic hydrogel decreased the size of pores inside the walls for all hydrogel systems and also fill the larger pores with diameters approx. 500 µm. The synthesized polymer systems belong to porous materials with pore diameters from a few micrometers to a few hundred micrometers. Nanopores have not been found in synthesized systems [8].

Experimental studies in rabbits showed that in the first 5 days after implantation of the hybrid hydrogel in the scleral sac, orbit and auricle, all animals had swelling of the postoperative suture and adjacent conjunctiva, as well as a slight serous-secretion from the conjunctival cavity. After five days, there was a decrease in edema and discharge from the conjunctival cavity and lasted for 8–10 days. It is important to note that when examining the postoperative wound of the skin and conjunctiva in the first days and in the following days with the implantation of a hybrid hydrogel, wound healing was the primary tension.

The obtained satisfactory result of clinical evaluation of soft tissues of the orbit and auricle to the implantation of a hybrid hydrogel, we found it appropriate to assess the response of cellular structures to the implant, the presence of germination of surrounding tissues in its structure and propensity to resorption.

Pathohistological studies showed that on the 10th day after the implantation of the hybrid hydrogel into the scleral sac, inflammatory infiltration of the sclera was noted in the site of the implant location. However, no inflammation was noted in the scleral portions distant from the implant.

In the infiltrate, in addition to lymphocytes, there is a fairly large number of eosinophilic leukocytes (**Figure 2a**).

An important requirement for the implant material is the ability to germinate the surrounding tissue structure of the implant, as well as its tendency to resorption. Therefore, it was expedient for us to study the influence of the surrounding biological tissues on the mesh-like structure of the implant (**Figure 2b**).

In **Figure 2b** it can be noted that the structure of the implant is preserved, and along the crossbars there is the formation of delicate bundles of collagen fibers, which are slightly infiltrated by lymphocytes. The composition of "cellular" structures is absent, possibly as a result of histological processing. We did not observe any changes on the side of the orbit walls.

In clinical practice, there is a need to fill the soft tissues after removal of tumors of the orbit, eyelids and oculoorbital area. In this regard, we found it appropriate to study the relationship of the implant - a hybrid hydrogel with soft tissues and cartilaginous structures. Pathohistological studies have shown that when the implant is placed in the tissues of the auricle after 10 days, a delicate fibrous tissue is formed around it, which is infiltrated by inflammatory cells. At the same time the

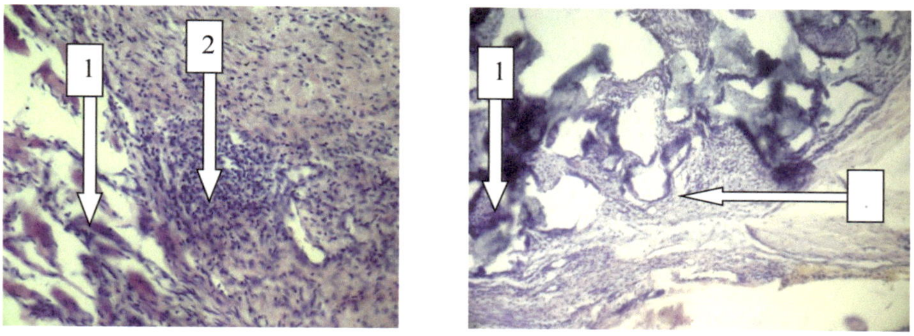

a b

Figure 2.
A and b. the tenth day after implantation of the hybrid hydrogel in the scleral sac; a - (1-implant; 2- inflammatory scleral infiltration) (hematoxylin–eosin; x 120), b - (1-implant; 2- fibrous capsule) (hematoxylin–eosin; x 70).

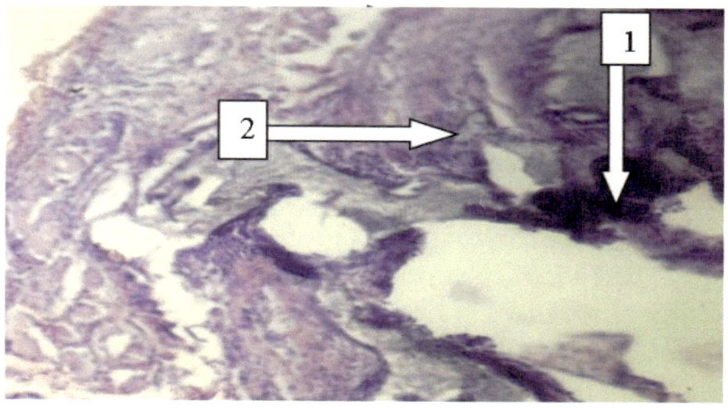

Figure 3.
Thirty days after implantation of the hybrid hydrogel in the scleral sac.

weak basophilic maintenance of "cellular" structures remains, and on partitions the initial phenomena of fibrotization are noted.

Thus, the assessment of clinical signs and the results of histopathological examinations after implant placement - a hybrid hydrogel in the scleral sac and tissues of the rabbit auricle allowed to draw preliminary conclusions, which were that within 8–10 days there was an inflammatory reaction from the tissues of the orbit and auricle, especially the first 5 days. It is important to note that in no case did we notice the implant being exposed and the wound healing was the primary tension. Pathohistological studies showed that around the implant, both in the scleral sac and in the tissues of the auricle there are all signs of inflammation (lymphoid and leukocyte infiltration, etc.), the presence of signs of germination surrounding the tissue structure of the implant and its tendency to resorption. Having obtained preliminary data, it was expedient for us to study the nature of the interaction of the implant - a hybrid hydrogel with the surrounding tissues in the longer term. Therefore, we decided to assess the nature of histopathological changes after 30 days.

When placing the implant in the scleral sac after 30 days, inflammatory phenomena around it is absent, but there was the formation of a fibrous capsule with the spread of fibrous tissue on the partitions of "cellular" structures. The fibrous layers are quite rough and do not contain inflammatory elements (**Figure 3**). Up to 30 days, the content of "cellular" structures was determined by the wall and in small quantities.

Formation of a fibrous capsule and massive growth of fibrous tissue along the partitions of "cellular" structures (1-implant; 2- growth of fibrous tissue along the partitions of "cellular" structures) (Hematoxylin–eosin; x 180).

A similar pathohistological picture was observed after 30 days of the implantation of a hybrid hydrogel in the tissues of the auricle, which consisted in fibrotization of the walls of the "honeycomb" structures of the implant without signs of inflammation. It should be noted that after 60 days we did not notice signs of inflammation around the implant except for the formation of a fibrous capsule.

The obtained experimental studies, which study the nature of the reaction of soft tissue bone structures of rabbits to the implantation of a hybrid hydrogel in the scleral sac and auricle tissue, allowed to answer a number of questions that arise in the development of implant materials.

The first and most important requirement for implants is their biocompatibility. As our studies showed, in all experimental rabbits there was a moderate inflammatory reaction, which disappeared by 8–10 days. It is important to note that in all groups of animals studied wound healing was the primary tension, and therefore in no case was the exposure of the implant, which indicates a very important positive indicator for implants. Pathohistological studies showed that up to 10 days there are final inflammatory phenomena close to the implant in the form of lymphoid and leukocyte infiltration, while in more remote areas relative to the implant, they were absent. The second important indicator we noted is the germination of the surrounding tissues in the implant structure and the formation of a delicate fibrous capsule by the tenth day after its implantation (**Figure 2b**), and by the 30th day - the formation of a massive fibrous capsule (**Figure 3**). The third important advantage of the implant is the lack of its tendency to resorption, which is very important to obtain a stable clinical result. It is also important to note that we did not observe changes in the bone structures of the orbit and in the cartilaginous plate of the rabbit auricle when placing the implant in the soft structures of the orbit and auricle.

Our in vivo experimental studies demonstrated that the high biocompatibility of the hybrid highly porous material based on polyvinylform developed by them, the lack of resorption and the ability to germinate the surrounding biological tissues. This indicates the high prospects of the developed material and provides grounds for further research aimed at improving its performance.

3. Influence of the structure of hydrogels hydrogel implants on dynamics of deposition and diffusion of doxorubicin

It should be noted that it is important to prevent the recurrence of the malignancy after its removal, so it is important that the implant materials contain antitumor drugs.

The hybrid hydrogels used are spatially crosslinked hydrophilic polymers that are characterized by a unique combination of properties such as high hydrophilicity, softness, flexibility and strength, as well as unique biocompatibility [9]. Due to their ability to absorb significant amounts of water and biological fluids, porosity and elasticity, they more than any other synthetic biomaterials resemble human tissues and have been successfully used for decades as a means of targeted transport and prolonged drug release [10], biosensors [11], anti-burn and hemostatic dressings [12], materials for tissue engineering and plastic surgery [13], etc. Given the possibility of using the proposed hybrid hydrogels in the creation of implants that will have the ability to deposit drugs, primarily antimicrobial and antitumor, we thought it appropriate to study the diffusion properties of hybrid hydrogels with different porosity and with immobilized drugs, in particular drugs.

Materials and methods. The research was conducted in the department of functional hydrogels of the Ovcharenko Institute of Biocolloid Chemistry, NAS of Ukraine using the following substances and materials:

Reagents for the synthesis of hydrogels: Polyvinyl alcohol (PVA) (AppliChem GmbH, 98%; 72 kDa); formaldehyde (LAB-SCAN, 37%); concentrated sulfuric acid (AAc); Triton X-100 (AppliChem GmbH); acrylic acid (99%, Sinbias); ammonium persulfate (PSA) (Thermo Fisher, 98%); N, N′-methylenebisacrylamide (Merck) was used without further purification.

Medicinal product: Doxorubicin "Ebeve" - concentrate for solution for infusion containing 2 mg/ml For saturation with pharmaceuticals, hydrogels of different densities were obtained, varying the mass fraction of PVA. The content of PVA in the liquid-crosslinked gel was 7.1 wt. %, and in a tightly crosslinked gel - 8.0%. For the manufacture of a hybrid hydrogel based on pre-synthesized polyvinylformal and acrylic acid, 0.6 g of PVF was placed in a medical syringe with a capacity of 10 ml and impregnated with a solution containing 0.6 ml of AAc, 0.2 ml of 3% MBA solution and 5.25 ml of 40% solution of PSA. After impregnation, 4.5 ml of liquid was squeezed out and the resulting polymerization composition was placed in an oven at 40° C for 1 hour.

Spectral analysis (FTIR) of wet samples was performed using a spectrometer Spectrum BX FT-IR (Perkin Elmer). The spectra were recorded using the method of disturbed total internal reflection (internal reflection spectroscopy) in the spectral range 4000–550 cm^{-1} with a resolution of 2 cm^{-1}. Each spectrum was recorded 8 times to prevent accidental artifacts.

The porosity of the samples was determined by gravimetric method according to the formula:

$$P = \left(1 - \frac{m}{V \cdot \rho}\right) \times 100\% \qquad (1)$$

where P is the total porosity [%], m is the dry weight of the sample, V is the volume of the dry sample, ρ is the density of the material used [14]. When measuring the pore size, an optical microscope SIGETA MB 140 LED Mono was used to study the drugs in transmitted, reflected and mixed light. Toup View 3.5 was used to process statistical data and video images of the microscope.

Detailed information on the structure of the pore space of polymer systems was obtained from the analysis of microphotographs taken using a scanning electron microscope JSM-6060 LA (JEOL, Japan) with a resolution of 4 nm. The polymer samples were freeze-dried in a sublimation unit UZV-10 (Kharkov, Ukraine), attached to standard holders with a double-sided conductive film and covered with a layer of Au/Pd with a thickness of 25 nm in the ion-spray unit Gatan 682 Precision Patching and Coating System Gatan, USA).

The kinetics of swelling of the samples of the proposed hydrogels was studied at a temperature of 25°C in distilled water and saline (0.9% aqueous sodium chloride solution), determining the degree of swelling of Q samples weighing 23.8–27.0 mg by gravimetric method according to the formula: $Q_t = (m_t - m_d)/m_d$, where Q_t and m_t are the degree of swelling and the mass of the swollen sample in a certain time interval, m_d is the initial mass of the dry sample [15, 16].

Diffusion of doxorubicin in hybrid hydrogels was studied as follows. Samples of dry hydrogels in the form of cylinders with a diameter of 12 mm and a weight of 50 mg (height varied from 5 mm to 8 mm depending on the composition of the hydrogel) for saturation were placed in 0.02% doxorubicin solution for

18 hours at a temperature of 25°C. After saturation, the mass of the drug was calculated taking into account changes in the initial concentration. Excess fluid was squeezed from the swollen samples using a disposable medical syringe, the squeezed samples were weighed and placed in vials of 20 ml of saline. Diffusion of doxorubicin was examined by UV spectroscopy using a spectrophotometer-fluorimeter DS-11 FX + (DeNovix, USA), analyzing the samples at certain intervals during the day at a temperature of 25°C and periodic stirring. The concentration of active substances was determined by the normalized peak absorption of doxorubicin at 480 nm.

Results and discussion. IR spectroscopy. Based on the obtained IR spectra, the functional groups of porous matrices based on PVF were characterized (**Figure 4**). Wide and intense peaks in the region of about 3362–3382 cm^{-1} can be attributed to the valence vibrations of hydroxyl groups. The expansion of these absorption bands is explained by the hydrogen bonds that the OH groups join. Bands at 1007 cm^{-1} on the spectrum of the matrix based on PVF are also characteristic of the valence vibrations of the hydroxyl group of primary alcohols C OH.

According to the calculations performed by formula (1), the high-density crosslinked hydrogel had a porosity of 91.8%, and the low-density crosslinked hydrogel - 95.0%. The calculated porosity of the hydrogel composition with acrylic acid was 85.9%.

According to light-optical and electron microscopy, the obtained hydrogels had a heterogeneous multilevel porous architecture. That is, the pores of the highest level were also formed from porous structures that were about two rows smaller. According to the calculations, the pores of the highest level had a diameter of 120–180 μm in a high-density crosslinked hydrogel (**Figure 5a**) and 460–670 μm in a low-density crosslinked hydrogel (**Figure 5b**). The pore size in the hybrid hydrogel with acrylic acid varied from 200 μm (**Figure 6a**) to 590 μm [15].

For small pores of the lowest level, which form the substructure of the walls of large pores (**Figure 6a**), regardless of the density of the hydrogel, their diameter was 3–5 μm (**Figure 6b**).

The porosity and pore size of the implant material play a significant role in tissue regeneration, so these parameters are widely studied and discussed in numerous studies. The porous structure of the matrix is necessary for tissue regeneration, because it depends on the adhesion, migration and proliferation of cells, as well as the diffusion of nutrients, oxygen and metabolites. It has been found that large pores provide nutrient delivery and removal of metabolic products, while small pores provide a larger surface area for cell adhesion [10, 17]. It should be noted that the influence of pore architecture on the behavior of cells also depends on

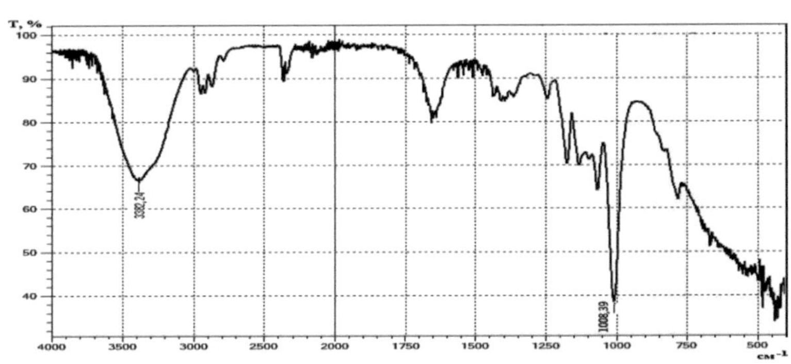

Figure 4.
IR spectrum of a porous matrix based on PVF.

DOI: http://dx.doi.org/10.5772/intechopen.95080

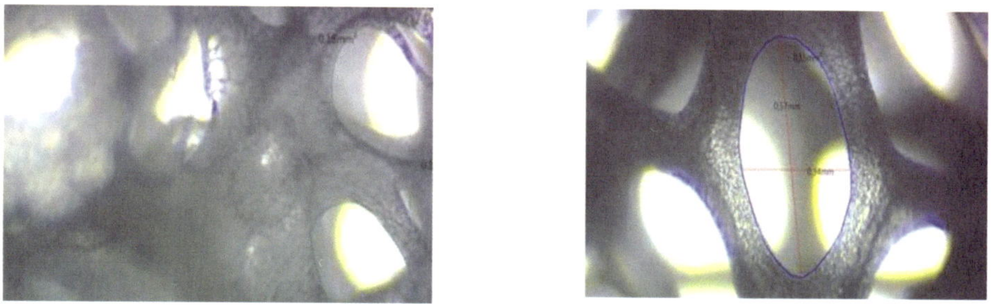

a b

Figure 5.
A and b. porous structure of high-density crosslinked (a) and low-density cross-linked (b) PVF hydrogels according to the processing of microscopic images 40x.

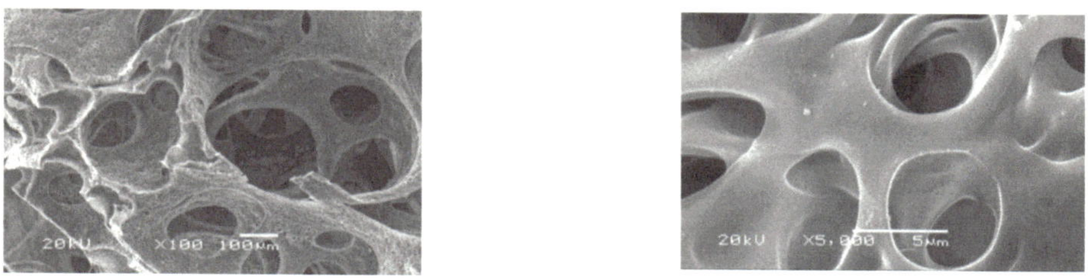

a b

Figure 6.
A and b. electron microscopic image of the pore architecture of PVF hydrogels: A - pores of the highest level, b - pores of the substructural level.

their nature. *In vitro* experiments have shown that 380–405 μm pores are best for chondrocytes and osteoblasts, while fibroblasts are prone to proliferation in smaller diameter pores (186–200 μm) [18]. Such preferences may be explained by the fact that, although large pores improve the diffusion of nutrients and oxygen, fibroblasts tend to cling to the substrate with smaller pores, as this increases the area of specific contact [17]. According to in vitro studies, greater porosity is accompanied by increased cell migration and infiltration [19, 20]. At the same time, in vivo it can be the cause of protein leaching [17, 21]. Also an important characteristic is the interporous connection, which depends not only on the diffusion properties of the matrix in relation to nutrients and oxygen, but also the possibility of ingrowth of newly formed vessels [21].

Based on this, it can be argued that our proposed hydrogels are able to accumulate and transport through a system of small pores of various metabolites and drugs, as well as serve as a matrix for attachment and migration of different cell types that ensure regeneration processes in biological tissues.

Kinetics of hydrogel swelling. From the analysis of the kinetics of swelling of hydrogels of different structure it can be concluded that all samples of hydrogels in water reach an equilibrium state of swelling in the first 30 minutes. In saline, the degree of swelling of the hydrogels was slightly lower (approximately 16%), but this had little effect on the high rate of swelling. Only in the composite hydrogel with acrylic acid, the equilibrium state in saline was reached within 3 hours. This pattern is inherent in hydrogels in general and is explained by a decrease in ionic osmotic pressure, which causes swelling of hydrogels, with increasing ionic strength of the solution. The obtained results were used to determine the period of saturation of hydrogel samples with drugs.

3.1 Diffusion of doxorubicin from hydrogels

The diffusion kinetics of doxorubicin are shown in **Figure** 7. The low-density cross-linked hydrogel sorbs twice as much doxorubicin as the high-density cross-linked hydrogel, possibly due to the absence of steric obstacles to penetration of the porous hydrogel structure by a large drug molecule (molecular weight is 544 g/mol). In *in vitro* experiments, the former hydrogel provided a 3–4-fold greater drug concentration in the environment compared to the latter hydrogel (**Figure** 7). The latter hydrogel, however, allows for a smoother and more prolonged drug release profile and therefore it is advisable to use for implants with a prolonged drug effect, while low-density crosslinked hydrogel - for urgent release of a shock dose of cytostatic preparation.

Hybrid hydrogels based on PVF and incorporated poly-AAc have a much greater - about an order of magnitude - the ability to deposit doxorubicin (compared to PVF). This effect may be due to the formation of ionic bonds between the active -COOH groups present in the hybrid hydrogel and the amine groups present in the structure of doxorubicin. The slow hydrolysis of these ionic bonds explains the prolonged (several days) release of doxorubicin from hybrid hydrogels (**Figure 8**).

This prolonged ability of hybrid hydrogel implants will facilitate their use for the deposition of antitumor drugs and maintain their effective concentration in the pathological focus.

Thus, studies have shown that the kinetics of diffusion of drugs from liquid-crosslinked hydrogel reaches a minimum therapeutic level within a few minutes, whereas in the case of densely crosslinked hydrogel diffusion begins with a delay of

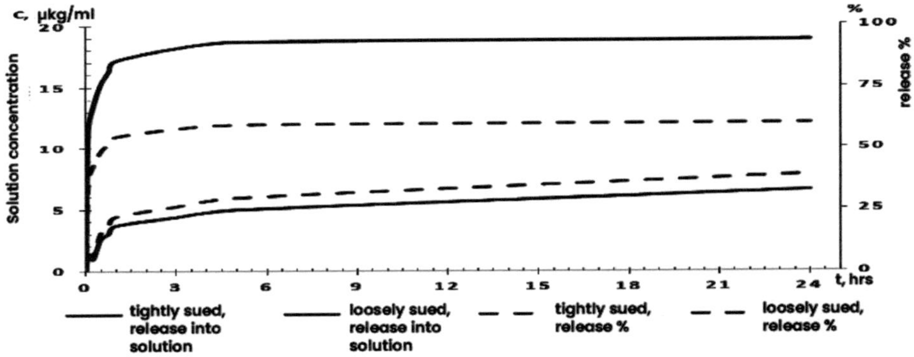

Figure 7.
Diffusion of doxorubicin from low-density crosslinked (1, 2) and high-density cross-linked (3, 4) hydrogel during the day (—— - release into solution; ------ -release percentage).

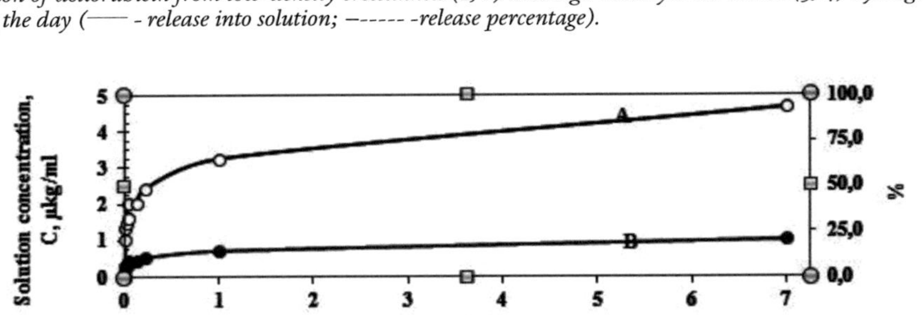

Figure 8.
Diffusion of doxorubicin from saturated samples of composite hydrogel containing polyacrylic acid during the week; A-concentration, μg/ml; B-percent release from sorbed.

several hours and the amount of drug released at equilibrium is much lower. Values (20–25%). It has also been found that the liquid crosslinked hydrogel absorbs twice as much cytostatics as doxorubicin, which may be due to the lack of steric barriers to the penetration of the bulk molecule of doxorubicin (molecular weight 544 g/mol) into its porous structure. This hydrogel provides *in vitro* experiments 3–4 times higher concentration in the environment compared to densely crosslinked polymer, and also provides a smoother, prolonged release of the drug.

It is important to note that the main factor in antitumor therapy is the temporary parameter of tissue saturation with drugs, in this regard, we continue to study in this direction. However, this direction of antitumor therapy is accompanied by surgery.

4. Nanoparticles, possible way of delivery of doxorubicin to tumor cells

Noteworthy is the delivery of doxorubicin to tumor cells through the use of nanomaterials [22].

In recent years, researchers have focused on the so-called "smart" therapeutic systems that are able to respond to minor changes in their environment by a sharp change in their physicochemical (primarily diffusion) characteristics [23]. The greatest attention is paid to thermo- and pH-sensitive hydrogels, which under the influence of minor, physiologically acceptable changes in temperature or pH are capable of controlled mass release of drugs, in particular, anticancer [21].

Even, doxorubicin is one of the most effective and widely used drugs against a wide range of cancers. But, its clinical use in parenteral administration is accompanied by such side effects as high cardiac toxicity and myelosuppression. The most serious long-term adverse effect of doxorubicin therapy is irreversible cardiomyopathy, which is based on the total cumulative dose [22]. In one clinical study, ~4% of patients receiving dosages of 500–550 mg/m^2 developed congestive heart failure, 18% with dosages of 551–600 mg/m^2, and 36% with cumulative dosages higher than 601 mg/m^2 [24]. This necessitates the development of new therapeutic systems for the transport of doxorubicin, increasing its therapeutic efficacy and minimizing side effects. Ideally, therapeutic transport systems of doxorubicin should inhibit the release of the drug in plasma and release it only after reaching the tumor site by actively targeting tumor cells through endocytosis.

As a trigger for targeting the therapeutic transport system of doxorubicin can be used a significant difference in the pH of plasma (pH = 7.4) and the microenvironment of the tumor (pH = 6.5) and lysosomes (pH = 4.8–5) [6, 9, 21]. In particular, this determines the prospects for the use of pH-sensitive hydrogels for controlled transport of anticancer drugs, primarily doxorubicin.

However, nanogels that are sensitive to changes in both pH and temperature, such as, for example, hydrogel copolymers synthesized by us based on N-isopropylacrylamide (NIPAm) and acrylic acid (AAc), seem to be especially promising.

The synthesis of nanogels based on NIPA was described in detail earlier [25, 26]. N-isopropylacrylamide, NIPAm (Sigma-Aldrich, 97%) was recrystallized from hexane and dried under vacuum; N,N′-methylenebisacrylamide (MBA) (Merck,98%), acrylic acid (AAc) was purified by distillation and subsequent fractional distillation, potassium persulphate, PSP (Sigma 98%)were used without additional purification, as well as sodium dodecylsulphate (SDS), polyethylenimine (Sigma-Aldrich MM 2000 Da) and iron salts ($FeSO_4$ and $FeCl_3$) used in magnetite synthesis. Briefly, 2,3 g of NiPAm, 0,0393 g of MBA, 0,1124 g of SDS, 5 mL of magnetite suspension, 0,115 g of AAc and 135 g of water were placed in the beaker.

After that the beaker was set on a magnetic stirrer to dissolve the reagents at room temperature. At the end of the mixing the solution in the beaker underwent purification with argon for 2 minutes. It was then transferred into the glass reactor equipped with a stirrer and thermometer. The reactor was placed in a water bath with that was maintained at constant temperature. The synthesis was carried out at 68–70°C. When the reactor temperature reaches these temperature, 10 mL of 0,93% solution of PSP in water was added. The mixing rate was 500 rotations per minute. The duration of the synthesis took additional 6 hours. The release kinetics of the antitumor drug doxorubicin were investigated using a UV spectrometer "Specord M 40" (maximum absorption 480 nm).

The size of the polymer carriers (transport systems) of anticancer drugs is of great importance, since nanoparticles with a diameter of less than 200 nm, on the one hand, are able to penetrate into cells, in particular, affected cells, and on the other hand, they are not captured by macrophages, which contributes to an increase in the duration of their circulation in the body. As can be seen from the Electronic Microphotographs (TEMs) shown in **Figure 9**, the synthesized nanogels are characterized by uniformity of shape and size and have an average diameter of about 100 nm. At magnification (see **Figure 9**, box), you can see incorporated into the nanopherogel nanoparticles of magnetite with a size of about 10 nm.

The obtained images correlate well with the results of dynamic light scattering measurements. It is shown that the average size of the synthesized hydrogels based on NIPAm and AAc is about 100–200 nm and depends on the temperature and pH value, as well as the value of the zeta potential of nanoparticles. Synthesized copolymer nanogels based on NIPAm and AAc combine thermo- and pH-sensitivity. When heated above the LCST (lower critical solution temperature, equal for NIPAm to a temperature of 32–34°C) and when the environment is acidified, the diameter of the nanoparticles decreases. Thus, it was found that the average size of nanoparticles of copolymer hydrogels based on NIPAA and AAc when heated from 25 to 50°C decreases by 3–5 times, which is a consequence of thermo-induced phase transition from swollen to collapsed state of the hydrogel (**Figure 10a** and **b**).

At the same time, in the acidic region, the pH of nanopherogels is about 10 nm, while in an alkaline environment increases by about an order of magnitude. Note that these processes are reversible and further cooling of the nanogels (as well as an

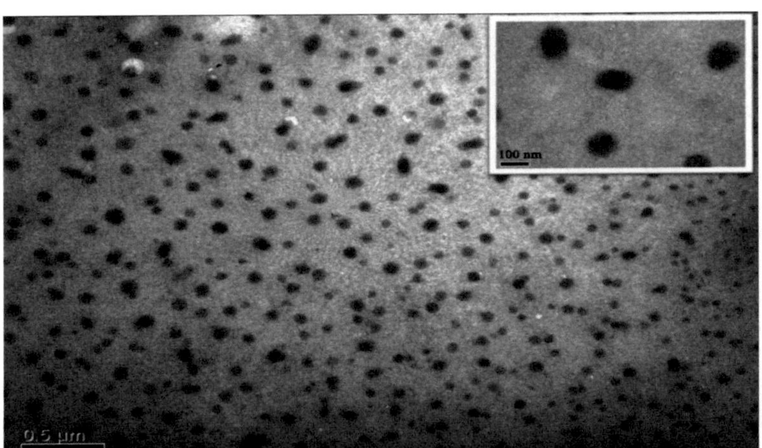

Figure 9.
Microphotographs (TEM) of synthesized nano(ferro)gels based on NIPAm - AAc copolymer with incorporated magnetite.

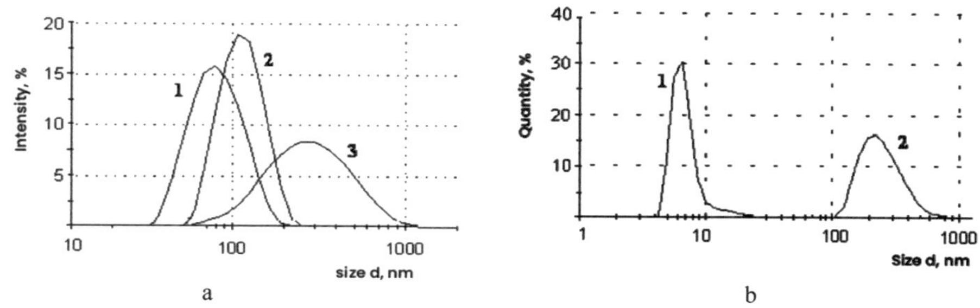

Figure 10.
A and b. size distribution of nano(ferro)gels based on NIPAm – AAc copolymer with incorporated magnetite depending on: A - temperature at 50°C (1), 37°C (2) and 25°C (3); b - acidity of the medium at pH = 1.1 (1) and pH = 12.0 (2).

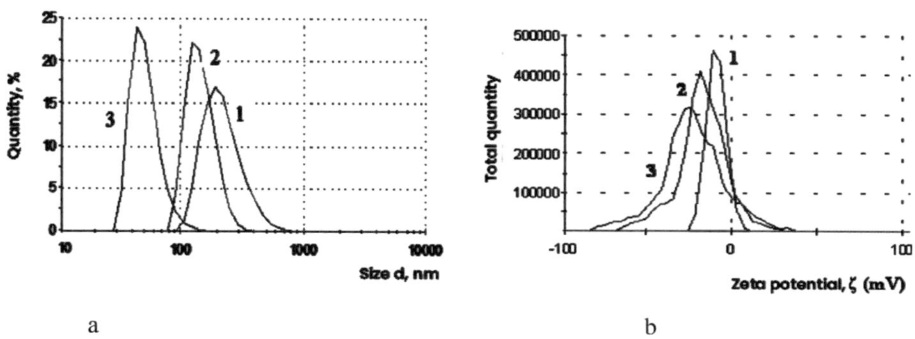

Figure 11.
A and b. size distribution (a) and zeta potential (b) of nano(ferro)gels based on NIPAm- AAc copolymer with incorporated magnetite and doxorubicin at temperatures of 25°C (1) 37°C (2) and 50°C (3).

increase in pH) leads to an increase in their size to the original values. This behavior of nanosized hydrogel matrices creates the preconditions for spontaneous targeted release of incorporated antitumor drugs, primarily doxorubicin when heated in a temperature-acceptable range, for example, in drug hyperthermia or in contact with affected cells, which are characterized by acidic pH.

Zeta potential as a function of the surface charge of a substance in a liquid is an excellent characteristic of electrostatic repulsion between particles. Zeta potential is usually used to predict and control the stability of the dispersion. Moreover, the characteristics of the solid–liquid interface can have a strong effect, in particular on adhesion, flotation, and in more concentrated systems on the rheological behavior of the system.

Thus, it shown that an increase in temperature in the range of 25°C to 37°C, up to 50°C leads to an increase (in absolute value) of the zeta potential and a decrease in the size of ferrogel nanoparticles, which indicates an increase in aggregate stability of the corresponding colloidal systems. This pattern can be explained by the rupture of intermolecular hydrogen bonds that promote aggregation, with increasing Brownian motion when heating NIPAm macromolecules.

Thermo- and pH-sensitive copolymer hydrogels based on NIPAm and AAc with incorporated magnetite and cytostatic doxorubicin were also characterized using a Zetasizer Nano ZS (Malvern Instruments) zeta-seiser. It was demonstrated (**Figure 11a** and **b**) that as the temperature increases (in the physiologically acceptable range), the size of nanoparticles decreases (to about 50 nm) and the zeta potential increases, which indicates an increase in the aggregate stability of nanosuspensions.

Taking in the account medical field of application of synthesized nano(ferro) gels, an extremely important problem is their washing from the unreacted monomers and other toxic pristine materials since the gelation reaction never proceeds with 100% conversion. Washing of medical nanogels from monomer residues and unreacted initiators is carried out by long-term extraction (for 4–10 days) with a suitable solvent (preferably water) with its repeated replacement.

As it can be seen from **Figure 12**, the immediately after synthesis, the concentration of NIPAm monomer significantly exceeds the maximum allowable level. After washing 5 times, the concentration of monomer decreases 50 times, and after seven times - more than 500. Analyzing the size distribution spectra of the crude nanogel samples and the corresponding samples after washing, obtained by dynamic light scattering using a Zetasizer Nano ZS (Malvern Instruments), we can conclude that due to washing using diafiltration the average size of nanoparticles increases slightly, which, in our opinion, is associated with the leaching of surface-active sodium dodecyl sulfate, which prevented the aggregation of nanoparticles [27].

It can be seen from **Figure 12**, the concentration of NIPAm monomer significantly exceeds the maximum allowable level immediately after the synthesis. While, after washing 5 times, the concentration of monomer decreases 50 times, and after seven times – drop down more than 500 times.

In the case of macrogels, the temperature of their phase transition between the swollen and collapsed state (which determines the possibility of controlling their physicochemical properties, primarily diffusion) is determined gravimetrically, which is almost impossible in the case of nanogels. However, it has been demonstrated that the phase transition temperature can be determined no less accurately by measuring light transmission. As can be seen from **Figure 13**, (□), at temperatures below 30°C hydrogels are in the expanded conformation, while when heated above 32°C (lower critical solution temperature, LCST) there is a phase transition to a compact collapsed state due to the destruction of hydrogen bonds between molecules water and hydrophilic amide groups of NIPAm caused by Brownian motion, as well as the strengthening of hydrophobic interactions of isopropyl groups of NIPAm. As a result, there was a sharp decrease in the light transmission of dispersions, and the phase transition temperature for nanopherogels was about 35°C. A small increase in the magnitude of the phase transition from the inherent NIPAm temperature of 32°C is explained by its copolymerization with hydrophilic acrylic acid. Due to the established effect of increasing the NIPA phase transition temperature when copolymerized with a more hydrophilic monomer (eg acrylamide or AAc) and decreasing the NIPAm phase transition temperature when copolymerized with a more hydrophobic monomer (eg acrylonitrile), therapeutic systems based

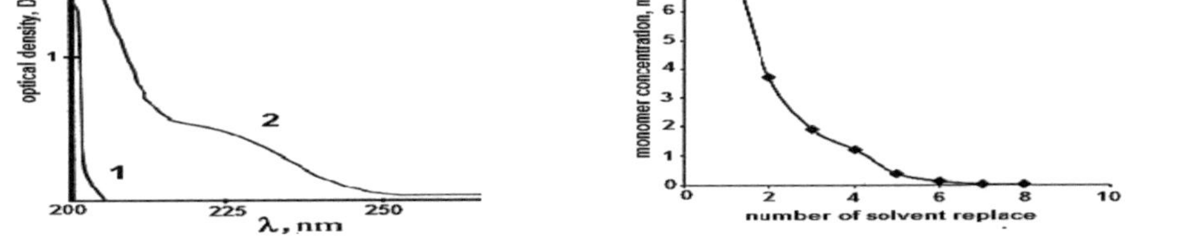

Figure 12.
A and b. reduction of absorption (a) of monomeric NIPAm in the UV region (1-after washing; 2-immediately after synthesis); change in the concentration of NIPAm depending on the number of washes (b).

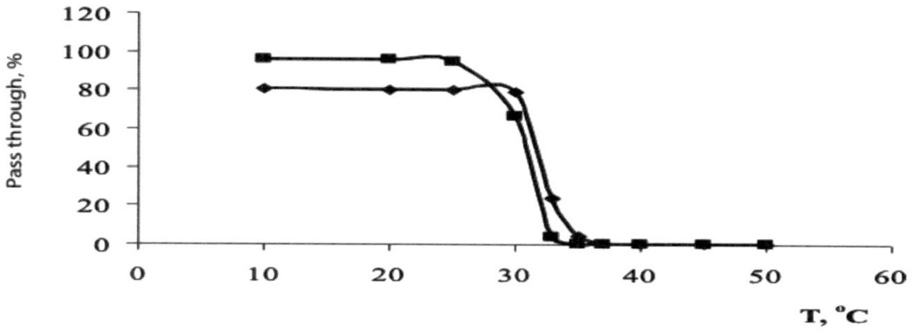

Figure 13.
The effect of temperature on light transmission for crude (□) and purified (◊)nano(ferro)gels based on NIPAm and AAc with incorporated magnetite at pH = 7.

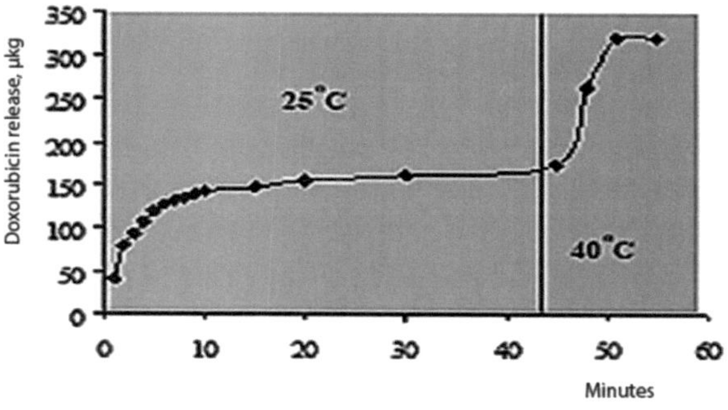

Figure 14.
Kinetics of release of doxorubicin from nano(ferro)gels based on NIPAm and AAc with incorporated magnetite at pH = 7 (nano(ferro)gel was saturated with a solution of the drug with a concentration of 2.5x10^{-2}*%).*

on delivery and controlled release at the desired temperature of various drugs, in particular doxorubicin.

The analysis of **Figure 14** shows that at 25°C the release of the antitumor drug doxorubicin is completed after 30–40 min, whereas heating above the LCST causes spontaneous release of the drug from the collapsed hydrogel. Thus, the synthesized nano (ferro) gels based on NIPAm, AAc and magnetite due to their unique properties are a promising material for the creation of therapeutic systems of targeted delivery and controlled release of drugs, in particular, in drug hyperthermia.

Incorporation of pre-synthesized nanosized magnetite into nanogels allows to give the corresponding nanopherogels magnetically controlled properties, namely - the possibility of targeted localization under the influence of a constant magnetic field of anticancer drug carriers in close proximity to the target organ, which is extremely important. Means and the need to minimize their overall impact on the body. Thus, the incorporation into the composition of hydrogel matrices of nanosized magnetite provides the possibility of targeted localization of the developed therapeutic systems in close proximity to the target organ by applying a constant low-intensity magnetic field with subsequent controlled release of incorporated drugs (primarily, cancer-free - or low-intensity alternating magnetic field.

For nano(ferro)gels on the base of NIPAm, biological studies were performed that showed that magnetic hydrogels with a magnetite content of up to 10% are not toxic to PTP cells (primary swine testicle) (**Figure 15a**). Moreover, upon contact of the original matrix with the cells, it was found that their activity tends to increase compared to the activity of control intact cells. Therefore, the result allows us to

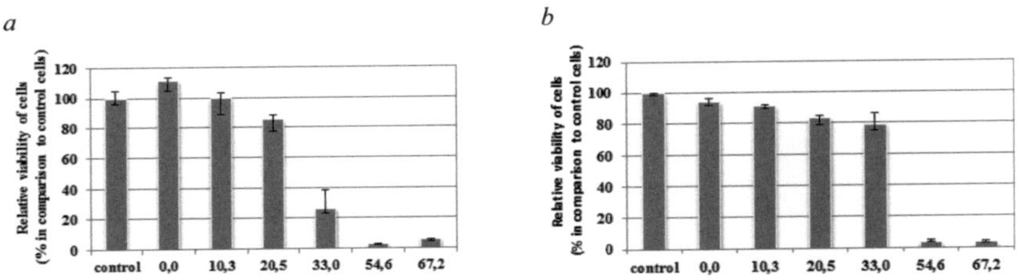

Figure 15.
a and b. Cytotoxicity of nano(ferro)gels based on NIPAm for PTP cells (a) and HEP-2 cells (b).

consider nano(ferro)gels based on NIPAm hydrogels, suitable for the development of hyperthermia of cancer cells, targeted delivery and controlled release of drugs, as well as objects for cell growth. Similar results were obtained in the study of cytotoxicity for HEP-2 cells (epidermal carcinoma of larynx) (**Figure 15b**).

For copolymer ferrogels with a 95% NIPAA content, biological studies performed showed that magnetic hydrogels with a magnetite content of up to 10% are not toxic to PTP cells (**Figure 15a**). Moreover, upon contact of the original matrix with the cells, it was found that their activity tends to increase compared to the activity of control intact cells. Therefore, the result allows us to consider ferrogels based on copolymer hydrogels, which contain 95% NIPAA and 5% AA, suitable for the development of hyperthermia of cancer cells, targeted delivery and controlled release of drugs, as well as objects for cell growth. Similar results were obtained in the study of cytotoxicity for HEP-2 cells (**Figure 15b**).

5. Conclusion

From the above points, it can be concluded that the hydrogel implant developed by us will allow to fill soft tissue structures quite effectively during tissue resection. However, this will partially solve the problem. The clinician always faces such an important task as to avoid tumor recurrence. Immobilization and diffusion of doxorubicin into the implant showed that the kinetics of diffusion of the drug from the liquid-crosslinked hydrogel reaches a minimum therapeutic level within a few minutes, whereas in the case of densely crosslinked hydrogel diffusion begins with a delay of several hours and the amount is released. Much smaller values (20–25%). It is also shown that the tightly crosslinked hydrogel has a higher ability to deposit doxorubicin, and therefore, it is advisable to use for implants with a prolonged antibacterial effect, while the liquid crosslinked hydrogel - for the immediate release of a shock dose of antiseptic. It is important to note that the liquid-crosslinked hydrogel absorbs twice as much cytostatics as doxorubicin, which may be due to the lack of steric barriers to the penetration of the bulk molecule of doxorubicin (molecular weight 544 g/mol) into its porous structure. This hydrogel provides in vitro experiments 3–4 times higher concentration in the environment compared to densely crosslinked polymer, and also provides a smoother, prolonged release of the drug.

The obtained preliminary experimental results allow us to conclude that our developed pathways for the delivery of drugs, in particular, doxorubicin to tumor cells will increase the effectiveness of antitumor therapy. We are faced with many questions that we will implement in further research.

Author details

Anatoliy Parfentievich Maletskyy[1]*, Yuriy Markovich Samchenko[2] and Natalia Mikhailivna Bigun[3]

1 The Filatov Institute of Eye Diseases and Tissue Therapy, NAMS of Ukraine, Odessa, Ukraine

2 Ovcharenko Institute of Biocolloid Chemistry, NAS of Ukraine, Kyiv, Ukraine

3 Lviv Regional Clinical Hospital, Lviv, Ukraine

*Address all correspondence to: maletskiy@filatov.com.ua

References

[1] Palamar O.I, Lukach E.V., Hooke A.P., Maletskyi A.P., Poliakova S.I., Kravets O.V., Serezhko Yu.O., Okonski D.I. Clinical, morphological, CT and MRI characteristies of anterior scul base and orbital tumors. Jornal of Ophthalmology (Ucraine) – 2020 – Number 5 (496). P. 62-74.

[2] Primary orbital tumors: A review of 122 cases during a 23-year period: A histo-clinical study in material from the ENT Department of the Medical University of Silesia/Jarosław Markowski, Estera Jagosz-Kandziora,Wirginia Likus, [et al]. // Med Sci Monit.- 2014;- 20: P. 988-994.

[3] Halli RC, Mishra S, Kini YK, et al. Modified lateral orbitotomy approach: a novel technique in the management of lacrimal gland tumors. J Craniofac Surg. 2011;22(3):1035-1038. [PubMed].

[4] Kim JW, Yates BS, Goldberg RA. Total lateral orbitotomy. Orbit. 2009; 28(6):320-27. [PubMed.].

[5] Discher D., Mooney D., Zandstra P. Growth factors, matrices, and forces combine and control stem cells // Science. – 2009. – № 324. – P. 1673-1677.

[6] Balakrishnan B., Banerjee R. // Chem. Rev. – 2011. – № 111. – P. 4453-4457.

[7] Maletsky AP, Samchenko YM, Vit VV, Bigun NM, Kernosenko LO. Peculiarities of the reaction of soft tissues of orbits, auricle in rabbits to the developed hybrid hydrogel implant // Archive of Ophthalmology 2018, Vol. 6, №2 (11), C-20-27.

[8] Samchenko Yu., Korotych O., Kernosenko L., Kryklia S., Litsis O., Skoryk M., Poltoratska T. Pasmurtseva Stimuli-responsive hybrid porous polymers based on acetals of polyvinyl alcohol and acrylic hydrogels // Colloids and Surfaces A 544 (2018), P. 91-104.

[9] Chai Q. Hydrogels for biomedical applications: Their characteristics and the mechanisms behind them. / Chai Q., Jiao Y., Yu X./ *Gels*. 2017;3(1):6. doi:10.3390/gels3010006.

[10] Overstreet D.J. Temperature-responsive graft copolymer hydrogels for controlled swelling and drug delivery. /Overstreet, D.J.; McLemore, R.Y.; Doan, B.D.; Farag, A.; Vernon, B.L./ *Soft Matter*. 2013; 11: 294-304.

[11] Yu X. Applications of gold nanoparticles in biosensors. /Yu X., Jiao Y., Chai Q./ *Nano LIFE*. 2016; 6: 1642001.

[12] Sugak OA, Panasenko OI, Knysh EG, Kamyshny OM Antimicrobial and antifungal activity of 3- (alkylthio) -4-R-5- (thiophen-2-ylmethyl) -4H-1,2,4-triazole derivatives. Current issues of pharmaceutical and medical science and practice. 2015, №3 (19): 67-70.

[13] Shapiro J.M. Hydrogel composite materials for tissue engineering scaffolds. /Shapiro J.M., Oyen M.L./ *JOM*. 2013; 65: 505. https://doi.org/10.1007/s11837-013-0575-6A.

[14] Brünler R, Aibibu D, Wöltje M, Anthofer AM, Cherif C. In silico modeling of structural and porosity properties of additive manufactured implants for regenerative medicine. Mater Sci Eng C Mater Biol Appl. 2017; 76: 810-817.

[15] Abureesh M.A. Facile synthesis of glucose-sensitive chitosan-poly(vinyl alcohol) hydrogel: drug release optimization and swelling properties. / Abureesh M.A., Oladipo A.A., Gazi M. /*International Journal of Biological Macromolecules*. 2015; 90: 75-80.

[16] Samchenko YM, Maletsky AP, Bigun NM, Dolinsky GA, Kernosenko LO, Pasmurtseva NO, Poltoratskaya TP, Mamyshev IE Dynamics deposition and diffusion of drugs (chlorhexidine, 5 fluorouracil and doxorubicin) when using hydrogel implants with different densities. // Journal of Ophthalmology (Ukraine). - 2020. - № 3. - P. 53-60.

[17] Murphy C.M. The effect of mean pore size on cell attachment, proliferation and migration in collagen–glycosaminoglycan scaffolds for bone tissue engineering. /Murphy C.M., Haugh M.G., O'Brien F.J./ *Biomaterials*. 2010; 31: 461-466.

[18] Oh S.H. In vitro and in vivo characteristics of PCL scaffolds with pore size gradient fabricated by a centrifugation method. /Oh S.H., Park I.K., Kim J.M., Lee J.H./ *Biomaterials*. 2007; 28: 166421671.

[19] Bulysheva A.A. Low-temperature electrospun silk scaffold for in vitro mucosal modeling. /Bulysheva A.A., Bowlin G.L., Klingelhutz A.J., Yeudall W.A. *J./ Biomed. Mater. Res.* Part A. 2012; 100: 757-767.

[20] Somo S.I. Pore interconnectivity influences growth factor mediated vascularization in sphere-templated hydrogels. /Somo S.I., Akar B., Bayrak E.S., Larson J.C., Appel A.A., Mehdizadeh H., Cinar A., Brey E.M./ *Tissue Eng.* Part C: Methods. 2015; 21: 773-785.

[21] Cuggino, J.C., Molina, M., Wedepohl, S., Igarzabal, C.I., Calderón, M., & Gugliotta, L. (2016). Responsive nanogels for application as smart carriers in endocytic pH-triggered drug delivery systems. European Polymer Journal, *78*, 14-24.

[22] Zhao N, Woodle MC, Mixson AJ. Advances in delivery systems for doxorubicin. J Nanomed Nanotechnol. 2018;9(5):519. doi:10.4172/2157-7439.1000519.

[23] Samchenko Yu., Ulberg Z., Korotych O. Multipurpose smart hydrogel systems//Advances in Colloid and Interface Science, 2011, V.168, P.247-262.

[24] Singal PK, Iliskovic N, (1998), Doxorubicin-Induced Cardiomyopathy, New England Journal of Medicine, 339:900-905.

[25] Korotych O. Samchenko Yu. Boldeskul I. Ulberg Z. Zholobak N. Sukhodub L. N-isopropylacrylamide-based fine-dispersed thermosensitive ferrogels obtained via in-situ technique// Materials Science and Engineering C, V33 (2013), P. 892-890.

[26] Samchenko Yu.M, Konovalova V.V., Kryklya S.O., Pasmurceva N.O., [et al] Synthesis and characterization of multi-responsive nano-sized ferrogel based on N-isopropylacrylamide and Acrylic Acid// Zurnal Hromatografichnogo Tovarystva. – 2016. – T. XV, № 1-4. – P. 30-40.

[27] Konovalova V. V., Samchenko Yu. M., Kryklya S. O., Scherbakov S. M., Burban A. F. Ulberg Synthesys and characterization of multi-responsive nano-sized hydrogel based on N-isopropylacrylamide and magnetite// Journal of Applied Chemical Science International 6(3): 132-140, 2016.

Chapter 13

The Paradigm of Targeting an Oncogenic Tyrosine Kinase: Lesson from BCR-ABL

Enrico Bracco, M. Shahzad Ali, Stefano Magnati and Giuseppe Saglio

Abstract

The aberrant tyrosine phosphorylation, either due to constitutive tyrosine kinases (TKs) or to inactivation of protein tyrosine phosphatases (PTPs), is a widespread feature of many cancerous cells. The BCR-ABL fusion protein, which arises from the Philadelphia chromosome, is a molecular distinct and peculiar trait of some kind of leukemia, namely Chronic Myeloid and Acute Lymphoblastic Leukemia, and displays constitutive tyrosine kinase activity. In the chapter, we will highlight the milestones that had led to the identification of the BCR-ABL fusion gene and its role as the only molecular pathogenic event sufficient to elicit and sustain chronic myeloid leukemia. We will also discuss the effort made to unveil the molecular mechanisms of action of the chimeric tyrosine kinase that eventually lead to aberrant cell proliferation and impaired cell-death. Furthermore, we will also review the lesson learned from the selective inhibition of BCR-ABL which currently represent a breakthrough in the treatment of several tumors characterized by defective tyrosine kinase activity.

Keywords: chromosomal translocation, fusion gene, tyrosine kinase, leukemia, tyrosine kinase inhibitors, targeted therapy

1. Introduction

The up-regulated enzymatic activity of tyrosine kinases (TKs) is one of the most frequent events in human cancers. Basically, it is attributable to three distinct molecular-genetic mechanisms covering either the overexpression, the activating mutations or eventually chromosomal translocations involving tyrosine kinase genes. Therefore, targeting the kinases harboring oncogenic properties has led to prominent changes in cancer clinical management. An outstanding contribute in achieving the goal has been offered by the BCR-ABL oncogene, whose story started more than half a century ago. In the 1960s a couple of scientists working in Philadelphia described a major chromosomal abnormality in patients affected by Chronic Myeloid Leukemia (CML) [1, 2]. The chromosomal aberration consisted of an acrocentric chromosome that was originally thought as the outcome of a chromosomal deletion. At that time, it was the first chromosomal abnormality unambiguously associated to a specific malignancy. With the improvement of the chromosomal banding techniques, it became clear that the chromosome abnormality was a shortened chromosome 22. Among a chorus of skepticism and wonder at the beginning of the seventies that short chromosome, that it is now known as Philadelphia chromosome (Ph), was identified as the product of a reciprocal translocation between the long arms of chromosomes 9 and 22, t(9;22). However, we had to wait until the eighties to know that the exact molecular consequence of the t(9;22) was a fusion gene encoding for a chimeric protein displaying constitutively tyrosine kinase activity. Altogether these discoveries delivered an outstanding message whereby a disease was tightly linked to a single oncogene, BCR-ABL. Since then, dozens of translocations have been found in other cancers, including acute promyelocytic leukemia.

BCR-ABL is a peculiar protein for several of reasons: 1) it is a chimeric protein that is encoded by a fusion gene deriving from a reciprocal chromosomal translocation; 2) it is a constitutively active tyrosine kinase eliciting oncogenic signals, 3) it has been the first oncogene associated to a disease displaying dual properties either as driver and in sustaining the neoplasm evolution, and 4) it has been the first kinase to be selectively targeted with small molecules, thus paving the way for the development of a number of tyrosine kinase inhibitors (TKIs).

In the present chapter we are going to discuss the milestones of a story, started 60 years ago, which has happily led to the selective pharmacological inhibition of BCR-ABL. Hence, CML, whose diagnosis was before a death sentence, is now successfully cured in the vast majority of the cases.

2. Is there any specific reason underlying the generation of the Ph chromosome?

Basically, every chromosomal translocations require DNA Double-strand breaks (DSBs) in two different locations and that the broken ends of non-homologous chromosomes are fused together. DNA double-strands breaks might be due to different causes (*e.g.* ionizing radiation, reactive oxygen species, DNA replication across a nick, malfunctioning of DNA metabolic enzymes such as type II DNA topoisomerase or RAG complex during illegitimate V(D)J recombination). Cells to preserve their genome integrity upon DNA damage respond by activating a repair machinery that should catalyzes the joining of the broken ends [3]. However, the outcome of the joining process leads to a variety of rearrangement. For instance, precise joining of broken ends can generate a normal chromosome. Inversions, deletions and duplications can occur when joining involves two broken ends on the same chromosome. Non-Homologous End Joining (NHEJ) is often imprecise; thus some nucleotides may be lost during the joining process. Eventually, translocations may occur when the broken ends of two non-homologous chromosomes are joined together thus leading to novel chromosomes containing part of normal chromosomes [4].

Aside these notions, currently our knowledge regarding the molecular mechanisms responsible for the reciprocal chromosomal translocation occurring between the chromosome 9 and the 22, t(9;22), generating the Philadelphia chromosome (Ph), remain still rather elusive. Fundamentally, it has been speculated that there are two plausible hypotheses. One view prefers to lean towards an entirely random "breaking and re-ligating process" occurring with relatively similar frequency between any two chromosomes within a cell. Chromosomal translocations that give and adaptive advantage are pretty rare and associated with negative consequences (*e.g.* cancer). The success of the t(9;22) can be explained by the fact that, the resulting fusion gene encodes for a protein with transforming properties conferring selective fitness advantages to the host cell. Conversely, by virtue of this, any other chromosomal rearrangement that does not satisfy the requisite for survival and expansion will be handicapped and thus will soon disappear. Though, at this time there are no experimental indications ruling out this view it is worthwhile to notice that the juxtaposition of the ABL and BCR genes has been observed in nuclei of human hematopoietic cells over the S/G2 phases and through the whole G2 phase up to the middle of the M phase (*i.e.* metaphase stage) [5]. Ultimately, there is no conclusive evidence that DNA sequences potentially relevant to chromosomal translocations, such as the Alu repeats or Chi-like octamers, are present around the BCR-ABL rearrangement [6]. Hence, by now the only trustable conviction is that the exchange between two chromosomal positions implies that they must be physically close to each other at the time the event occurs. However, besides the external triggering events (*e.g.* ionizing radiation) the details about what are the molecular players and how they cooperate to the birth of such aberrant chromosome remain to be mechanistically elucidated.

3. What is the consequence of the t(9;22)?

The results of the chromosomal translocation occurring between the chromosome 9 and 22, t(9;22), are a longer chromosome 9 (9q+) and a smaller derivative chromosome 22, the Ph [7, 8]. By the eighties of the past century the molecular characterization of the Ph led to the identification of a novel chimeric gene, BCR-ABL, which later on has been found to encode for a chimeric protein with a constitutive tyrosine kinase activity and with potent oncogenic properties [9, 10]. The c-ABL and Breakpoint of Cluster Region (BCR) loci are localized on the long arm of the chromosome 9 and 22, respectively [11]. Depending on the different breakpoints occurring on the two chromosomes resulting in different BCR-ABL variants. Though, all BCR and c-ABL DNA breakpoints fall within intronic regions those occurring in the BCR gene are highly variable and thus responsible for defining the major differences among the different variants. The variation in the BCR part of the fusion transcript contrasts with the constant c-ABL part. Indeed, all the breakpoints so far identified within the c-ABL gene occur in a large (300-kb) region in the 5′ portion of the gene, localized upstream of the exon 2, and generally falling in the intron sequences restricted between the two alternative first exons (1b and 1a). Regardless the structure of the different fusion genes the BCR exons directly fuse to the second c-ABL exon (a2). The most frequent BCR-ABL fusion variant is the p210 in which the BCR exon 13, or 14, is fused downstream of the alternative exons 1 of the c-ABL gene and thus leading to a fusion protein with approximately the first half from BCR and the remaining second half from ABL. Mostly this variant is found in CML patients accounting for approximately 95% of the BCR-ABL fusion gene in all the CML cases. A second frequent variant, p190, is found in approximately 20–30% of adult patients with Acute Lymphoblast Leukemia (ALL) [12] and, very rarely, also in Acute Myeloid Leukemia (AML) [13]. When compared to the p210 variant, in this case the breakpoint within the BCR locus is localized in the 3′ half of the first BCR intron, thus encoding for a shorter BCR portion (approximately 425 aminoacids). The third most common BCR-ABL variant, p230, is the largest and is defined by a breakpoint cluster region encompassed between the exons 19 and 21. Whereas the p190 characterizes a more acute form of leukemia usually of lymphoid origin, the latter variant is peculiar of neutrophilic CML. Besides, there are additional BCR-ABL variants, though they have been observed less frequently. Interestingly, some of them are peculiar because they are the results of alternative splicing leading to truncated chimeric proteins that are all lacking tyrosine kinase activity [14]. Furthermore, in hematopoietic malignancies, the BCR gene has been identified fused to multiple tyrosine kinases encoding genes, other than ABL, including Fibroblast Growth Factor Receptor1 (FGFR1) -t(8;22)- [15, 16], Platelet Derived Growth Factor Receptor A (PDGFRA) -t(4;22)- [17, 18], RET -t(10;22)- [19] and Jak2 -t(9;22)-[20–22] producing different fusion transcripts that are all encoding for cytoplasmic chimeric proteins displaying dysregulated tyrosine kinase enzymatic activity and onocogenic properties. The causal reason behind the commonality of BCR as fusion partner is not well understood. As we have previously discussed it has been speculated that genes such as BCR are located near chromosomal fragile sites that show breaks or gaps on metaphase chromosomes due to replication stress which are prone to breakage and translocation as result. Interestingly, though BCR fusion genes have also been detected in solid tumors, to date BCR fusion proteins that behave as cancer drivers have solely been identified in hematological cancers.

4. Structural features of the different BCR-ABL protein variants

Both c-ABL and BCR are rather large proteins with molecular sizes ranging from 145 to 160 kDa, respectively, and harboring numerous well defined structural conserved domains. The cABL is a non-receptor tyrosine kinase harboring several motifs that are required for its own enzymatic activity and to signal to other molecules. Intramolecular interactions occurring between the SH3 domain and the linker peptide connecting the SH2 and the tyrosine kinase domain, alongside with that occurring between the kinase and the SH2 domain, keep c-ABL in a close inactive state [23]. The central part of the protein is characterized by proline-rich (PxxP) stretches acting as docking sites for SH3 containing proteins and a DNA binding domain (DBD). Eventually the carboxy-terminal region contains an actin binding domain (ABD) which allows the interaction either with the monomeric- (G) and with the filamentous- (F) actin. Within cells, the ABL is distributed either in the nucleus and, to a lesser extent, in the cytoplasm where it plays distinct roles. The shuttling between the two compartments it steered by its nuclear-localization and nuclear-export signals and it is depending on different extracellular cues (*e.g.* cell to substratum adherence) [24]. While cytoplasmic c-ABL regulates several actin-dependent cellular processes, for example by positively controlling the filopodia exploration and the membrane ruffling [25], the nuclear c-ABL is a pivotal proapoptotic play-actor, playing a role in the cellular response to genotoxic stress (*e.g.* ionizing radiation) [26].

Alike c-ABL, BCR is a multidomains protein with a peculiarity consisting of a Dbl homology (DH) and a Rho-GAP domain that are localized in the central region and at the C-terminus of the protein, respectively. These domains act as Guanine Exchange Factor (GEF) and GTPase Activating regulatory elements (GAP) for some members of the Rho superfamily, including Cdc42, Rac1, Rac2 and RhoA. Additionally, BCR protein harbors other structural regions, including two lipid binding domains namely Pleckstrin Homology (PH) and Calcium-dependent lipid-binding domain (C2), which is localized in the central part of the protein, and an N-terminal 63 aminoacids long coiled-coil oligomerization peptide that is followed by a Serine/Threonine kinase domain. BCR expression is rather ubiquitous and enriched in brain. Differently from c-ABL, the subcellular localization of BCR is predominantly restricted to the cytoplasmic compartment [27].

The structural composition of BCR-ABL proteins may vary quite a lot depending from which fusion gene breakpoint one refer to (**Figure 1**).

However, the variation is always restricted to the BCR part, while the c-ABL part remains constant in all the different transcript variants. This is in itself an indication that c-ABL is mostly responsible for its transforming properties. Briefly, all BCR-ABL proteins share the same c-ABL part with all the prominent structural

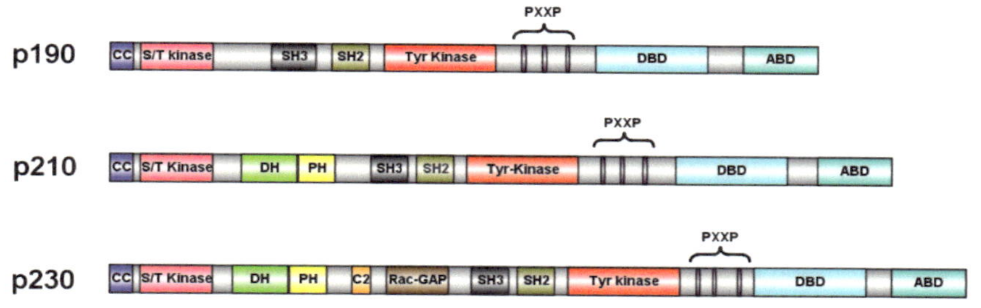

Figure 1.
Structural features of the different Bcr-Abl protein variants. Linear depiction of the functional motif composition of the different BCR-ABL proteins: p190, p210 and p230. CC: Coiled-coil; S/T kinase: Serine/threonine kinase; DH: Dbl-homology; PH: Pleckstrin homology; C2: Ca^{2+}-dependent membrane-targeting module; Rac-GAP: Rac GTPase; SH3: Src Homology3; SH2: Src Homology2; Tyr kinase: Tyrosine kinase: DBD: DNA binding domain; ABD: Actin binding domain; PXXP: Proline rich region, where X indicates any aminoacid.

features of c-ABL, including SH3, SH2, tyrosine kinase, proline rich regions, DNA-binding and Actin Binding Domains. By contrast, the distinguishing part is represented by the BCR peptide. In the shortest BCR-ABL variant (p190) or alternatively named p185, the BCR portion encodes for a peptide of approximately 490 amino-acids encoded by the first BCR exon, encompassing the very N-terminal coiled-coil oligomerization domain and the serine/threonine kinase domain, fused to the ABL. Conversely, in the longest BCR-ABL variant, p230, the BCR portion harbors all BCR structural domains with the exception of the GAP that is truncated. Eventually, the most common BCR-ABL variant, p210, encodes for a chimeric protein in which the BCR portion comprises the coiled-coil, Ser/Thr, Rho-GEF and PH domains. Crucial for the constitutive activation of the c-ABL tyrosine kinase is the BCR oligomerization domain that promotes either the dimerization or tetramerization of the protein [28]. In this way the BCR-ABL proteins can cross-phosphorylate each other on tyrosine residues in their kinase-activation loops. BCR-ABL phosphorylated tyrosine residues usurp the physiological functions of the normal ABL and can act as docking sites for SH2-domain containing proteins that contribute in activating downstream signaling pathways. On the whole this leads to clear readouts comprising deregulated cellular proliferation, decreased adherence of leukemia cells to the bone marrow stroma and reduced apoptotic response to mutagenic stimuli. Alike the BCR, but differently from the c-ABL protein, strikingly all the BCR-ABL chimeric proteins display a cytoplasmic localization, though all retain both the nuclear-localization and nuclear-export peptide sequences. The main reason for its cytoplasmic localization is its constitutively activated tyrosine kinase activity that thus allows to the chimeric tyrosine kinase to interact and cross talk with a number of proteins, thus exerting its leukemogenic effect. Interestingly, upon BCR-ABL pharmacological inactivation (*i.e.* Imatinib) and concurrent blocking of its nuclear export (*i.e.* leptomycin B) the protein re-localizes within the nuclear compartment and it is trapped there. Astonishingly, upon Imatinib removal and the tyrosine kinase activity of the nuclear BCR-ABL is reactivated it is converted from an antiapoptotic to proapoptotic protein thus inducing cell death [29].

5. "In-vitro" and "in-vivo" tools for the assessment of the BCR-ABL leukemogenic properties

The importance of BCR-ABL in leukemogenesis/neoplastic transformation has been examined in numerous "*in-vitro*" and "*in-vivo*" biological systems, including immortalized fibroblast cell lines, growth-factor-dependent hematopoietic cell lines, primary bone marrow cells and mice. Though all these models represent very important tools that have significantly contributed to elucidate the molecular mechanisms of CML formation and to identify potential therapeutic targets, each of them display pros and cons either in term of their tractability and physiological relevance. Many cancer cell lines, including leukemia, have been excellent models for "*in-vitro*" studies because of their relative ease in obtaining a large number of cells for biochemical analysis, genetic manipulation and biological examinations. However, they display remarkable limitations, including their failure to recapitulate the physiology of the disease. By contrast animal models are excellent in term of physiological relevance, thus allowing to recapitulate the disease and to assess its potential evolution, but rather deficient in tractability. The product of BCR-ABL is a constitutively active tyrosine kinase that is more active than c-ABL, thus the expression of BCR-ABL transforms established mouse fibroblast cell lines, factor-dependent hematopoietic cell lines and primary bone-marrow cells. Usually, under physiological conditions normal hematopoiesis requires a strict balancing among cellular-proliferation, –growth and –survival, which are all tightly regulated by growth factors and cytokines (e.g. IL-3, IL-7, GM-CSF and erythropoietin) [30], which upon binding to their cognate receptors activate a number of intracellular signaling pathways. By making use of different cell lines it has been determined that the constitutively active BCR-ABL tyrosine kinase abrogates this growth factor dependency [31] by activating essential downstream molecules in a ligand independent manner. Hence, the expression of BCR-ABL, likewise v-ABL, confers immortalizing properties to the cells. In summary, cellular models have been extremely useful to dissect the molecular pathways activated by BCR-ABL and to determine which parts of the protein are required to confer transforming properties. Nonetheless, transgenic murine models offer additional benefits thus allowing to ascertain and further validate which parts of the protein are mandatorily required for the induction of a CML-like disease, to study the role of the environment in leukemogenesis and eventually to identify therapeutic target for pre-clinical investigations. The "*in-vivo*" convincing experimental evidence validating the leukemogenicity of BCR-ABL were provided only around the 1990s by using transgenic murine models [32, 33]. In this respect, the initial development of transgenic and knock-in murine CML models displayed major drawbacks. Indeed, the generation of conventional BCR-ABL transgenic knock-in mice, through the expression of the chimeric gene under the control of the BCR promoter, caused embryonic lethality due to the toxicity of the activated tyrosine kinase during embryonic development. Afterwards, the use of murine stem-cell retroviral vector and mice created through expression of BCR-ABL under the control of a tetracycline-responsive promoter allowed to overcome that problem and revealed that to develop a CML-like disorder it is crucial to express this oncogene in proper tissue/cell type. With the help of these models it was also shown that the expression of the p210 BCR-ABL variant in bone marrow caused a CML-like disease. Remarkably, the progression of the p210 associated disease was consistent with the apparent indolence of the human CML chronic phase. Interestingly, mice models expressing the p190 variant at levels similar to that of the p210, allowed to uncover that they displayed clinically distinct conditions consisting in a de-novo development of acute leukemia with a short period of latency [34]. Furthermore, these studies allowed to functionally dissect the BCR-ABL protein and to determine to what extent the different domains of the BCR-ABL protein are required for the onset of the different kind of leukemia. The tyrosine-kinase activity of BCR-ABL is essential for its oncogenic properties, but not sufficient. Indeed, although the transduction of v-ABL in a helper virus-containing system causes a murine hematopoietic disease it is distinct from the

CML-like syndrome elicited by BCR-ABL developing only modest splenomegaly and malignant disease of several hematopoietic cell types [35]. In addition to its tyrosine kinase domain the *in vivo* molecular dissection of the protein led to the identification of another domain that is apparently required for the induction of the CML-like disease. This domain turned out to be the SH2. Remarkably, the SH2 domain requirement is peculiar only for myeloid but not for the lymphoid leukemogenesis. Notably, this later issue has been rather debated due to some discrepancies between different studies [36, 37]. Additionally, in mice model for the induction of the chronic leukemia-like disease the Grb2 binding site (Tyr-177) is required [38].

6. Molecular mechanisms conferring oncogenic properties to BCR-ABL

Once BCR-ABL has been identified as the molecular pathogenic event in CML and other leukemia related disorders, significant effort has been addressed to unveil the molecular mechanisms of action of the chimeric tyrosine kinase through the identification of signaling pathways that are impacted by BCR-ABL. The most prominent feature of the BCR-ABL fusion protein is its potent and constitutive tyrosine kinase activity. The tyrosine phosphorylation is a vital mechanism of intracellular signal transduction, used by many growth factor receptors. Usually, approximately less than 2% of total cellular tyrosine residues are phosphorylated, and the activity of tyrosine kinases is counterbalanced by the activity of tyrosine phosphatases. In cells that express a constitutively active tyrosine kinase, this finely-tuned regulation is subverted, leading to a situation that resembles chronic growth factor stimulation.

Actually, BCR-ABL displays a tyrosine kinase activity amazingly higher than that of to the c-ABL counterpart [39] and differences among the different variants have been assessed, being the p190 more potent than that of the p210 and the latter more potent than p230 [40]. Though the BCR-ABL oncoprotein can activate a large number of different signal transduction pathways they appear to target few crucial cellular functions, including increased cellular proliferation, reduced apoptosis and autophagy combined with a deregulated interaction with the bone marrow stromal cellular matrix (**Figure 2**).

Whereas in BCR-ABL transformed cell the PI3K/AKT signaling has been shown to have a pivotal role in mediating both the activation of cell survival and anti-apoptotic signaling, the activation of the Ras/Raf/MEK/ERK cascade has been implicated in the BCR-ABL-dependent uncontrolled cell growth [41]. To the latter purpose the adaptor protein Crk Like (CrkL) has shown to be an important player, being constitutively bound to and a substrate of BCR-ABL [42, 43]. Noteworthy, BCR-ABL itself, through the phosphorylated Tyr-177 can activate the Ras/Raf/MEK/ERK pathway by interacting with Grb2 which in turn recruits SOS that activates Ras [44, 45]. Eventually, Ras triggers the downstream signaling cascade leading to the activation of ERK1/2 [46]. The BCR-ABL dependent pathways leading to apoptosis resistance involve the aberrant expression of the apoptosis regulators proteins of the Bcl2 family including Mcl1, Bcl2 and BclXL along with the proapoptotic members Bim and Bad [47, 48]. Their regulation is mediated by the BCR-ABL-activated PI3K/AKT pathways [49]. The AKT-dependent phosphorylation of Bad leads to its dissociation from Bcl2 and to its sequestering by the adaptor protein 14-3-3, hence leaving less free Bad available to heterodimerize with the anti-apoptotic BclXL proteins. Therefore, more BclXL and Bcl2 remain in the cytoplasm exerting their antiapoptotic role by preserving the mitochondria outer membrane integrity. In addition, it is likely that BCR-ABL also negatively regulates c-ABL, whose function in regulating the apoptotic process is central. The constitutive

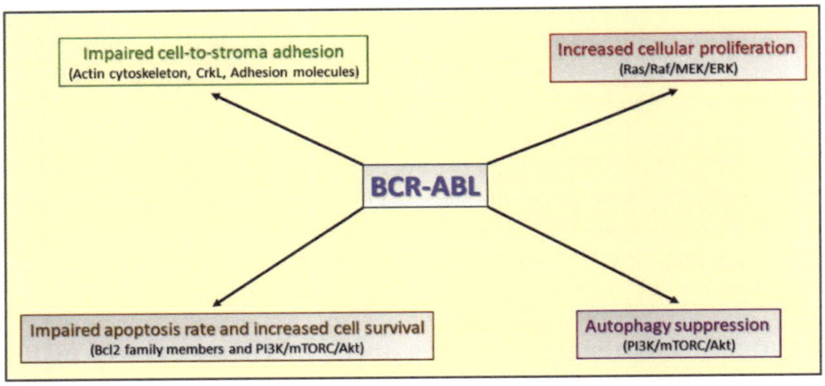

Figure 2.
BCR-ABL exerts its leukemogenic effects by impacting diverse cellular processes: the constitutively active BCR-ABL tyrosine kinase triggers a numbers of signaling pathways, including the Ras/Raf/MEK/ERK and PI3K/mTORC/Akt pathways. On the whole their enhanced activation leads to increased cell-survival and –proliferation, and impaired apoptosis rate. Meanwhile, the oncogenic tyrosine kinase impacts also the cellular autophagy rate and eventually the interaction of the BCR-ABL positive leukemic cells with the stromal microenvironment.

tyrosine kinase activity of BCR-ABL impacts also on the cell-to-substratum adhesion. Indeed, the BCR-ABL-transformed cells display an impaired adhesion to the extracellular matrix. Mostly this behavior is due to the CrkL protein that is one, among many, substrate on the chimeric protein BCR-ABL [42]. Interestingly, CrkL is constitutively binds to BCR-ABL through its first SH3 domain and, at least *in-vitro*, CrkL supports and even potentiates the c-ABL tyrosine kinase activity. CrkL plays a pivotal role in adhesion and cell motility through its association with paxillin, Crk-associated substrate (Cas), Focal Adhesion Kinase (FAK) and the Cbl proto-oncogene. Furthermore, BCR-ABL itself can directly affects the actin cytoskeleton via its actin binding domain localized at its very carboxy-terminal tail and by regulating crucial proteins, such as Rho, Rac and Cdc42 responsible for the cytoskeletal actin dynamics [50–52]. The gene expression of several cell adhesion molecules encoding genes, either mediating the cell-to-substratum and cell-to-cell adhesion including the integrin subunit α-6 and the L- and P-selectins, is under the control of BCR-ABL [53, 54]. Eventually, BCR-ABL suppresses autophagy, an intracellular degradative process allowing cells to adapt to developmental changes and/or unfavorable environmental conditions. Remarkably, autophagy has been shown to provide a survival mechanism to cancer cells [55]. The BCR-ABL-mediated suppression of autophagy occurs via the PI3K/mTORC/Akt signaling pathway since by pharmacologically inhibiting the PI3K in BCR-ABL expressing cells the autophagy is induced again [56].

Alike CrkL some downstream BCR-ABL downstream effectors might play dual role, such is the case of Stat5 that is directly tyrosine phosphorylated by BCR-ABL in a JAK independent way [57, 58]. The Stat5 transcription factor mediates the transcription of several pro-survival and pro-proliferative, as well as anti-pro-apoptotic protein encoding genes [59].

Interestingly, though all BCR-ABL variant proteins are collectively characterized by constitutive and enhanced tyrosine kinase activity they still differ in their binding partners, substrates and as a consequence in their elicited signals. For example, while both p190 and p210 can activate the Ras/Raf/MEK/ERK through the Grb2/SOS complex that binds to the phosphorylated tyrosine residue at position 177 (Tyr-177), the activation of Stat5 is exclusively triggered by the p210. Conversely, the p190, when compared to the p210, shows higher affinity towards the tetrameric

Adaptor Protein Complex 2 (AP2), the adaptor protein DOK1 and the tyrosine kinase Lyn [60]. Overall, the signals triggered by the constitutively active BCR-ABL tyrosine kinase are promiscuous affecting several aspects of the components of the cellular machinery.

7. BCR-ABL inhibitors: paving the way for novel tyrosine kinase inhibitors

Amazingly, in the 1980s and 1990s both the scientific community and pharmaceutical industry were rather skeptic about the issue of pharmaceutically inhibiting protein kinases. Much of their skepticism was lying in the prevailing perception that ATP-binding competitive inhibitors would have had a rather limited target specificity to be translated into useful clinical drug. Moreover, some of the early transgenic animals, in which the genes encoding for tyrosine kinases were inactivated, displayed embryonic lethal phenotypes. Altogether these observations led to the acceptance that tyrosine kinase inhibitors would have been enormously toxic, thus inadequate either for scientific and clinical use. Last but not least, it was assumed that the selective targeting of a single defect would not be sufficient to treat a highly heterogeneous disease such cancers. However, by the end of the 1980s and the beginning of 1990s the first selective tyrosine kinase inhibitors (TKIs) were developed, tyrphostins also known as benzene malononitrile derivatives. Outstandingly, these compounds were found to effectively inhibit EGFR [61]. Afterwards, with crucial reagents in hands, including phospho-tyrosine specific antibody coupled to time-consuming approach such as high-throughput screens of chemical libraries, a team of scientists at Giba-Geigy (now Novartis) seeking for compounds with kinase inhibitory activity identified a promising class of compounds: the 2-phenylaminopirimidine series. Surprisingly, among these molecules one displayed very high selectivity towards the receptor for the platelet derived growth factor (PDGFR), ABL and the stem cell factor receptor (c-kit) [62, 63]. In the first half of 1990s a single molecule the Signal Transduction Inhibitor 571 (STI571) (Gleevec, Glivec, Imatinib™) was shown to be the most specific at selectively suppress the growth of BCR-ABL expressing cells either from CML patients or cell lines [64]. Afterwards, following these *in-vitro* encouraging results pre-clinical data were produced with the help of BCR-ABL transgenic animal models [65, 66]. Consistent with the "*in-vitro*" evidence the animal studies showed that Imatinib treatment led to a dose dependent selective inhibition of BCR-ABL-expressing cells without significant effects against v-SRC-expressing tumors. On the whole, in 1998 these encouraging and promising data prompted a handful of scientist led by B. Druker to set-up the first clinical trial using Imatinib in CML patients. However, before clinical trials could start scientists had to overcome some difficulties concerning the toxicity of the molecule, whether targeting a single kinase would have been an effective and successful strategy and most important whether the pharmaceutical company would realize a return on its investment due to the fact that CML is a pretty rare disease and thus representing a small market. At the end of the 1990s a phase I dose escalation study using Imatinib in CML patients' refractory to IFNα-based therapy started. Surprisingly, within one year the vast majority chronic phase patients who had failed IFN-α therapy and treated with Imatinib 300 mg once a day achieved a complete hematological response. These promising data paved the way for a phase II study and eventually in 2001, three years later after the phase I, Imatinib received the final approval from the Food and Drug Administration (FDA) [67]. The dramatic success in the treatment of CML by an inhibitor of the BCR-ABL kinase is due to a mechanism involving a single biochemical defect a special characteristic that is missing in nearly all the other forms of malignancy. Indeed, conversely from other cancers, in which each genotype encodes diverse phenotypic traits, CML displays an unambiguous genotype–phenotype relationship. However, although most of patients responded excellently to Imatinib therapy a minority relapsed. Especially those patients with advanced CML phases initially respond to Imatinib but then progressed to accelerated or blast crisis. The reason for the relapse is straightforward: while in the patients that respond to Imatinib the BCR-ABL tyrosine kinase activity is abrogated, in those that relapse the tyrosine kinase is reactivated due to mechanisms that either prevent Imatinib to reach the target or render the target insensitive to Imatinib. A combination of approaches, including functional studies that have been then validated by the crystallization of the ABL tyrosine kinase domain with Imatinib coupled with the sequencing of the ABL tyrosine kinase domain, allowed to identify and determine critical contact points between the protein and the inhibitor [68, 69]. Indeed, most of the patients who developed Imatinib insensitivity harbor ABL tyrosine kinase point mutation, especially in the P-loop decreasing its flexibility and therefore its capability to bind to Imatinib. The resistance to Imatinib has led to the development of second generation of tyrosine kinase inhibitors (Nilotinib™, Dasatinib™ and Bosutinib™) and the boost of pharmacogenomics [70]. Imatinib is effective also in the treatment of various malignancies, other than CML. For example, it has shown significant activity in patients with Acute Lymphoblastic Leukemia Ph + (ALL Ph+) [71], in a significant proportion of people with Gastrointestinal Tumor (GIST) that harbor c-KIT mutations [72] and those disorders characterized by translocations involving the PDGFRB gene, including myeloproliferative and myelodysplastic syndromes [73, 74]. The demonstration that small molecule inhibitors could effectively treat chronic myeloid leukemia opened the door to the development of new tyrosine kinase inhibitors and to the blooming era of targeted cancer therapies (**Figure 3**).

Though cancer is the predominant indication for tyrosine kinase inhibitors (TKIs), currently the disease targets are extensively growing. For example, Tofacitinib™ is a Jak3 inhibitor that is currently approved for the treatment of rheumatoid arthritis [75, 76] and Nintedanib™ is a FGFR/multikinase inhibitor that is approved for the treatment of pulmonary fibrosis [77]. Furthermore, Pegaptanib, Ranibizumab and Aflibercept that act by inhibiting the VEGF receptor tyrosine kinase activity are currently used for the treatment of the age-related

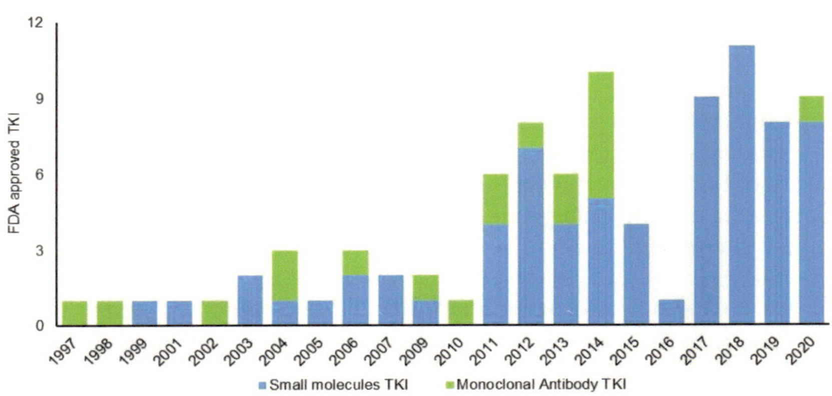

Figure 3.
The FDA approval timeline of tyrosine kinase inhibitors (TKIs): Upon the approval of the Imatinib for the treatment of CML other TKIs have been developed and nowadays small molecules TKIs are dozens. Though, originally they have been designed for neoplasms in the last decade we have also witnessed to an amazingly growth of the diseases, other than cancers, that significantly benefit from TKIs treatment.

macular degeneration, which is a common cause of visual impairment and blindness in elderly adult [78–80].

8. Conclusions

Advances in our understanding in tumor biology have encouraged not only the reassessment of the tumors classification by the site of origin in favor of molecular alterations but also in terms of oncogenic drivers (e.g. tyrosine kinases) amenable for treatment. Since Imatinib has been approved by FDA in 2001 as small molecule competing with ATP, dozens of orally effective small molecule protein kinase inhibitors have been subsequently approved. This is also due to the significantly shortening of the timelines of drug development, as it happened in the case of a record time for the Crizotinib™. The approval of Imatinib for the successful treatment of leukemia (CML) definitively chased away the notion targeting the ATP-binding sites of protein kinases was not selective or efficacious because of the large number of protein kinases, thus leading to copious side effects.

Conflict of interest

The authors declare no conflict of interest.

Author details

Enrico Bracco[1*], M. Shahzad Ali[2], Stefano Magnati[2] and Giuseppe Saglio[2]

1 Department of Oncology, University of Turin, Italy

2 Department of Clinical and Biological Sciences, University of Turin, Italy

*Address all correspondence to: enrico.bracco@unito.it

References

[1] Nowell P, Hungerford D. A minute chromosome in human chronic granulocytic leukemia. Science (80-). 1960;132:1497-1497.

[2] Nowell, P.C., Hungerford DA. Chromosome studies in human leukemia. II. Chronic granulocytic leukemia. J Natl Cancer Inst . 1961;27:1013-1035.

[3] Lieber MR, Ma Y, Pannicke U, Schwarz K. Mechanism and regulation of human non-homologous DNA end-joining. Nat Rev Mol Cell Biol. 2003 Sep;4(9).

[4] Rowley JD. Chromosome translocations: dangerous liaisons revisited. Nat Rev Cancer. 2001 Dec;1:245-250.

[5] Neves H, Ramos C, da Silva MG, Parreira A, Parreira L. The nuclear topography of ABL, BCR, PML, and RARalpha genes: evidence for gene proximity in specific phases of the cell cycle and stages of hematopoietic differentiation. Blood. 1999 Feb;93(4):1197-1207.

[6] Chissoe SL, Bodenteich A, Wang Y-F, Wang Y-P, Burian D, Clifton SW, et al. Sequence and Analysis of the Human ABL Gene, the BCR Gene, and Regions Involved in the Philadelphia Chromosomal Translocation. Genomics. 1995 May;27(1).

[7] Rowley JD. A New Consistent Chromosomal Abnormality in Chronic Myelogenous Leukaemia identified by Quinacrine Fluorescence and Giemsa Staining. Nature. 1973;243:290-293.

[8] Rowley JD. Ph1-positive leukaemia, including chronic myelogenous leukaemia. Clin Haematol. 1980 Feb;9(1):55-86.

[9] de Klein A, van Kessel AG, Grosveld G, Bartram CR, Hagemeijer A, Bootsma D, et al. A cellular oncogene is translocated to the Philadelphia chromosome in chronic myelocytic leukaemia. Nature. 1982 Dec;300(5894).

[10] Ben-Neriah Y, Daley GQ, Mes-Masson AM, Witte ON, Baltimore D. The chronic myelogenous leukemia-specific P210 protein is the product of the bcr/abl hybrid gene. Science (80-). 1986 Jul 11;233(4760):212-214.

[11] Groffen J, Stephenson JR, Heisterkamp N, de Klein A, Bartram CR, Grosveld G. Philadelphia chromosomal breakpoints are clustered within a limited region, bcr, on chromosome 22. Cell. 1984;36(1).

[12] Faderl S, Kantarjian HM, Talpaz M, Estrov Z. Clinical significance of cytogenetic abnormalities in adult acute lymphoblastic leukemia. Blood. 1998 Jan;91(11):3995-4019.

[13] Neuendorff NR, Burmeister T, Dörken B, Westermann J. BCR-ABL-positive acute myeloid leukemia: a new entity? Analysis of clinical and molecular features. Ann Hematol. 2016 Aug 14 95(8).

[14] Volpe G, Cignetti A, Panuzzo C, Kuka M, Vitaggio K, Brancaccio M, et al. Alternative BCR/ABL Splice Variants in Philadelphia Chromosome–Positive Leukemias Result in Novel Tumor-Specific Fusion Proteins that May Represent Potential Targets for Immunotherapy Approaches. Cancer Res. 2007 Jun 1 67;(11).

[15] Gallo LH, Nelson KN, Meyer AN, Donoghue DJ. Functions of Fibroblast Growth Factor Receptors in cancer defined by novel translocations and mutations. Cytokine Growth Factor Rev. 2015 Aug;26(4).

[16] Montenegro-Garreaud X, Miranda RN, Reynolds A, Tang G,

Wang SA, Yabe M, et al. Myeloproliferative neoplasms with t(8;22)(p11.2;q11.2)/ BCR-FGFR1 : a meta-analysis of 20 cases shows cytogenetic progression with B-lymphoid blast phase. Hum Pathol. 2017 Jul;65.

[17] Yigit N, Wu WW, Subramaniyam S, Mathew S, Geyer JT. BCR-PDGFRA fusion in a T lymphoblastic leukemia/ lymphoma. Cancer Genet. 2015 Jul;208(7-8).

[18] Baxter EJ, Hochhaus A, Bolufer P, Reiter A, Fernandez JM, Senent L, et al. The t(4;22)(q12;q11) in atypical chronic myeloid leukaemia fuses BCR to PDGFRA. Hum Mol Genet. 2002 Jun 1 11(12).

[19] Ballerini P, Struski S, Cresson C, Prade N, Toujani S, Deswarte C, et al. RET fusion genes are associated with chronic myelomonocytic leukemia and enhance monocytic differentiation. Leukemia. 2012 Nov 19 26(11).

[20] Cirmena G, Aliano S, Fugazza G, Bruzzone R, Garuti A, Bocciardi R, et al. A BCR-JAK2 fusion gene as the result of a t(9;22)(p24;q11) in a patient with acute myeloid leukemia. Cancer Genet Cytogenet. 2008 Jun;183(2).

[21] Griesinger F, Hennig H, Hillmer F, Podleschny M, Steffens R, Pies A, et al. A BCR-JAK2 fusion gene as the result of a t(9;22)(p24;q11.2) translocation in a patient with a clinically typical chronic myeloid leukemia. Genes, Chromosom Cancer. 2005 Nov;44(3).

[22] Cuesta-Domínguez Á, Ortega M, Ormazábal C, Santos-Roncero M, Galán-Díez M, Steegmann JL, et al. Transforming and Tumorigenic Activity of JAK2 by Fusion to BCR: Molecular Mechanisms of Action of a Novel BCR-JAK2 Tyrosine-Kinase. PLoS One. 2012 Feb 27 7(2).

[23] Pluk H, Dorey K, Superti-Furga G. Autoinhibition of c-Abl. Cell. 2002 Jan;108(2).

[24] Taagepera S, McDonald D, Loeb JE, Whitaker LL, McElroy AK, Wang JYJ, et al. Nuclear-cytoplasmic shuttling of C-ABL tyrosine kinase. Proc Natl Acad Sci. 1998 Jun 23 95(13).

[25] Woodring PJ. Regulation of F-actin-dependent processes by the Abl family of tyrosine kinases. J Cell Sci. 2003 Jul 1 116(13).

[26] Shaul Y. c-Abl: activation and nuclear targets. Cell Death Differ. 2000 Jan 6;7(1).

[27] Wetzler M, Talpaz M, Van Etten RA, Hirsh-Ginsberg C, Beran M, Kurzrock R. Subcellular localization of Bcr, Abl, and Bcr-Abl proteins in normal and leukemic cells and correlation of expression with myeloid differentiation. J Clin Invest. 1993 Oct 1 92(4).

[28] McWhirter JR, Galasso DL, Wang JY. A coiled-coil oligomerization domain of Bcr is essential for the transforming function of Bcr-Abl oncoproteins. Mol Cell Biol. 1993 Dec;13(12).

[29] Vigneri P, Wang JYJ. Induction of apoptosis in chronic myelogenous leukemia cells through nuclear entrapment of BCR–ABL tyrosine kinase. Nat Med. 2001 Feb 1 7(2).

[30] Kaushansky K. Lineage-Specific Hematopoietic Growth Factors. N Engl J Med. 2006 May 11 354(19).

[31] Jonuleit T, Peschel C, Schwab R, van der Kuip H, Buchdunger E, Fischer T, et al. Bcr-Abl kinase promotes cell cycle entry of primary myeloid CML cells in the absence of growth factors. Br J Haematol. 1998 Feb;100(2).

[32] Daley G, Van Etten R, Baltimore D. Induction of chronic myelogenous leukemia in mice by the P210bcr/abl gene of the Philadelphia chromosome. Science (80-). 1990 Feb 16;247(4944).

[33] Heisterkamp N, Jenster G, ten Hoeve J, Zovich D, Pattengale PK, Groffen J. Acute leukaemia in bcr/abl transgenic mice. Nature. 1990 Mar;344(6263).

[34] Voncken J, Kaartinen V, Pattengale P, Germeraad W, Groffen J, Heisterkamp N. BCR/ABL P210 and P190 cause distinct leukemia in transgenic mice. Blood. 1995 Dec 15 86(12).

[35] Scott ML, Van Etten RA, Daley GQ, Baltimore D. v-abl causes hematopoietic disease distinct from that caused by bcr-abl. Proc Natl Acad Sci. 1991 Aug 1 88(15).

[36] Zhang X, Wong R, Hao SX, Pear WS, Ren R. The SH2 domain of Bcr-Abl is not required to induce a murine myeloproliferative disease; however, SH2 signaling influences disease latency and phenotype. Blood. 2001 Jan 1 97(1).

[37] Roumiantsev S, de Aos IE, Varticovski L, Ilaria RL, Van Etten RA. The Src homology 2 domain of Bcr/Abl is required for efficient induction of chronic myeloid leukemia-like disease in mice but not for lymphoid leukemogenesis or activation of phosphatidylinositol 3-kinase. Blood. 2001 Jan 1 97(1).

[38] Million RP, Van Etten RA. The Grb2 binding site is required for the induction of chronic myeloid leukemia-like disease in mice by the Bcr/Abl tyrosine kinase. Blood. 2000 Jul 15 96(2).

[39] Lugo T, Pendergast A, Muller A, Witte O. Tyrosine kinase activity and transformation potency of bcr-abl oncogene products. Science (80-). 1990 Mar 2;247(4946).

[40] Li S, Ilaria RL, Million RP, Daley GQ, Van Etten RA. The P190, P210, and P230 Forms of the BCR/ABL Oncogene Induce a Similar Chronic Myeloid Leukemia–like Syndrome in Mice but Have Different Lymphoid Leukemogenic Activity. J Exp Med. 1999 May 3 189(9).

[41] Hazlehurst LA, Bewry NN, Nair RR, Pinilla-Ibarz J. Signaling Networks Associated with BCR–ABL–Dependent Transformation. Cancer Control. 2009 Apr;16(2).

[42] Sattler M, Salgia R. Role of the adapter protein CRKL in signal transduction of normal hematopoietic and BCR/ABL-transformed cells. Leukemia. 1998 May 29 12(5).

[43] Bhat A, Kolibaba K, Oda T, Ohno-Jones S, Heaney C, Druker BJ. Interactions of CBL with BCR-ABL and CRKL in BCR-ABL-transformed Myeloid Cells. J Biol Chem. 1997 Jun;272(26).

[44] Pendergast AM, Quilliam LA, Cripe LD, Bassing CH, Dai Z, Li N, et al. BCR-ABL-induced oncogenesis is mediated by direct interaction with the SH2 domain of the GRB-2 adaptor protein. Cell. 1993 Oct;75(1).

[45] Puil L, Liu J, Gish G, Mbamalu G, Bowtell D, Pelicci PG, et al. Bcr-Abl oncoproteins bind directly to activators of the Ras signalling pathway. EMBO J. 1994 Feb;13(4).

[46] Sattler M, Mohi MG, Pride YB, Quinnan LR, Malouf NA, Podar K, et al. Critical role for Gab2 in transformation by BCR/ABL. Cancer Cell. 2002 Jun;1(5).

[47] Datta SR, Katsov A, Hu L, Petros A, Fesik SW, Yaffe MB, et al. 14-3-3 Proteins and Survival Kinases Cooperate to Inactivate BAD by BH3 Domain Phosphorylation. Mol Cell. 2000 Jul;6(1).

[48] Neshat MS, Raitano AB, Wang H-G, Reed JC, Sawyers CL. The Survival Function of the Bcr-Abl Oncogene Is

Mediated by Bad-Dependent and -Independent Pathways: Roles for Phosphatidylinositol 3-Kinase and Raf. Mol Cell Biol. 2000 Feb 15 20(4)

[49] Bedi A, Zehnbauer B, Barber J, Sharkis S, Jones R. Inhibition of apoptosis by BCR-ABL in chronic myeloid leukemia. Blood. 1994 Apr 15 83(8).

[50] Harnois T, Constantin B, Rioux A, Grenioux E, Kitzis A, Bourmeyster N. Differential interaction and activation of Rho family GTPases by p210bcr-abl and p190bcr-abl. Oncogene. 2003 Sep 25 22(41).

[51] Thomas EK, Cancelas JA, Zheng Y, Williams DA. Rac GTPases as key regulators of p210-BCR-ABL-dependent leukemogenesis. Leukemia. 2008 May 20 22(5).

[52] Durand-Onaylı V, Haslauer T, Härzschel A, Hartmann T. Rac GTPases in Hematological Malignancies. Int J Mol Sci. 2018 Dec 14 19(12).

[53] Wertheim JA, Forsythe K, Druker BJ, Hammer D, Boettiger D, Pear WS. BCR-ABL–induced adhesion defects are tyrosine kinase–independent. Blood. 2002 Jun 1 99(11).

[54] Gordon MY, Dowding CR, Riley GP, Goldman JM, Greaves MF. Altered adhesive interactions with marrow stroma of haematopoietic progenitor cells in chronic myeloid leukaemia. Nature. 1987 Jul;328(6128).

[55] Dikic I, Johansen T, Kirkin V. Selective Autophagy in Cancer Development and Therapy. Cancer Res. 2010 May 1 70(9).

[56] Bellodi C, Lidonnici MR, Hamilton A, Helgason GV, Soliera AR, Ronchetti M, et al. Targeting autophagy potentiates tyrosine kinase inhibitor–induced cell death in Philadelphia chromosome–positive cells, including primary CML stem cells. J Clin Invest. 2009 May 1 119(5).

[57] de Groot RP, Raaijmakers JAM, Lammers J-WJ, Jove R, Koenderman L. STAT5 Activation by BCR-Abl Contributes to Transformation of K562 Leukemia Cells. Blood. 1999 Aug 1 94(3).

[58] Hoelbl A, Schuster C, Kovacic B, Zhu B, Wickre M, Hoelzl MA, et al. Stat5 is indispensable for the maintenance of *bcr/abl* -positive leukaemia. EMBO Mol Med. 2010 Mar 3 2(3).

[59] Wingelhofer B, Neubauer HA, Valent P, Han X, Constantinescu SN, Gunning PT, et al. Implications of STAT3 and STAT5 signaling on gene regulation and chromatin remodeling in hematopoietic cancer. Leukemia. 2018 Aug 27 32(8).

[60] Reckel S, Hamelin R, Georgeon S, Armand F, Jolliet Q, Chiappe D, et al. Differential signaling networks of Bcr–Abl p210 and p190 kinases in leukemia cells defined by functional proteomics. Leukemia. 2017 Jul 23 31(7).

[61] Yaish P, Gazit A, Gilon C, Levitzki A. Blocking of EGF-dependent cell proliferation by EGF receptor kinase inhibitors. Science (80-). 1988 Nov 11;242(4880).

[62] Buchdunger E, Zimmermann J, Mett H, Meyer T, Muller M, Regenass U, et al. Selective inhibition of the platelet-derived growth factor signal transduction pathway by a protein-tyrosine kinase inhibitor of the 2-phenylaminopyrimidine class. Proc Natl Acad Sci. 1995 Mar 28 92(7).

[63] Buchdunger E, Zimmermann J, Mett H, Meyer T, Müller M, Druker BJ, et al. Inhibition of the Abl Protein-Tyrosine Kinase in Vitro and in Vivo by a 2-Phenylaminopyrimidine Derivative. 1996 Jan;56(1):100-104.

[64] Druker BJ, Tamura S, Buchdunger E, Ohno S, Segal GM, Fanning S, et al. Effects of a selective inhibitor of the Abl tyrosine kinase on the growth of Bcr–Abl positive cells. Nat Med. 1996 May;2(5).

[65] le Coutre P, Mologni L, Cleris L, Marchesi E, Buchdunger E, Giardini R, et al. In Vivo Eradication of Human BCR/ABL-Positive Leukemia Cells With an ABL Kinase Inhibitor. JNCI J Natl Cancer Inst. 1999 Jan 20 91(2).

[66] Wolff NC, Ilaria RL. Establishment of a murine model for therapy-treated chronic myelogenous leukemia using the tyrosine kinase inhibitor STI571. Blood. 2001 Nov 1 98(9).

[67] Druker BJ, Talpaz M, Resta DJ, Peng B, Buchdunger E, Ford JM, et al. Efficacy and Safety of a Specific Inhibitor of the BCR-ABL Tyrosine Kinase in Chronic Myeloid Leukemia. N Engl J Med. 2001 Apr 5 344(14).

[68] Nagar B, Hantschel O, Young MA, Scheffzek K, Veach D, Bornmann W, et al. Structural Basis for the Autoinhibition of c-Abl Tyrosine Kinase. Cell. 2003 Mar;112(6).

[69] Hantschel O, Nagar B, Guettler S, Kretzschmar J, Dorey K, Kuriyan J, et al. A Myristoyl/Phosphotyrosine Switch Regulates c-Abl. Cell. 2003 Mar;112(6).

[70] Gillis NK, McLeod HL. The pharmacogenomics of drug resistance to protein kinase inhibitors. Drug Resist Updat. 2016 Sep;28.

[71] Towatari M. Combination of intensive chemotherapy and imatinib can rapidly induce high-quality complete remission for a majority of patients with newly diagnosed BCR-ABL-positive acute lymphoblastic leukemia. Blood. 2004 Dec 1 104(12).

[72] Demetri GD, von Mehren M, Blanke CD, Van den Abbeele AD, Eisenberg B, Roberts PJ, et al. Efficacy and Safety of Imatinib Mesylate in Advanced Gastrointestinal Stromal Tumors. N Engl J Med. 2002 Aug 15 347(7).

[73] Apperley JF, Gardembas M, Melo J V., Russell-Jones R, Bain BJ, Baxter EJ, et al. Response to Imatinib Mesylate in Patients with Chronic Myeloproliferative Diseases with Rearrangements of the Platelet-Derived Growth Factor Receptor Beta. N Engl J Med. 2002 Aug 15 347(7).

[74] Cools J, DeAngelo DJ, Gotlib J, Stover EH, Legare RD, Cortes J, et al. A Tyrosine Kinase Created by Fusion of the *PDGFRA* and *FIP1L1* Genes as a Therapeutic Target of Imatinib in Idiopathic Hypereosinophilic Syndrome. N Engl J Med. 2003 Mar 27 348(13).

[75] Fleischmann R, Kremer J, Cush J, Schulze-Koops H, Connell CA, Bradley JD, et al. Placebo-Controlled Trial of Tofacitinib Monotherapy in Rheumatoid Arthritis. N Engl J Med. 2012 Aug 9 367;(6).

[76] van Vollenhoven RF, Fleischmann R, Cohen S, Lee EB, García Meijide JA, Wagner S, et al. Tofacitinib or Adalimumab versus Placebo in Rheumatoid Arthritis. N Engl J Med. 2012 Aug 9 367;6.

[77] Richeldi L, du Bois RM, Raghu G, Azuma A, Brown KK, Costabel U, et al. Efficacy and Safety of Nintedanib in Idiopathic Pulmonary Fibrosis. N Engl J Med. 2014 May 29 370;22).

[78] Gragoudas ES, Adamis AP, Cunningham ET, Feinsod M, Guyer DR. Pegaptanib for Neovascular Age-Related Macular Degeneration. N Engl J Med. 2004 Dec 30 351;27).

[79] Rosenfeld PJ, Brown DM, Heier JS, Boyer DS, Kaiser PK, Chung CY, et al. Ranibizumab for Neovascular

Age-Related Macular Degeneration. N Engl J Med. 2006 Oct 5 355;(14).

[80] Brown DM, Kaiser PK, Michels M, Soubrane G, Heier JS, Kim RY, et al. Ranibizumab versus Verteporfin for Neovascular Age-Related Macular Degeneration. N Engl J Med. 2006 Oct 5 355;(14).